35100

OXFORD MEDICAL PUBLICATIONS

The Senescence of Human Vision

The faculty of accommodating the eye to various distances, appears to exist in very different degrees in different individuals. . .

A young lady of my acquaintance can see at 2 inches and at 4; the difference being equivalent to 4 inches focus. A middle aged lady at 3 and at 4; the power of accommodation being only equal to the effect of a lens of 12 inches focus. In general, I have reason to think, that the faculty diminishes in some degree, as persons advance in life; but some also of a middle age appear to possess it in a very small degree.

I take out of a small botanical microscope, a double convex lens, of eight-tenths radius and focal distance, fixed in a socket one-fifth of an inch in depth; securing its edges with wax, I drop into it a little water, nearly cold, till it is three-fourths full, and then apply it to my eye, so that the cornea enters half-way into the socket, and is everywhere in contact with the water. My eye immediately becomes presbyopic. . .

Thomas Young (1801)

(Permission to reproduce kindly given by the Royal Society)

The Senescence
of Human Vision

R.A. WEALE

Age Concern Institute of Gerontology
King's College London
and
Professorial Unit
Moorfields Eye Hospital
London

Oxford   New York   Tokyo
OXFORD UNIVERSITY PRESS
1992

Oxford University Press, Walton Street, Oxford OX2 6DP

Oxford New York Toronto
Delhi Bombay Calcutta Madras Karachi
Petaling Jaya Singapore Hong Kong Tokyo
Nairobi Dar es Salaam Cape Town
Melbourne Auckland

and associated companies in
Berlin Ibadan

Oxford is a trade mark of Oxford University Press

Published in the United States
by Oxford University Press, New York

A catalogue record for this book is available from the British Library

Library of Congress Cataloging in Publication Data
Weale, R. A. (Robert Alexander)
The senescence of human vision / R.A. Weale.
(Oxford medical publications)
Includes bibliographical references and index.
1. Vision disorders in old age. 2. Eye—Aging. I. Title.
II. Series.
[DNLM: 1. Aging—physiology. 2. Retina—physiology. 3. Vision—physiology. WW 103 W362o]
RE48.2.A5W43   1992   612.8'4'0846—dc20   92-13162
ISBN 0-19-262034-7 (H'bk)

Typeset by
Advance Typesetting Ltd, Oxford
Printed in Great Britain by
Biddles Ltd, Guildford and Kings Lynn

Preface

The life expectancy of the human race continues to grow. This progress will not persist forever, but has lasted long enough to have led to a number of projections, for example as regards the health expectancy of our eyesight.

Purely from the mathematical point of view, it could be said that the prolongation of life promotes blindness. It is not surprising, therefore, that the subject of ocular and visual ageing is receiving a great deal of experimental attention. This has led in the last decade or so to the appearance of a number of texts on these subjects (Cullinan 1986; Lumbroso and Sciuto 1988; Platt 1989; Rosenbloom and Morgan 1986; Sekuler *et al.* 1982; Weale 1982*a*), but none of them has related the subject in any but a general sense to contemporary gerontological thinking. Part of the explanation may be that the eye lends itself to accurate experimentation, with results which may disagree with roughly sketched hypotheses. It is, however, more likely that the hypotheses are inadequate. The need to continue studying the properties of the ageing eye has, however, become progressively more urgent.

A number of ideas in the science of ageing have recently started to be formed. I was invited to inaugurate at the Florida State University, Tallahassee, USA, a series of lectures on the topic of the ageing eye, commemorating William Rushton, late of the Physiological Laboratory, Cambridge, UK. The above authors and, indeed, other writers have devoted much effort to describing the senescence of many anatomical and histological features; therefore it seemed a good idea to confine oneself to the *raison d'être* of the eye, namely vision. I was given five lectures in which to deal with the subject, and this is also a suitable number of chapters in which to cover the subject.

> This book will perhaps appeal not only to eye specialists but also to those interested in ageing in general. It may attract the attention of some who dislike to be reminded that, once upon a time, they knew more algebra than they remember now. To stop them from putting the book down just for that reason, and, because others may be happier to see some of the arguments expressed in analytical terms, I have made a vain attempt to please everyone. Each algebraic argument is enclosed in a box like the one which surrounds this paragraph. You will not lose the thread of the story if you skip these boxes.

It may be prudent to declare one's position as early in an argument as possible. I have heard it said that senescence can be useful both in the biological sense and in a social context. My good friend Laszlo Bito stated at the International Congress on Eye Research in Helsinki (1990) that monkeys produce a significantly greater sperm count when some older members of their clan are around than when they are alone. He saw this as a fructifying biological influence on the part of the elderly. It is, however, possible to view this result in terms of competition. In 1991, a 92-year-old man was reported as having fathered his sixth child, and it is not inconceivable that an elderly male monkey may be seen as a threat by a younger one, whose hormones are thereby spurred to improve his potential.

Again, on the social side, the elderly are seen as purveyors of information (Mergler and Goldstein 1983). We probably think of Homer as old because he was blind, and the notion that old age allows communication of knowledge between one generation and the next is attractive. However, it overlooks the fact that children can only kneel in rapt attention at their parents' or grandparents' feet if the older generation is still alive. This has not been possible without a widespread increase in our life expectancy, and is unlikely to have played a significant role in the course of our evolution. I also have to be convinced, both as a son and as a father, that the transmission of such information, even when it is on offer, is either valued or accepted.

My thanks are due to Mrs C.S. Lawrence, Librarian, Institute of Ophthalmology, University of London, UK, for her unremitting help in meeting my requests for original material, the staff of Oxford University Press for helpful advice, and to my ever-patient wife who read the text and did more than just dot i's and cross t's.

London   R.A.W.
May 1992

Contents

3. Retinal senescence

4. Senescent vision

1. Theories

1.1 Introduction

Procreation, not recreation, is the probable reason for the excellent development of our various visual abilities. We use our eyes more often than our ears or nose in selecting our mates-to-be. Moreover, most occupations, even in societies which are not based on modern technology, require the possession of eyesight for the provision of those necessities of life which serve for the protection and development of the subsequent generation.

Biologists do not deny the role played by civilization in our development: indeed, Young (1968) suggested that man-made factors would condition the future of evolution because, he felt, that we had all but brought our environment under control. (Although the greenhouse effect had been mentioned before then, at that time few considered the risk to be serious.) But, until now, it has been simpler to look upon the various characteristics of mankind as the results of natural selection rather than as the outcome of man-made factors. Indeed, Kirkwood and Holliday (1986) doubt whether we have yet arrived at an evolutionary plateau: the world population is growing very rapidly, and it may be that the genes, if any, determining our modes of senescence have yet to reach their optimum. The possibility of a deterioration in our natural environment cannot be overlooked: there is enough evidence even from cursory comparisons of different ethnic groups that physical factors must have played, and probably still are playing, an all-important role.

If the fittest are selected to survive, why is Nature's work undone by their being permitted to age and die? There are some who would replace the word 'permitted' with 'programmed' or 'destined'. Comfort (1979) has said that the number of theories of senescence exceeds the facts available to support them, or words to that effect. Since the systematic study of ocular and visual gerontology is a relatively young discipline, existing surveys are inevitably, at best, taxonomies tacked onto the time-scale of senescence, and, at worst, litanies of pathological decay. With one exception, the works listed above represent collections of contributions by many authors; which makes it virtually impossible to use them in support of any general ideas.

It is, however, feasible to survey recent work on human vision so as to form a picture, not of design, but of a tentative pattern of the rise and fall of our eyesight which can be understood in terms of a wider biological framework.

But, to try to understand the broad outlines of ocular and visual ageing, it is indispensable to familiarize oneself with contemporary ideas bearing on the subject in general.

New and broad generalizing concepts are beginning to enter into gerontological thinking, for example non-adaptive theories of ageing. These theories are distinguished from older, adaptive ones; for example, the notion that we age and die to make room for others, who might perhaps benefit from new mutations, is adaptive. The idea, however, that we exhibit senescence because it would be biologically too costly to maintain ourselves as individuals once we have produced offspring is non-adaptive (Kirkwood 1984). To perceive a design in senescence is to adopt an adaptive view, but to consider it from the aspect of the availability of biological resources follows a non-adaptive one. In terms of modern economics, one would class adaptism with planned economy, and non-adaptism with one propelled by market forces.

It may be that one theory is better at predicting one set of phenomena, while another succeeds with a second set, and so on. It is probable, however, that those who support the theory of evolutionary pressures will be slow to stress notions of biological design. Our eyes function well during a definite, but significantly restricted, period of our life span: there are deficits at both ends. Some theories of senescence may be more plausible than others; however, it is unlikely that the eye and vision are so special as to need specific theoretical attention. More than one of the many theoretical frameworks may be usable, and looking at the problem from a biological point of view may lead to verifiable predictions.

1.1.1 Senescence – is it definable?

The very definition of ageing has been problematic (Kirkwood 1984), partly because the process has been identified with an increase in mortality. This can be seen experimentally, because cells can be 'aged' artificially, for example by irradiating them; they are then more likely to die than equally old unirradiated ones.

Ocular ageing can be defined fairly reliably during the first half of our life span on the basis of the amplitude of accommodation, but after the first five decades the value of this index lapses (Chapters 2 and 5). While it is a truism to say that those who can no longer accommodate are nearer to death than those who can, the observation can scarcely be quantified.

The attributes of senescence may precede adulthood and even puberty. From the strictly evolutionary point of view, senescence may be said to be characterized by the loss of faculties necessary not just for the generation of viable offspring, but also for their rearing, their protection, and their successful attainment of an age when they, in turn, can carry out their biological lot.

1.2 Ideas on senescence

1.2.1 Is senescence planned?

Using the language of earlier theorists, Beutler (1986) is the latest of a long line of adaptive thinkers to examine the possibility that human ageing is planned. Emphasizing that it is easier to replace damaged proteins than to repair them, he suggests that the planned destruction of the human biosystem is a sensible point of view from which to study ageing. Like Kirkwood and Holliday (1986), he has considered the matter of the biological cost/benefit ratio but, unlike those authors, he has not attempted to define it. He postulates that the absence of ageing phenomena, for instance in erythrocytes, is the result of a decision on the part of natural selection to allow an erythrocyte to exist, in the case of man, for four months, rather than to endow it with a repair mechanism. This obsolescence is said to be planned. Medvedev (1972) notes that avian erythrocytes have inert nuclei, and that hence a change, for example in the constitution of DNA, could not exert a significant effect on their senescence.

It is not clear from Beutler's ideas how ageing is planned, and the notion of decision-making opposes that of trial-and-error which some authors believe to underlie the random element that makes natural selection potent. In terms of biological cost/benefit, it might be thought more economical to programme growth and development, which seems to be essential if an organism is to achieve a biological objective, and to curb that investment once the objective has been reached. In thermodynamic terms, this would lead to an increase in entropy and disorganization without any planning being required.

In this connection attention ought to be drawn to the manifold contexts in which the word 'programme' is commonly used and which may colour our perception of the concepts to which it is applied. For example, it may convey the notion of intent, which is unacceptable in evolutionary terms. The only observable entities are consequences, consequences, not of any intentional planning or programming, but probably of chance mutations and development. To the extent to which the consequences are repeated from one generation to the next and hence form a pattern, the existence of a genetic programme may be inferred. On the basis of well-known and generally accepted premises, genetic attributes manifesting before the termination of the reproductive period are passed on from generation to generation, which is why late mutations are not thought to be able to affect the genome. This is a reason for doubt about the existence of genes specific for the transmission of senescence, a feature of life which can be pictured as achievable by simpler concepts, such as a failure in the well-documented repair processes which have evolved.

1.2.2 *Organ-based concepts of senescence*

Beutler's example of erythrocytes raises an interesting question met repeatedly in gerontology, and one which is relevant also in the specific case of the eye. The problem of erythrocytes ageing is of general gerontological interest. In theory, ageing and, finally, death could be achieved by an age-related deterioration of the blood, which could ultimately become toxic. Such a possibility falls within the ambit of so-called organ-based theories discussed below.

It is the quality of erythrocytes that is central to Beutler's hypothesis. Their fragility increases slightly with age both in human beings (Bowdler *et al*. 1981) and in rats (Nicak 1986), probably because of an increase in membrane rigidity, as determined indirectly by polarization spectrofluorimetry (Gareau *et al*. 1991). The adenosine triphosphate (ATP) content of bovine erythrocytes decreases with age in spite of a concomitant drop in ATPase activity (Bartosz *et al*. 1982). Human glutathione, which plays an important antioxidant role (see p. 238) and also protects the cells from free radicals and cytotoxic agents, varies in human beings in an untypical manner. It rises from its infant values to a peak between 25 and 40 years of age (p. 37), and then returns to its original value. Glutathione S-transferases, which catalyse the conjugation of glutathione with a variety of noxious agents, follow a similar course, as does glutathione reductase (Stohs *et al*. 1984) which preserves glutathione in its reduced, that is its functional form.

These observations would lead to the conclusion that blood might act as an agent of senescence. However, apart from the fact that non-primate species were involved in those studies, it would appear that obtaining blood from 'healthy' donors, as stated by the above authors, does not provide an unambiguous description of its quality.

Corberand *et al*. (1987) studied this by taking blood samples from elderly donors and young controls. For each age two groups were selected − A, on the basis of stringent criteria of health, based on the Senieur Protocol (Lightart *et al*. 1984), and B, consisting of other age-matched volunteers considered as healthy by their own general practitioners. On admission, group B was screened less thoroughly than group A.

Detailed haematological tests revealed that there was no significant difference between young and elderly group A males. But leukocyte numbers were lower, and the erythrocyte sedimentation rate was higher for elderly females in that group than for young controls. In contrast to these observations, the differences between control and test were greater for both sexes in group B in comparison with group A, and the variability was greater amongst the elderly in group B. Moreover, elderly women in group A had higher erythrocyte counts, and both haemoglobin and haematocrit were higher: no such difference was found between the young control groups.

The problem with Beutler's view on planned obsolescence is therefore the following. The type of erythrocyte that exemplifies it is obtained from medically superior persons — those considered healthy by their own general practitioners fail to reach this standard. Yet, as reported by Borkan and Norris (1980), the general practitioner's subjective judgment regarding the patient's clinical appearance is valuable as an index of biological age. The exclusion of pathology has been correctly stressed whenever it has been sought in most gerontological, and visual, studies. But mortality statistics are not confined to the healthiest members of a given nation or population. This makes the potential use of bio-gerontological data to predict life expectancy and mortality of doubtful value, and possibly even misleading.

Elites spoil the figures

The question of clinically exemplary senescence is raised in connection with another potentially fundamental investigation, namely the variation of potassium levels in body tissues as a function of age (Cox and Shalaby 1981). A multiple isotope dilution technique involving radioactive sodium, potassium, tritium and sulphur was used for the determination of the total exchangeable sodium, potassium, and the total body water and extracellular fluid volume. Potassium was found to decrease with age absolutely and also in relation to dry body weight and fat-free body weight. Between the ages of 27 and 95 years, the rate of loss of sodium was only one third that of potassium.

However, these measurements were made on a hospital population, and particularly the elderly amongst them might have been suffering from dietetic deficiencies. The authors speculate that senescent cells may leak potassium, or that a damaged ATP production may lead to an impairment of cellular membrane mechanisms. They leave it as a moot point whether a leakage of potassium is normal, or normal for the type of population which they studied: they speculate whether the same results would have been obtained if the study had been conducted on very healthy elderly people. Perhaps, in gerontology, it is not only hypotheses that create problems for those who are trying to generalize.

At the same time, the dilemma made manifest in these and other studies needs to be dealt with. A given physiological or morphometric characteristic probably exhibits a normal distribution at any one calendar age (Fig. 1.1). It is not uncommon for the variance of a measure to increase with age (Fig. 1.2a), though there are also examples showing it to be constant (Fig 1.2b). In the former case, it is probable that there is a sequential influence of earlier variabilities upon later ones — an example of the 'drunkard's walk'. If a variable, for example, a visual threshold, rises with age, and the standard deviation does so in much the same way, though the average increases, a measurable elite among the elderly may retain a virtually unaltered threshold value. The characteristics of a defined population as a whole and those indicating

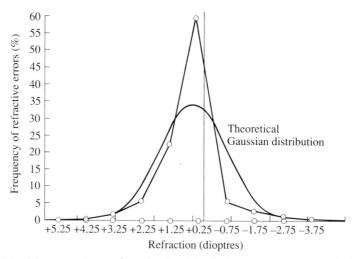

Fig. 1.1 Many anatomical and physiological variables obtained for one age-group can be approximately described by a Gaussian curve. This is illustrated for the distribution of refractive errors. After Trevor Roper (1974).

what may be possible *in extremis* therefore need to be distinguished from each other.

Not even such a distinction is, however, likely to provide any information on the genetic potential unless the influence of the environment is fully understood: it is conceivable that it might modify the characteristics of the population surveyed. The environment acts on specific organs, of which the above-mentioned erythrocytes provide one of many examples and the musculature another.

The ageing of muscles, their function being modifiable by training, i.e. by voluntary intervention, bears not only on these ideas but is also relevant to ocular performance insofar as the involuntary (ciliary and pupillary) musculature is concerned; the (external) oculo-motor system appears to be more resilient. Grimby and Saltin (1983) state that the progressive reduction in muscle mass with age is due more to a reduction in the number of fibres than to one in their size. They point out that these results need to be interpreted with caution, since, in recent decades, factors such as nutrition, physical activity, disease and selective mortality may have varied with age. The reduction in muscle mass with age is greater in men than in women, and may even proceed from birth onward. The motor-neuronal system exhibits considerable plasticity, in that the territory of a motor unit increases with age. This suggests not only that there is likely to be a loss of innervation, but also that fibres that have lost their innervation may atrophy, a point well illustrated in the ciliary muscle (Stieve 1949), and

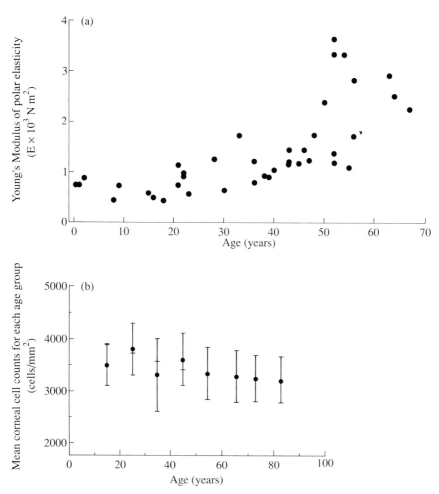

Fig. 1.2a The variance of lenticular elasticity (p. 80) increases with age. After Fisher (1971), **b** that of endothelial cell counts in the cornea remains constant. After Reim (1984).

discussed in Chapter 2. Neurogenic losses are more frequent in distal than in proximal muscles, and Grimby and Saltin attribute this tentatively to the risk of nerve fibre atrophy increasing with the length of the nerve trunk.

The well-attested change in muscular performance with age appears to be due not to a change in the nature of the motor supply but in its distribution. The loss of motor units with age, amounting to some 33 per cent between the ages of 30 and 70 years, appears to prevail amongst the largest and fastest-conducting units which innervate high-threshold fast-twitch fibres (see also p. 000). The drop in isometric and dynamic muscle power parallels the fall in muscle mass, and this may mean that there is no qualitative age change in muscle composition or fibre morphology. Extended over a period of 12 weeks, training appeared to increase both slow-twitch and fast-twitch fibres in subjects up to 65 years of age, but the increase in muscle strength was only slight. This is not surprising, as the dominant age-dependent variable is to be found in stochastic changes in the motor neurons in the central nervous system.

That an all-embracing theory can be developed to account for every aspect of senescence (see p. 238) is unlikely. It is worth noting, however, that some of the aspects of muscular ageing outlined by Grimby and Saltin (1949) can be formally represented by Doubal's theory of reliability (Doubal 1982), which was presented later in a slightly different way, and elaborated by Witten (1983, 1984), as well as having been explored independently earlier by Abernethy (1979).

Based in essence on systems analysis and engineering concepts, Doubal's theory of reliability presents ageing in terms of the breakdown of hypothetical modules which are endowed with a certain amount of redundancy and repair potential: only when a critical number of them has broken down will the organism traverse the point of no return. Like many other theories, Doubal's version views death as the pinnacle of ageing rather than as an event that interrupts it for good. That hypothesis is considered later (p. 240).

Another aspect of elitism in gerontology is underlined by Parsons (1978). The fact that the expectancy of life is rising in most industrialized countries is attributable to an improvement in our control of the environment, although a reduction in infant mortality has also made a great contribution to this statistic (Warnes 1989). The amelioration in the Western world since the Second World War has led to better nutrition and provided an increase in heated accommodation, where previously houses were damp and cold. Parsons emphasizes that many gerontological studies refer to individuals in protected environments. Reading and Weale (1991) have recently shown that there is not only a difference in putative life span of some 15 years between people in the rich and poor countries, but that inhabitants of the latter also have a poorer physical constitution.

The possible benefit of an 'ideal' environment can be studied even at the cellular level. Using human diploid fibroblasts, Mayer *et al.* (1987) studied the effects of slight cooling and slight warming on assays of spontaneous and gamma-ray induced single-strand and double-strand breaks in the DNA and their repair at temperatures of 34, 37, and 39 °C. In what the authors refer to as the first cytogerontological study, they examined the response to both ionizing and non-ionizing radiation, the former being a well-known 'ageing' factor. Note that Lindop and Rotblat (1961) found that exposing mice to ionizing radiations led to a shortening of life because a few weeks were lost in early life. Maynard

Smith (1962) suggests that radiation and ageing differ in that the former causes somatic mutations, which are largely recessive in their influence, whereas normal ageing is due to causes other than somatic mutations.

Similarly, Giess (1980), irradiating *Drosophila melanogaster* with 25 kr of ^{60}Co, found that radiation-induced death varied with the insect's age, and stated categorically that ionizing radiation failed to accelerate the process of ageing. However, Mayer *et al.* (1987) used temperature as an additional monitor of ageing. It will be recalled in this connection that Hayflick (1965) made the following seminal observation.

When embryonic lung tissue is dissociated in tissue culture, the multitude of cells can be separated by centrifugation. If subsequently incubated at body temperature in a suitable nutrient, they proceed to divide, and, after a week, they begin to coalesce to form a monocellular layer, and further division is inhibited by contact. The process of division can be made to resume if some cells are removed from the parental culture and transferred in equal numbers to unused bottles containing fresh nutrient. This subcultivation leads to an approximate doubling of the number of cells removed from the parental bottle once con-fluence is reached yet again. The doubling is only approximate because some cells may not divide at all, while others may do so more than once.

Originally, this procedure could be repeated about 50 times under optimal conditions; more recently, however, appreciably higher figures (approximately 100 subcultivations) have been reported. When the parental tissue is obtained from an older donor, the number of doublings (**D**) is found to be reduced. **D** is therefore a cellular index of the age of the parental cells (but see Martin *et al.* (1981) for a possible role played by the considerable variance recordable in such measurements).

Mayer *et al.* (1987) found that the cumulative value of **D** at 37 °C was greater than the values at either 34 or 39 °C ($P < 0.01$). Moreover, the so-called thymidine-labelling index, which is a measure of the number of cells capable of synthesizing DNA, rose up to 70 at 37 °C, while reaching the lower 50s at 34 °C, and the higher 50s at 39 °C. Spontaneous breaks in DNA were at their lowest at 37 °C, but at 39 °C cells performed better in repairing single-strand breaks than was true at 37 °C. No effect specifically linked to temperature was identified in the response to ionizing radiations. As this study relates to cells in tissue culture, it is arguable whether or not enough stress was produced to be comparable with the *in vivo* situation. Parsons (1978) has shown that, in a population exposed to extreme environmental stresses (including physical, biological, and social stress) longevity differences between genotypes will be increased in comparison with those prevailing under optimal conditions. Evidently the stresses have to act before the end of the procreative period to be of evolutionary significance.

Modern medical advances have led to a progressively more varied genetic pool since the virtual disappearance of the unhygienic conditions which, as recently as the nineteenth century, led to frequent juvenile and young adult deaths of the type described by Charles Dickens; but the presence of some of these phenotypes is now conditional on an environment relatively free from stress. If, in a few decades, the environment should change, perhaps as a result of the rise in temperature, the pattern of senescence might well begin to approximate again to what is now observable in warmer climates. Though mortality may not be affected, some aspects of senescence, such as presbyopia are: the age of its onset drops approximately by 8 months for every °C rise in temperature (Weale 1982a). A reduction in this age is unlikely to be vitally significant, even though more than one author (Bernstein and Bernstein 1945; Helps 1973; Steinhaus 1932) have sought to justify it as a biomarker or, more aptly, as a necromarker.

On the face of it, there appears to be some correlation between the age of onset of presbyopia and life expectancy, if one makes for example a crude comparison between climatically temperate and hot countries. A misleading correlation is sometimes put forward between the incidence of presbyopia and that of cataract (which both happen to be age-related), and there appear to be correlates between environment and the incidence of cataract (see Chapter 5). More recently, there have been two studies linking cataract and mortality (Hirsch and Schwartz 1983; Benson *et al.* 1988) understandably without regard to environment, a pointer to the caution with which correlative studies need to be approached.

However, there are other vital properties of our bodies that depend closely on temperature (see p. 21); the biosystem being pushed beyond its present limit of tolerance may lead to homoeostatic readjustments or to selective pressures which some genotypes may be better able to adapt to than others. The point made by Parsons (1978) is that natural selection will become more apparent, given that many of today's survivors have been rendered medically fit for their present environment; but a rougher future may no longer suit their genetic make-up.

One cannot deduce from this that the mortality of those genotypes who may be fit to cope with a new environment will remain unchanged. Indeed, Parsons amalgamates the notion of stress as regards our physical, biological, and also social environments, and, like Young (see p. 1), he sees natural selection less as something that progresses than as a phenomenon that happens to test homoeostasis.

Toxicity as an ageing factor

The above-mentioned biological environment can be looked on as including the internal biosystem. It is, therefore, perhaps somewhat artificial to distinguish organ-based theories of senescence from environmental ones. Presumably the environment affects one or more organs, otherwise it would not be noticed and could not play a role. The issue would appear to be rather whether devolution of an organ in parallel with ageing is endogenous or exogenous (Grimley Evans

1988): if the former, then a cellular and genetic explanation may be expected, if the latter, then toxicity, neglect, starvation, etc. offer useful semantic models. Note the use of the words 'in parallel': it is important to disregard the idea that a particular phenomenon 'is due to ageing'. For example, Brock (1985) speaks of 'a direct effect of age on the circadian pacemaker . . .'. This can lead only to circular arguments. The calendar is a useful correlate with, but not an explanation of, senescence (see p. 28).

The notion that waste products may be noxious and agents of senescence goes back to the early years of this century (Hayflick 1965) when the age-related accumulation of the so-called age-pigments was first reported. The best-known of these are melanin and lipofuscin, and both are found in the eye (Chapter 3).

The conventional wisdom is that the age-pigments systematically increase in various human and animal tissues. For example, Nandy and Bourne (1966) and Mann *et al.* (1978) noted this as regards lipofuscin in nervous tissue, Davies *et al.* (1983) in the adrenal cortex, Strehler *et al.* (1959) in the myocardium, and Wing *et al.* (1978) and Feeney-Burns *et al.* (1984) in the retinal pigment epithelium. Associated by some authors with stress (Aloj Totaro *et al.* 1986; but see Davies *et al.* 1983), and with dietary deficiency by others (Katz *et al.* 1984), lipofuscin may result from auto-oxidation.

Ethnic differences have also been observed. Mann and Yates (1982) studied the presence of both lipofuscin and melanin in British and Sri Lankan brains, and found that the former was lower in inferior olives obtained from Sri Lankan rather than from British brains. Lipofuscin increased with age at a rate almost twice as fast in the tissue from British brains as in that from Sri Lankan brains. However, there was no difference, not was there any variation with age, in the amount of melanin found in other cerebral tissues, such as the substantia nigra and the locus caeruleus. The difference between the lipofuscin concentrations is tentatively attributed to the greater fat consumption in Britain compared with that in Sri Lanka; as discussed later (p. 160), this offers a cautionary tale.

Hayflick's reservation (1985) that the association between pigment accumu-lation and the increasing concentration of waste products is intuitive rather than substantiated is, therefore, well taken. Lipofuscin in the retinal pigment epi-thelium could be due to light exposure (Weiter 1987), which, admittedly, does not rule out the accumulation of undisposed retinal debris (p. 157), but it is striking that an age-pigment should accumulate mainly during the first two decades of our lives (Weale 1989*b*). In the retinal pigment epithelium, vitamin E deficiency leads to an increase in lipofuscin (Katz *et al.* 1984), but no other sign of senescence has been reported. Conversely, the administration of vitamin E fails to decrease the concentration of the pigment or to play a significant role in connection with the length of the life span.

The increase of lipofuscin concentration in human neural tissue not exposed to light is well documented, but it is noteworthy that, just as happens in the retinal pigment epithelium (Chapter 3), the accumulation in the human stellate

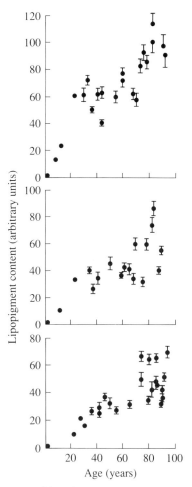

Fig. 1.3 The distribution of lipofuscin in three human cerebral ganglia as a function of age. After Koistinaho *et al.* (1986).

ganglion, the superior mesenteric ganglion, and the frontal cortex (Fig. 1.3) occurs in two phases (Koistinaho *et al.* 1986): the rise to a plateau in middle life occurs far more slowly than is true of the retinal pigment epithelium, but the onset of the final phase at the age of about 60 years is similar (see Chapter 3).

Mann *et al.* (1978) studied, in addition to the age variation of lipofuscin in, the RNA content and nucleolar volume of, human dentate, olivary and the Purkyně and pyramidal cells of the hippocampus. The ribosomal RNA and the size of the nucleolus are linearly related, and various pieces of evidence point to these quantities being reliable indices of the rate of protein synthesis and function. But though the rate of accumulation of lipofuscin differs drastically (by almost 10:1 in the two extremes) as amongst the four types of cell, the losses in RNA and nucleolar volume with age are remarkably constant. The authors believe that, if lipofuscin is noxious, it is more likely to act in a mechanical manner — just by being there in the cell — than in any other way.

This view may be contrasted with one put forward by Buchanan and Sidhu (1986) who noted that autofluorescence, used as an index of the presence of lipofuscin, increases exponentially with the falling doubling capacity of cultured fibroblasts. They observed that cells with a raised cumulative doubling capacity, i.e. possibly aged cells, do not respond to agents that raise it in cells where it is low to begin with. Moreover, autofluorescence rises in cells with a low capacity treated, for example, with increasing concentrations of aminogly-coside, known to accumulate in lysosomes. It also appears that there is an upper limit to the intensity of autofluorescence that can accumulate in cell cultures. Aminoglycoside and other substances such as streptomycin, the antibiotic G418, and ammonium chloride all increase the rate of increase of autofluorescence, but, with the exception of G418, they do not change the life span. Thus, even though higher doubling numbers are associated with a larger putative con-centration of lipofuscin, the reverse, namely that lipofuscin could promote senescence, does not appear to be true.

In any case, in order to act as an ageing factor rather than simply as a sort of cellular calendar, lipofuscin would have to be shown to affect the function of the cells that contain it. Davies and Fotheringham (1981) and Davies *et al.* (1983) argue on the basis of observations on mice that, although for example the amount of pigment in the supra-optic nucleus rises with age, it occupies only a very small part of the cellular volume. The findings that the volume of the neurosecretory granules in this nucleus decreases without being accompanied by an increase in lipofuscin, and that, under osmotic stress, the granules remain unchanged while the amount of lipofuscin is reduced lead the authors to question whether any cellular damage follows pigment accumulation.

Free radicals

A guarded attitude as regards correlational evidence also needs to be taken with another idea based on toxicity, namely the free-radical theory of ageing (Harman 1984). This states 'that free radical reactions, arising largely in the course of normal metabolism, are responsible for the progressive accumulation of the changes with time associated with or responsible for the ever-increasing likelihood of disease or death that accompanies advancing age'. The formation of the free radicals results therefore from everyday enzymatic reactions pro-moting or accompanying the maintenance and function of the individual. When scavengers are available to dispose of them, and hence to prevent their accumu-lation to hazardous levels, no question of toxicity is likely to arise. However, other reactions induced by free radicals, perhaps in a random manner, and others, arising from leakage of these ions during their normal metabolism, may be less benign. Deleterious reactions linked to the excessive presence of free radicals include, for example, cumulative oxidation in such stable molecules as collagen, elastin, and chromosomal material; the breakdown of polysaccharides; the accumulation of age-pigments, especially the above-mentioned lipofuscin; modifications of cell membrane characteristics in mitochondria and lysosomes consequent upon lipid peroxidation; and others. Free radicals are believed to play a signal role in the senescence of the human crystalline lens because they are produced, *inter alia*, by ionizing radiation (such as the all-pervasive cosmic rays) and also by ultraviolet radiation. Glutathione, present in the lens, decreases with age (Harding 1970) which may increase the risk from free radical reactions. The predominant presence of the free compound in the cortex and its progressive age-related reduction may help to explain why senile cataract frequently assumes a cortical form (see Chapter 5).

In listing reactions involving free radicals, Harman (1984) sees them as precursors to a long range of ultimately fatal diseases, and, in this respect, many of his arguments are valid and accepted (see also Hayflick 1985). It is also noteworthy that both the superoxide anion and hydrogen peroxide (Sohal *et al.* 1989, 1990) are related hyperbolically to the so-called maximum life span potential, a figure that for captive animals, has shown a tendency to increase with our ability to maintain their health.

But the simple fact that the rate of accumulation of some of the noxious factors can be controlled, for example by dietary means, seems to vitiate Harman's generalizing approach. It could be that some free radicals accumulate merely because their precursors are being continually ingested. According to DeLong and Poplin (1977), there is sparse evidence to show that free radicals actually accumulate, and they may react in only an intermittent way, rather than in the continuous manner which would make them ageing agents. On the other hand, von Zglinicki (1987) postulates that free radicals attack mitochondrial membranes with a consequential and age-related loss of water from the organelles, a point which is elaborated later (p. 16).

In a development of the above ideas, Hayflick (1985) emphasizes that, for all their well-documented noxiousness, free radicals cause, by the very enfeebling of the organs that contain them, a reduction not in life span, but in life expectancy. Delaying death and prolonging life are not equivalent in gerontological theory.

It is also possible that some of the evidence quoted in support of the free radical hypothesis could be in error. For example, contrary to Harman's view, lipofuscin does not always increase linearly with age in humans (Figs 1.3 and 3.20). Its correlation is not inevitably linked to neuronal losses even when it occurs in a neural tissue such as the retina. As regards melanin, in connection with which 'a similar effect has been noted', the contrary has also been observed: in the retinal pigment epithelium and in the iris (Weiter *et al.* 1986; Weale 1989*b*) the rate of decrease in melanin concentration is almost equal to the rate of increase in lipofuscin concentration.

Membranes as gates to senescence

Free radicals are regarded as having special significance in the ageing of mitochondrial membranes (Siliprandi *et al.* 1979). The authors found that diamide mimics and accentuates the effect of free radicals, and that the supply of dithioerythritol can counteract this. Many authors believe that ageing is the principal multifactorial aspect of the organism (see Olson 1987), and are reluctant to allocate priorities to a group of organs rather than protein synthesis or vice versa; but others tend to focus on what they see as almost overriding influences. Scientific objectivity does not oblige authors to renounce the importance of what may well be their life's work and achievement. Sun and Sun (1979) consider the membrane deterioration theory as 'the most basic factor in explaining the aging process in general', attributing to free radicals (p. 13) an important destructive role, and seeing the accumulation of, for example, lipofuscin (p. 152) as evidence of senescence based on membrane defects.

It is not unreasonable that great importance should be attached to membranes. The point is that some 50 per cent of a membrane consists of lipids, which provide the fundamentals for a proper functioning of antigens, enzymes and receptors, such as the retinal photoreceptors. They are also important for the conduction of nervous impulses, because they form impermeable bilayers in conjunction with hydrocarbon chains. During ageing, pliable structures are replaced by more rigid ones owing to an increase in cholesterol, sphingolipids, etc. Zs.-Nagy (1978, 1979) attributed an increase in rigidity of the membranes of the brains of rats and rabbits with advancing years to the progressive increase of the cholesterol/phospholipid ratio. In addition there is a reduction in membrane lipid fluidity. The composition of membrane proteins changes only late in life, which suggests that the earlier changes are reversible (Shinitzky 1987). Lipid tissue hardening may be due to the formation of cross-linkages between the constituent macromolecules, and explain the observed increase of intracellular potassium. A further result would be a slow-down in transcription and a retardation in enzymatic processes.

These observations have been extended to human beings (Rivnay *et al.* 1980): the serum cholesterol/phospholipid ratio and membrane microviscosity rise systematically with age, and are correlated with each other in the higher age groups. This is seen as a possible cause for a reduction in immune responses in advancing years.

The membrane of mitochondria receives special attention from von Zglinicki (1987) who suggests that the decrease of phospholipids and the rise of cholesterol in these organelles, the reverse of the above-mentioned cases of brain and of serum, is due to free radical activity. The rise in the phospholipid/cholesterol ratio both modifies the interaction of the mitochondrial proteins with the surrounding lipid phase and causes phase segregations in the organelles; the permeability to small ions is likely to increase, and ultimately an efflux of water will occur. This would explain a reduction in the activity of certain transport enzymes, and von Zglinicki also attributes the accumulation of lipofuscin in postmitotic cells to this cause. He concludes that 'alterations in the energy metabolism of mitochondria are very likely to play a central role in the aging process'.

In their careful review, Sun and Sun (1979) analyse the possible effects of the passage of time on such membrane-dependent processes as neurotransmission and hormonal activity (see p. 19), and they emphasize the changes in membrane lipids − essential for the conduction of nervous impulses − and their metabolism. Because it can be obtained in a relatively pure form, myelin received a great deal of attention: for example, significant alterations were observed in the phospholipids of the human frontal cerebral cortex (though Grinna (1977) reports that the total lipid or phospholipid content of human and murine brains remains constant), but no functional correlation appears so far to have been established with these changes. Some metabolic alterations were observed in the ageing murine brain.

Other changes include increases in cell size, both *in vivo* and in cultured cells, including human fibroblasts (Grinna 1977), but this may be no more than a manifestation of cell death (see p. 20) with surviving cells filling the vacuum left by those that have died. The number of mitochondria in the human liver decreases with age, but their increase in volume is more likely to be due to an increase in water content resulting from osmotic (and membranous) changes. Protein synthesis (pp. 23, 26) linked to membrane function may also play a role. Numerous age-related changes in membrane composition have been reported, their absence in erythrocyte membranes (see p. 3) receiving mention. However, human erythrocytes reveal an age-related increase in cholesterol: it is not established whether this is a genetic result or due to dietary causes during the donor's lifetime. The increase in extrinsic proteins on the plasma membrane surface of erythrocytes is similarly unexplained. The synthesis of membrane lipid and protein constituents appears to be independent of age (see above). But while membranes in some tissues exhibit morphological changes, the relation between cause and effect is unresolved, and the effect on function unknown. Indeed, Choe and Rose (1976) emphasize that changes in ageing membranes are not obvious, and it is worth repeating that erythrocytes are stable and that this is also true of their membranes.

Some immunological and neuroendocrine factors

The line between organ-based and cellular theories of ageing starts wearing a little thin when it comes to allocating responsibility for a deterioration in function or diminished prospects of survival on the basis of immunological properties and hormonal activity of the organism. Taking issue with Hayflick's view (1985) that cellular ageing is likely to underlie that of the neuroendocrine system, Meites *et al.* (1987) note that, in even the simplest of organisms, hormones may control such cellular functions as growth, metabolism, and reproduction. This situation is accentuated in more highly organized animals whose survival depends on extracellular homoeostatic mechanisms governed, *inter alia*, by the neuroendocrine and immune system and the associated transporting mechanisms.

This is not to deny the importance of the role played by the senescence of cells of the immune system, notably of lymphocytes, carefully reviewed by Leech (1980). Unlike macrophages, the main classes of lymphocytes are marked by senescence, but in different ways. The cells in question are the cytotoxic T cells and the B cells, the effectors of the antibody response and the precursors of plasma cells producing immunoglobulin. Both types are responsible for immune responses, but the former have a shorter life. According to Beregi *et al.* (1991), the number of T cells increases between the ages of 70 and 100 years whereas that of the B cells remains constant. The magnitude of their effect is modulated by helper T_h, and suppressor T_s cells. Although the number of T lymphocytes, for example in 'healthy' people aged 65 years and over is normal (but is liable to rise as age approaches 100 years) their proportions are liable to change. Also the *in vitro* response of cells to antigens or mitogens (which stimulate mitosis) is decreased (Phair *et al.* 1988). Much of the work done in the field relates to mice, but, when age is replaced by life span, similarities with human cells become clear (Fig. 1.4). The immuno-traffic system (Fig. 1.5) provides a useful ground plan on which to sketch senescent effects.

It is worth noting that the difference which care in patient selection can produce, for example to an analysis of erythrocytes (p. 4), is reflected also in lymphocytes, in the specificity of auto-antibodies, and monoclonal gammopathies. Patients selected in accordance with the Senieur Protocol appeared to have fewer signs of senescence than was true of those not conforming to it (Lightart *et al.* 1990).

The efficiency of the immune system peaks during puberty and declines thereafter (Walford 1983), but human peripheral blood lymphocyte counts show a decline from $5000/mm^3$ in early infancy to $2000/mm^3$ in the adult. The suggestion (Polednak 1978) than an increase in leucocytes observed in women, exposed to ionizing radiations, may compensate for the drop in lymphocytes makes little biological sense; Polednak's sample was postmenopausal.

Data for T and B cells are contentious, perhaps for the reasons outlined above (p. 5). The loss of T cells, observed by some authors, was attributed for a long time to the involution of the thymus during childhood, a view that has proved untenable. More recent work has shown that the thymus interacts with the neuroendocrine system: it is its involution immediately after puberty that has

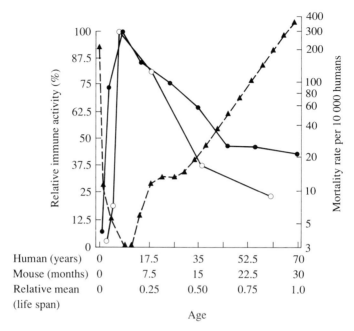

Fig. 1.4   When the differences in life span are allowed for, the time courses of human and murine immunological activities are found to be similar. After Leech (1980). ●, Natural serum isoagglutinin titres in human beings; ○, peak serum antibody response of mice to SRC (sheep red cells); ▲, mortality rate in human beings.

led to the suggestion that it controls immunosenescent events (Meites *et al.* 1987).

Lymphocytes can be made to proliferate following stimulation by antigens or mitogens, but do so less with advancing age (see above). The qualitative explanation advanced for this observation is that metabolic and/or structural changes prevent lymphocytic transformation and proliferation. It is supported by results of studies involving anti-immunoglobulin: in young mice, B cells do not respond to it, whereas those in old mice do: it inhibits them poorly.

Traffic of suppressor B cells, acting nonspecifically, seems to occur from bone marrow to peripheral lymph organs during ageing. Also T_h cell activity may weaken, although an increase has been observed in special circumstances. More generally, it has been suggested that auto-antibodies result from the failure of homoeostatic mechanisms. For example, Fixa *et al.* (1975) examined 483 persons, who were 'believed to be healthy', in the age range of 19 to 97 years for eight types of antibodies. They found a systematic and age-related (and sex-linked) rise, particularly in thyroid antibodies; however, the question of whether

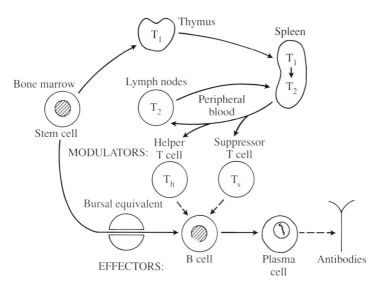

Fig. 1.5 The pathways of lymphocyte differentiation and traffic. The dashed lines represent activities by soluble factors. T_h and T_s modulate the activity of B cells. After Leech (1980).

this might be due to an inadequate immunological reaction to antigens, released perhaps owing to nonspecific damage, is unanswered.

But our knowledge of the traffic between immunological systems and neuroendocrine mechanisms is poor (Meites *et al.* 1987). This is also true of the correlates with age. The development of mammary and pituitary tumours apart, there are some universal and, therefore, fully gerontological links between the two mechanisms to be found in the decline of reproductive function, the diminution in the secretion of the growth hormone, and in protein synthesis (Makrides 1983).

Both growth hormone and sometomedins, which serve to stimulate the growth in many tissues, were found in smaller concentrations in elderly than in young persons. In rats, similar observations have been linked to a reduction in the hypothalamic release of both norepinephrine and dopamine, well-known to occur also in man. There is some indication that the decline in tissue protein synthesis in the liver, kidneys, heart, thymus and spleen of both rats and mice can be partly counteracted by daily injections of growth hormone. But Makrides (1983) warns that the literature on protein synthesis and ageing is contradictory for reasons that he has carefully analysed. Meites *et al.* (1987) are aware that tissue-specific cellular changes may play a role, but believe that the decline in growth hormone secretion is dominant.

Hypothalamic control, for instance of body temperature, weakens in later years (Collins and Exton-Smith 1986), and it may be that this is not due to genetic causes, but rather to toxic hormonal factors. Meites *et al.* (1987) suspect that the devolution of the reproductive system may be due to this, resulting from neuronal death in the hypothalamus and in the arcuate nucleus, mediated by oestrogen. The accumulation of lipofuscin is one of the signs; once again, its character as an age-pigment appears to be purely adventitious (p. 13). There is no implication here that all neuronal loss is due to a putative hormonal toxicity. It occurs throughout life, for example in the cerebellum (Hall *et al.* 1975), and during fixed developmental periods in the retina (Silver 1978) (but see p. 118).

There is increasingly compelling evidence to support the view that immunological senescence is under genetic control which is more than marginal (Walford 1983). A murine example is provided by the major histocompatibility complex (MHC) which controls that part of the immune system which depends on the thymus. The MHC determines the maximum life span by two sets of links: (a) via the developmental and differentiation programmes (which include the maturation of the immune response and which, as we saw on p. 17, occurs very early), and/or (b) via loci that code for biochemical mechanisms linked to senescent processes. In this, the H-2 complex exerts an overriding role. The degree of autoimmunity (in mice) correlates with the MHC, and demonstrates the notion of pleiotropy (Kirkwood 1984), since, polymorphic and protective early on, it may become a hazard late in life, because individuals with an age-related formation of antibodies have a shorter life expectancy than those without them. The MHC also appears to be in control of the degrees of DNA repair (pp. 28 and 235), the decay in which is likely to promote processes associated with senescence (Gottesman *et al.* 1982; Nette *et al.* 1984).

The fact that the maximum potential life span of chimpanzees is half that of man, but the two species differ in their DNA and amino acid sequences and proteins by less than 1 per cent also supports the idea that regulatory genes are important, and vary developmental patterns.

Though dominant, the MHC is unlikely to be the only supergene system to control immune regulation and ageing via developmental templates and biochemical routes (Gottesman *et al.* 1982) in spite of the control it exerts on the level of DNA repair and other functions as outlined above. Using seven different species, Hart and Setlow (1984) showed that there is a high correlation between their maximum life span and the rate and degree of unscheduled DNA synthesis in their fibroblasts exposed to damaging ultraviolet radiation. It is important to note that the relation refers to the maximum, and not the mean, life span: environmental and other non-genetic influences are less likely to affect the maximum than the mean. However, to some extent, the correlation is determined by the choice of species, even though it applies to man (Francis *et al.* 1981).

Hart and Setlow's work was thought to have been disproved by Kato *et al.* (1980) who examined 34 species in 11 different orders of mammal. Although the authors say that 'it is obvious that the majority of the species does not show correlations (sic) between the two parameters', statistical analysis of their results denies this. The correlation coefficient is low, at 0.3443, but significant, with $P = 0.025$. It might have been higher had the authors used gerontologically equally old phenotypes. To be able to do this it is necessary to study the degree of DNA repair for a given species as a function of age: Nette *et al.* (1984) have shown for human epidermal cells that this important property decreases linearly with age. Extrapolated to the age at which repair would be zero, the function may offer a definition of the life span of the species. In the human data, it appears to lie between 120 and 130 years (see Chapter 5).

There is evidence to suggest the MHC controls DNA repair by genes of the H-2 complex. Since the number of genes believed to be involved in this type of control is small, one would not expect all diseases characterized by impaired DNA capacity to mimic all characteristics associated with senescence. This is, indeed, the case, and lends further support to the notion that the MHC controls the intactness of those systems which, once its rule is relaxed, manifest characteristics of ageing.

Studies on biological clocks also reveal a genetic influence, for example in that the circadian control of mitosis weakens with age. It is important to distinguish endogenous entrained rhythms that are determined by circadian environmental stimuli, such as light or temperature, from free-running ones; these can manifest in a constant environment even though they may have approximately circadian or circannual periods. In general, only the latter are liable to vary with age.

Functionally, these free-running rhythms may be accompanied by partial or complete desynchronization, but there is no evidence to suggest that the two are related by cause and effect (Brock 1985). A subtle circannual effect was described by Dartnall *et al.* (1961), who found that the retina of the rudd (*Scardinius erythrophthalmus*) contains more of the visual pigment absorbing maximally at 507 nm in the summer, but more of one peaking at 535 nm in the winter. Bridges and Yoshikami (1970) showed that this is due to the light environment, as the effect could be mimicked in one eye by occluding it. This excluded humoral intervention, and proved that light acts in this respect directly on the retina. Old fish failed to show the change in pigment, and were left with the 'winter' pigment. However, the explanation of this result may be wholly physical, for Villermet and Weale (1972) showed that the suppression of the change coincided with a yellowing of the animal's crystalline lens, which created photic winter within the eye so that the circannual environmental change remained without effect as the photic stimulus could not penetrate to the retina in sufficient intensity.

There are two lessons to be learned from this episode. First this seems to be the edge of a phylogenetic development: an overtly circannual rhythm appears to be due to a local retinal action that can be stopped and started at the experimenter's will. Free- running mechanisms are likely to have started in an analogous manner, but have developed into automatic systems under the force of evolutionary advantage. Secondly, neither the neuroendocrine system nor specific genetic directives appear to be involved in the above example, which could be mimicked by the action of a photographic shutter. The yellowing of the lens of the rudd may yet be a coincidence, and a more complicated biochemical explanation may be required. But Occam's Razor is on the side of the lens, and other similar situations may be found that provide relatively simple solutions to involved observations.

1.2.3 *Cellular senescence*

Some of those who harbour reservations about waste theories, such as the free-radical one, stress the lack of experimental evidence with which to support them. This is neatly exemplified by Hirsch (1986) who has attempted to show by means of a theoretical model that the senescence of cells in tissue culture is subject to the accumulation of waste products within them. On the one hand, he quotes data showing a clear relation between mitotic function and the amount of fluorescent waste in human fibroblasts, and commends his analysis as useful in a simulation model which tests the relation between waste-product and ageing. He derives an expression for the rate of accumulation of sterile cells in terms of events leading to sterility, a function of the generation time of cells, real time, and some constants. On the other hand, owing to some of the prem-isses underlying the analysis, the author's regrettable conclusion is that this work cannot be used to verify or invalidate the waste-product hypothesis of cellular ageing. Its formulation is more complex than that of the reliability functions mentioned on p. 8, but it has the merit of being a hypothesis describing ageing rather than dying.

Hirsch achieves this by virtue of considering cell populations. One of the most important aspects of Hayflick's discovery (1965) of the phenomenon of tissue culture doubling capacity has been underestimated in the past. Hayflick has offered us an independent variable replacing time in the cytogerontological context. The state of a cell population can be expressed in terms of the average number of divisions it has undergone, and, in principle, it does not matter what is the mean time interval between two successive divisions. The life 'time' of a cell population may be 50, 70, or even 100 divisions, but the dimension of time is not the essence of it.

Mention has already been made of the notion that time serves as a framework for our observations, but is useless when one tries to explain them (p. 11). Operationally, this is obvious when correlations are made between two age- or time-related phenomena: their success or otherwise frequently resides in the elimination of time as the independent variable. The elucidation of mechanisms that underlie our observations is sought in terms of cellular changes, not as functions of time, but of the concentration of such and such an ion. In senescence what matters is the volume density of vital molecules, enzymes, proteins, etc., as Hirsch has clearly shown. This is probably one of the reasons why Adelman (1987) condemns the pursuit of collecting biomarkers: they are, indeed, little better than local calendars.

At present it is not practicable to extend this notion to a whole organism, and to say in a quasi-Aristotelian or Laplacean manner: 'Tell me how many cell divisions you harbour, and I will tell you how long you are going to live'. There is no need to dwell on environmental influences in this context, as they are conceptually taken care of in the above idea. What is important to establish is a, if not the, bridge between cellular changes and senescence and that of the next order in biological hierarchies, presumably an assembly of cells.

In an attempt to determine the relevance or otherwise of *in vitro* senescence to the *in vivo* situation, Mets *et al.* (1983) compared the division capacity of human stromal bone marrow with that of subcultured cells. These were of two kinds. First, a comparison was made between cells obtained from young and old donors with cells in early and late subcultivations of embryonic fibroblasts. Secondly, the authors obtained biopsic material from a young donor, cloned it *in vitro*, and the two patterns of division could again be compared.

Cell populations from young donors and early *in vitro* passages were similar to each other. There were also analogous changes to be seen in material obtained from middle-aged and old donors with middle and late *in vitro* passages, but they were more pronounced in the latter. This is attributed in part to the fact that the cultured cells had been driven to their maximum human life span (MHL) levels, whereas the oldest group of donors was 74 years old, which was estimated as more than 60 per cent of the MHL. In this example, then, senescent processes seen in tissue culture appeared to be relevant to those observed in the tissue itself.

Error hypotheses

Why should the number of divisions be finite? If the genetic programme can control large sequences, what stops the process of cell division? In a way, this question returns to the problem faced earlier (p. 3) in connection with a programme for senescence. In this case, there would be a genetic sequence, possibly analogous to an emptying cistern, allowing a cell to perform its function until the last drop has dripped away.

Another possibility, envisaged by Orgel (1963), might be that there is a deterioration in the ability of the gene to transcribe instructions, if not from cell generation to generation, but at least now and then. A transcription error can lead to the production of a faulty amino acid. This, in turn, will modify the protein of which it forms a component which could lead to the development of a structural defect and a change in the activity of the protein. This would persist until the elimination of the faulty messenger RNA or protein. However, positive feedback might reinforce the process in a random manner. In a later addendum, Orgel (1973) envisaged an exponential increase which such a feedback would promote '. . . the greater the number of errors that have accumulated in the macromolecular constituents of the cell, the faster the accumulation of further errors'.

It is possible (Laughrea 1982) that failure may occur not because there are too many errors for the repair mechanisms to deal with but because the latter consume too much energy for the successful continuation of cellular function.

When the number of errors has increased beyond what repair mechanisms can set right, a local catastrophe occurs and the cell stops functioning. Evidently, if this happens often enough, particularly within a compressed interval of time, the cell assembly and, later, the organ will fail. ˙

The importance of the hypothesis has been minimized by some authors (see Burch and Jackson 1976), but it has nonetheless been subjected to extensive tests. For instance, Gershon and Gershon (1970, 1976) have been unable to demonstrate the occurrence of cumulative damage: their study of senescent enzymes points to inactivation rather than alteration. Using the nematode *Caenorhabditis elegans*, Johnson and McCaffrey (1985) studied protein synthesis *in vivo*. In this species, some 16 per cent of proteins are under developmental control. The authors reasoned that, given that the processes occurring in senescence are similar to those found in development, this might be detected in the range of proteins synthesized during the life span of the species. But if an error catastrophe overtakes the protein(s) or more levels of gene expression underlie ageing, it should be possible to detect the faulty amino acids in newly synthesized protein.

Although some changes were detected, they were not such as to point to a change in gene control leading to senescence, nor was there any evidence of any faulty incorporation of amino acids into the newly synthesized proteins.

In a detailed review of the relevant literature, Laughrea (1982) examined the question of fidelity of translation decreasing with age, the formation of abnormalities in macromolecules, the possible misincorporation of amino acids in senescence (see above), and related problems. His conclusion is that at least a small increase in error frequency does occur during information transfer from nucleic acids to protein. This implicates messenger RNA, although it is conceivable that old proteins may fail to receive the message. But the changes appear to be too modest to enable the scale of their significance to be determined.

A different form of positive reinforcement of genetic messages has been postulated by Medvedev (1972), which, contrary to the above-mentioned positive feedback, is unlikely to be random. Impressed by the observation that polyploid cells are stable and long-lasting, and their proportion increases with age in a fair number of tissues, he asks whether an increase in the ratio between cell functions dependent on duplicated or multiple genes and on single, unique genes, respectively, is accompanied by a slow ageing rate and a longer life span in the case of highly differentiated post-mitotic cells. If the answer is yes, then there are not only evolutionary but also gerontological implications. From the point of view of evolution, the stabler the gene the more likely it is to survive phylogenetically (see Dawkins 1989); and from that of gerontology, a similar argument applies to the survival of the phenotype in its struggle against hostile external factors.

Repetition (**R**) serves to reduce the chance of molecular accidents. It can assume in the DNA of the gastropod *Nassaria obsoleta* as many as four figures: if the chance of a molecular accident were as high as 0.5, that is half of the nucleotide sequences were at risk during a given period, repetition of this magnitude reduces the probability to one with 301 noughts between the decimal point and the first significant figure. But even with a value of **R** of approximately 30, postulated by Medvedev for some tRNA genes, a probability of destruction of 0.5 is reduced to one in one thousand million.

This hypothesis is supported by several important observations. For example, in *Drosophila melanogaster*, the mutation which reduces the number of genes for ribosomal RNAs is accompanied by the process initiating the build-up of repetition in tRNA genes. The significance of this is that ribosomal RNA is conservative and is to be found in different species. However, tRNAs are species and tissue specific and exhibit considerable evolutionary variations. Another example between gene repetition and evolutionary change is to be found in a comparison between histones and haemoglobins: the mRNA of the former is short-lived, while that of haemoglobins is long-lived. This explains why, during the formation of erythrocytes, histone synthesis decreases and that of haemoglobin prevails.

Medvedev deduces from this that the senescence of cells must be linked to the loss of, or change, in non-repeated information. In the above numerical examples 'non-repeated' may be replaced with 'little repeated', where the magnitude of 'little' is linked to the probability of the occurrence of a molecular accident. He goes on to generalize to the effect that the evolution of the life span of an organism may depend on the availability (**A**) of non-repeated information in the genome and in specialized tissues of the mature body. A relative increase in **A** is liable to reduce the life span.

It is particularly interesting from the point of view of later parts in this chapter and also Chapter 2 that Medvedev addresses the problem of how long repetition has to be preserved. As the preservation of all order has to be paid for, the maintenance of repetition becomes uneconomical once the next phenotypic generation is capable of looking after itself. Medvedev postulates that the liberalization of unique genes of later post-embryonal or adult stages in an individual life initiates ageing and thereby promotes the deterioration of non-repeated information.

This extraordinary passage was written in the Soviet Union during the Cold War in manifest ignorance of Medawar (1952) having suggested in his Inaugural Address at University College London that natural selection acting on genes expressing at definite biological ages would inhibit the expression of noxious genes. If this inhibition is so strong as to delay expression to an age when the chances of survival in the wild were nil, natural selection would have nothing whereon to act. In the long run, a pool of noxious genes would be generated, and, given the human conquest of the natural environment, noxious factors could begin to harm the phenotype, and senescence could start.

This was echoed in a discussion of ageing of poikilotherms by the distinction between the two periods of ageing and dying (Maynard Smith 1963). Dell'Orco *et al.* (1986) obtained evidence in support of Medvedev's hypothesis in measurements of the nucleosome spacing, that is, the DNA repeat length of human diploid fibroblast cells derived from neonatal foreskin. They observed a marked heterogeneity, which is not peculiar to this system, and attributed the varied nucleosome spacings to the presence of linker regions of different sizes. The size distribution of DNA lengths, which are identifiable with Medvedev's 'redundant' repetitions **R**, changed systematically with increasing age: the proportion of short repeats was greater in older cells than in young ones.

Replication, clocks and DNA repair

This is relevant to the suggestion that somatic cells lose at each replication a terminal segment of DNA in a replicon, that is, the unit component of the source of the information needed for protein synthesis (Choe and Rose 1976). If this proved to be the case, there would be a blueprint for a biological clock or, per-haps more appropriately, a biological sandglass: either the loss of vital informa-tion contained in terminal units or that of a crucial number of similar DNA segments might spell the end to the sequence of events normally controlled by them. It does not follow that the existence of a clock implies a programme for ageing (see Choe and Rose 1976); it would be more economical to see it as a programme for the maintenance of cellular function even though it may be seen as based on gene depreciation. This may be contrasted with the notion that ageing cells synthesize an inhibitor of DNA synthesis, located within the senescent cell itself (Stanulis-Praeger 1987), and implies the existence of a programme which the cytoplasm would have to spend energy on maintaining throughout the life of the cell (see p. 37).

The mode of cellular senescence, of which the above may provide an example, has received a great deal of attention. It may help to note that there are three types of proliferating cell. There are the so-called cycling cells, deriving their name from the fact that they run through the cell cycle, namely from a gap, G1, through a period of DNA synthesis, S, to another gap, G2, terminated by the period of mitosis, M. The gaps each serve a different purpose. Protein synthesis occurring during G1 promotes the synthesis of DNA during S, whereas in G2 it prepares for cytokinesis or movement of the cell. There are also two types of non-cycling cell, depending on whether they are blocked at G1 or G2, and cycle only in response to stimulation. An ageing cell is hall-marked by an increased quiescence in G1; this points to protein synthesis suffering when this happens, and the conformational changes then taking place in a variety of proteins bear witness to this (Makrides 1983). The three types of proliferating cell may coexist in one tissue, but their proportions are liable to differ; in particular, the pro-portion of cycling to non-cycling cells is liable to increase in parallel with age (Gelfant and Smith 1972). This process is reversible and the rate and degree with which this occurs depend both on the parent tissue and its age. Good (1975), however, has cast doubt on the validity of a number of conclusions on the ground that they are vitiated by the lack of a variety of corrections.

The statement about proportions disguises a more fundamental aspect than a mere comparison of ratios would permit. The number of cycling cells will appear to be reduced when the length of the cycle increases (but see Good 1975, for traps). This can happen statistically when a fraction of cycling cells is blocked at either gap. In this case DNA will not be synthesized, and the cells are liable to remain in this state until they are stimulated into proliferation, for example owing to injury to the tissue, or until they die.

The apparent increase in period is well illustrated in a study in which biopsy material from female patients ranging in age from 17 to 77 years was irradiated with ultraviolet radiation, which damages DNA. The rate of repair, if any, was estimated on the basis of autoradiography of the dissociated epidermal cells, labelling having been achieved by means of tritiated thymidine (Nette *et al.* 1984). The results are clear (Fig. 1.6): unirradiated cells used as controls provide a baseline. Irradiated cells manifest in the form of photographic grains, and their population density decreases systematically as a function of age. This shows that isolated human epidermal cells, exposed to damaging ultraviolet irradiation, can repair the damage at all ages, but the extent of the repair greatly depends on the age of the tissue donor and possibly also on the *in vitro* age, a view not wholeheartedly subscribed to by Good (1975) who seems to be isolated in this respect (Stanulis-Praeger 1987).

The original tight correlation between the life span of a species and un-scheduled DNA synthesis, a measure of the excision repair system (Hart and Setlow 1974), is subject to a variety of technical influences, but remains broadly speaking valid (Francis *et al.* 1981).

It may be noted that extrapolation of the regression line in Fig. 1.6 leads to a zero value at an age of approximately 130 years (see Chapter 5); somewhere near this age, then, one might encounter a situation when damage to DNA is no longer repaired.

Schneider *et al.* (1979) who, amongst others, analysed some of the drawbacks of this experimentally difficult subject, noted that the frequency with which old colonies produced cloned cells was appreciably smaller than was true of young

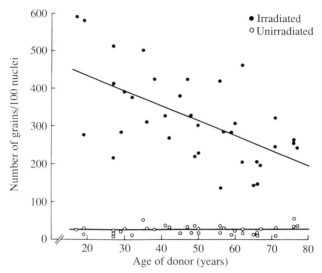

Fig. 1.6   The age-related variation of DNA repair in ultraviolet-irradiated epidermal cells. Modified from Nette *et al.* (1984).

ones. They saw this as a reliable index of the *in vitro* life span of the cultured human fetal lung fibroblasts, and showed that its validity could be extended to relate to the age of the *in vivo* donor (Fig. 1.6). This creates a problem, as the proliferative span of cell populations may exceed that of their parent tissues (Aufderheide 1984). The view of Schneider *et al.* that we do not die from a failure in cell replication, may well be belied one day by the extrapolation mentioned in the previous paragraph.

Cytogerontology, as exemplified by the above and many other studies, has led to the introduction of more definitions of senescence. Stanulis-Praeger (1987) expresses it in terms of the prolonged sterility in proliferation that precedes cell death. It is arguable that it is hard to distinguish between a relative and an absolute increase in quiescence, and that ageing could be identified with any such increase. In some restricted sense the process is reversible. For example, the presence of epidermal growth factor delays terminal differentiation, and the life span of corneal epithelial cells has been extended by fibroblast growth factor. Hydrocortisone has also been shown to exert a positive effect. However, an insulin-like growth factor equally affected human middle-aged and senescent lung fibroblasts as regards the inhibition of protein breakdown; protein synthesis was slightly stimulated in the oldest cells (Ballard and Read 1985).

Other evidence shows that immortality does not seem to have any survival value, for it is a recessive feature, making the life-limit of normal cells genetically dominant. Even the response to growth factors may vary with the age of the cell beneficiary (Stanulis-Praeger and Gilchrest 1986).

In contrast with the above body of opinion, there is the view that defects characteristic of ageing may not be entirely cell-specific (Tollefsbol and Cohen 1986). As above, the assumption is made that there is a genetic slowing-cycle, but that it affects not just G1 but also transcription, translation, and enzymatic induction. The decline in immune performance was mentioned on p.20, and this leads to a variety of immune-related diseases. The specific causes may be cellular, for example mitogenesis is reduced; and/or there may exist also an impairment of metabolic pathways, that is, the level is biochemical; and/or protein molecules may suffer from synthesizing errors and be degraded (p. 24). It is furthermore possible that the lifelong ingestion of potentially noxious metal ions may play an adverse role (Eichhorn 1979). The combination of two or more of these factors, not all of which are cellular, would manifest ultimately as senescence. It should be noted that, although mitogenesis and immunosenescence are used as examples, the authors extend their belief in the validity of a genetic cycle of deceleration beyond these fields. They, too, hold that for example the slow-down in protein synthesis is programmed genetically. The stricture made above, as regards economic aspects of genetic planning for ageing, would seem to apply also the this ultra-cellular hypothesis.

Aufderheide (1984) returns in this connection to a question addressed earlier by Maynard Smith (1962), namely whether ageing effects are to be seen only in rapidly growing cell assemblies. Evidence is quoted to show that such highly differentiated entities as neurons bear clear marks of ageing, which are supported by identified molecular changes, for example in the rat cortex. Bellamy (1986), however, holds the view that the important factor in senescence is not so much cell alteration as cell loss (see p. 112). Lymphoid organs, such as the thymus (p. 42), skeletal muscle (p. 6), brain (p. 118), and kidney, provide important examples. But the most promising human tissue to experiment on, as regards the relation between cell loss, structure and pathology, appears to be the gastric epithelium. It is accessible to the environment via diet and to therapeutic and protective drugs alike. And, by virtue of the dominant role played by degenerative disease in the alimentary tract, it transcends mere academic interest. If Bellamy is right, then the non-random loss of cells leading, in a manner as yet undetermined, to organ dysfunction, would make senescence a sort of delayed continuation of embryology: this, too, is characterized by non-random, patchy losses of cells that have fulfilled their biological purpose (p. 20).

Dietary restriction

The effect of diet, notably of its restriction, on longevity has been the subject of a great deal of work. Dietary restriction implies a reduction in energy intake in the absence of malnutrition. One of its more impressive effects is the reduction of a variety of murine tumours, and on atherosclerotic and autoimmune involvement (Yu 1985). Apart from its influence on the autoimmune system, dietary restriction may reduce the metabolic rate per unit body mass, but qualitative rather than quantitative metabolic changes are thought to promote an increase in mean life span. The use of the word 'mean' should be noted: the examples quoted indicate that dietary restriction appears to act primarily on life expectancy, rather than on life span. However, if, as has been observed, the restriction is applied to young animals so that selection may act, the life span itself may conceivably be modified (see Yu 1985). More precisely, when restriction is confined to the first year of life, and unrestricted feeding allowed during the second year, the increase in the rate of survival is maximized (see Young 1979).

Ross and Bras (1973) studied the food preferences of rats in relation to survival rate, and Young (1979) derived two Gompertz constants (see Chapter 5) from their data. However, these do not inform directly on the life span. Reading and Weale (1991) obtained expressions for **a'** and **a(max)**, approximating to life expectancy and estimates of the life span, respectively. Applied to the Young–Ross–Bras data, the constants are shown in Table 1.1.

The maximum potential life span of the rat quoted by Rosen *et al.* (1981) is 1150 days, which corresponds to the values in the column marked **a'**. The extrapolation to twice this value in **a(max)**, amounting to almost seven years, is less excessive than might appear; when the author visited F. Verzar in the Institute of Gerontology in Basle in 1959, he was shown a rat which was said to be 10 years old (i.e. 3650 days). The relevance of dietary restriction, free from malnutrition, to man is unestablished. In the special case of eyes and their development, a host of known pathologies contingent on dietary deficiency illuminate the difficulties which research on man may encounter (McLaren 1982).

1.2.4 *From senescent cells to genes for ageing*

There are several conditions, such as Down's and Werner's syndromes, which have well-established chromosomal substrates, and the signs of which are reminiscent of those of ageing (Martin 1979). Down's syndrome, a birth defect in which there is a supernumerary small autosomal chromosome, that is, one other than the sex chromosomes X or Y, ranks top in a listing of progeroid syndromes with a variety of early potential neuropathologies, hypogonadism, cataract, etc. Werner's syndrome has been seen in many ways as a paradigm of early ageing: this autosomal recessively inherited condition includes osteoporosis, atherosclerosis, diabetes, premature greying of hair, cataract, etc., but cerebral involvement is virtually never present. Even the neoplastic characteristics differ from those encountered amongst the elderly.

This raises an interesting point. When symptoms and even signs are similar in two conditions we tend to conclude that this also holds for their causes. Yet

Table 1.1 Putative life expectancy and life span (days) for the rat following two different modes of food supply

Food supply	Casein (%)	a′	a(max)
Unrestricted	10	697	1472
	22	676	1298
	51	762	1649
Restricted	10	1033	2153
	22	1066	2482
	51	1151	2532

we know that we can shed tears for joy, relief, in anger, and in agony. Admittedly the case for the association is strengthened as the number of different signs increases. But, as mentioned on pp. 2 and 9, ageing and dying have to be distinguished from each other in spite of the former increasing the probability of the latter. Gene regulation (Martin 1979) may be of prime importance in the control of longevity, but it does not follow that it also controls ageing. Structural gene evolution and morphological evolution (speciation) appear to follow independent rates: the coefficients of variation of the maximum life spans of a number of mammalian groups are an approximately linear function of the rate of chromosomal evolution. The tentative conclusion to be drawn from this is that longevity, like speciation, is a function of the speed of chromosomal rearrangement.

By logical extension to these observations, it seems that the association of genetically caused progerias with accelerated 'normal' senescence may be less than helpful to the development of concepts of ageing. The possibility of common mechanisms need not be ruled out by this caveat. Thus, Brown and Wisniewski (1983) picture two types of inherited characteristics specific to each species to be involved in senescence. The first is developmental and relates to rates of maturation (see Fig. 1.10). The second involves protection of the individual. There are, for example, enzymatic systems the levels of which vary with the species and which are determined genetically. They may involve DNA-repair processes, and the regulation of the expression of such enzymatic complexes may have mediated an increased life span, thus permitting an individual to survive for longer than would otherwise be the case. One or more of such enzymatic components may be modified in a progeria, but it is a moot point whether this turns these conditions into models of ageing.

If there is a relation between the longevity of a species and its chromosomal constitution, it would seem to follow that the so-called progerias would fit better into a biological system that does not dwell on aspects of their reputedly premature ageing. We do not attribute progeria to mice even though their life span is shorter than ours. It would probably be more appropriate to look on the phenotypes as heterotypic, as distinct from the homotypic possessors of the chromosomal complement associated with the majority in a given population.

The chromosomal restructuring observed in some of the above inborn disorders has led to the suggestion that ageing involves specific genes. This is not surprising because, in some of the conditions, an extra gene is involved. For example, in Down's syndrome, there is an autosomal supernumerary (third) copy of the gene for the amyloid precursor protein on chromosome 21 (Katzman 1988), and the condition is associated with a greatly reduced life span. However, it is not just chromosomal structure that is altered simply by the addition of a gene: the topology of the pre-existing genes is also altered, and it may be this, rather than the addition itself, that is responsible for the ultimate manifestation.

This is not merely a semantic problem of the type which tries to distinguish between half full and half empty vessels. What is involved is the fundamental principle of bio-economics: expenditure is unlikely to be incurred if thermodynamics and chance may be made to do the work for nothing. Of course, the addition of genes in progerias requires an explanation; but to seek in it an explanation of senescent processes in general would not appear to be the most economical way of proceeding.

Hart and Turturro (1985) have reservations about generalizations relating to the maximum achievable life span (MAL), on the just ground that it is not possible to know when a maximum is reached. In any case, the variety of MALs is perplexing, but beginning to be resolved in an extension of the ideas first advanced by Medawar (1952). He suggested that noxious genes cannot act in the wild, where species do not survive on environmental grounds long enough for the effects of those genes to appear. However, once a species is sufficiently protected, the situation can change, and even genes that proved of advantage to the individual when young, may change to become a hazard (p. 26).

It would seem that the concept of genes specially evolved to promote senescence might well be redundant given the proven existence of a variety of repair processes. If the latter run down because of the inadequate evolution of resources for their maintenance the end product will be the same. Hart and Turturro (1985) quote Sacher as saying that theories postulating the existence of senescence genes may be leaning on (subconscious) religious preconceptions in favour of an immortal existence as modified by evolution. This may be exaggerated, but it indicates that the postulate of the existence of such genes is tainted with redundancy.

A role for maintenance

A wider context for this concept is introduced by Holliday (1988) with his emphasis on the failure of maintenance. He writes: 'The adult organism maintains itself successfully for a major part of its total life-span, but its basic biological organisation and construction ensure that maintenance will be ultimately unable to cope with all accumulated damage and defects in cells, tissues, and organ systems'.

The wording of this important passage echoes, however unintentionally, the adaptive theories of yesteryear. The basic biological organization and construction must be deemed to ensure that the adult organism can procreate and look after its progeny so successfully that the latter, in turn, can occupy the parental place. After this, nothing matters. After this, maintenance does not have to try and cope; it is biologically cheaper if it is switched off. The problem with adaptive theories is not that they run counter to the accepted Darwinian wisdom and modern evolutionary ideas; it is rather that they ignore that evolution is run on a shoe-string. This is, indeed, inevitable. If a rare heritable characteristic is of advantage to a species, then it will be this characteristic and nothing else which leads, in the given circumstances, to an increase in the numbers of the species. The situation is strictly quantized; there is no waste. Any surplus would be within the prerogative of another heritable trait.

This can be extrapolated from a consideration of Fig. 1.1. Assume that the extreme left-hand part of the Gaussian (theoretical) curve could be of great survival value. This is more than a hypothesis: the positive end of the refraction distribution covers long-sightedness, which could have been of advantage to a race of people dependent on hunting. If a mutation occurred which greatly increased the frequency of positive refractions (because they were useful), the Gaussian curve would move to the left, unless negative refraction, that is myopia, also proved to have a significant survival value. In this case observations would be described by two separate distributions. Any other heritable trait mentioned above would be represented in another dimension. This is the algebraic way of saying that there is no waste.

On this view, the biological organization and construction relate only to the development of the organism and to its maintenance between the onset of its puberty and that of its offspring. In iteroparous species, the interpubertal period may evidently be prolonged, but this raises another issue. In the long run, it may be more economical for the organism to be apparently overendowed in certain aspects (see Chapters 2 and 5), because allowing a supply capacity to be run down stochastically may be cheaper than developing a means to stop it.

Olson (1987) puts the problem of bio-supplies succinctly, if not grammatically: 'Longevity is optimized such that reproduction is maximized'. In fact, the statement should be reversed; longevity has extent, not quality. It is important to tailor it to the optimization of reproduction. On a large scale, the latter is pointless if the young cannot be protected (as, for example, for turtles). Olson shows that the reproductive velocity of short-lived species is greater, and occurs earlier in the relative life span than for long-lived ones. Marked environmental causes of death favour short-lived species and vice versa (see Medawar 1952).

The economics of the situation is touched upon at the end of Olson's defence of a multi-factorial basis for ageing, when he diagnoses the cause of ageing as due to wear and tear not being irreparable but too costly in comparison with the benefit likely to be derived from repair. We must, however, be clear about who benefits and who bears the cost.

The stochastic nature of the physical environment demands adaptation if a species is to survive. Components which are structurally permanent are useful for the survival of the individual: memory is helpful but hard to imagine in the presence of frequently changing bio-chips. Variability, however, can be achieved only by changing the individual members of a species, that is by endowing them with death. The cost for development and growth is borne by the world's energy budget. The exchequer will therefore provide only so much metabolic cash as is necessary, not for the individual deriving pleasure from being alive, but for the survival of the species. This is the beneficiary, and that is the existential and financial bottom-line.

The relation between the investment of resources and longevity is embodied in the 'disposable soma theory' (Kirkwood 1984), recently presented on an analytic basis (Kirkwood 1988).

On the assumption that ageing is non-adaptive, Kirkwood suggests that the explanation is to be sought either in a failure of natural selection to prevent it, or in its resulting from other adaptive traits. Underlying the importance of reproductive success (see above), there is postulated a trade-off between the resources devoted to reproduction, **m**, and to the maintenance (of the reproducer), ϱ, respectively. Given a finite budget, there is bound to be an inverse relation between the two. But the lines are fairly finely drawn: if ϱ is too low, the individual may be killed off before reaching the stage at which a prolific **m** can operate. However, if ϱ is overfinanced and the individual can take on all (environmental) comers, the use of the relatively sparse resources for **m** may be greatly delayed. It can also be noted that, in principle, there is no reason why a young animal should not have sturdy, many-yeared parents, but such a delay runs counter to the notion of the variability of the gene-pool mentioned earlier. In other words, the demands of the maintenance (a) of the prospective parents, (b) of the maturing offspring, once born, and (c) of the changes in each generation requires fine bio-economical tuning.

On the basis of a mathematical model, Kirkwood and Holliday (1986) have shown that the balance struck always involves an investment of resources that is insufficient for somatic immortality. Hence (iteroparous) species will accumulate unrepaired physical damage, which will manifest as ageing. Arachnid males, in whom consummation and consumption are almost coincident, die without ageing (see p. 9). This, then, is the nub of the disposal-soma theory.

Consequently, what is programmed is repair, not senescence (see Walford 1981). It may well be that the number of repair facilities and that of their availability may also be programmed much as there is a zero rate of replenishment of the huge number of brain cells, a limited provision for the production of ova, and of dental replacements. Indeed, Walford and Crew (1989)

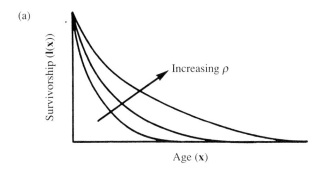

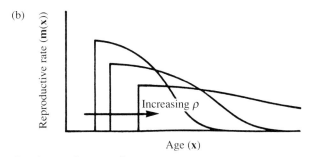

Fig. 1.7 The disposal-soma theory. How investment ϱ in somatic main-tenance and repair affects *a* survivorship $l(x)$ and *b* the rate of reproduction $m(x)$. After Kirkwood and Holliday (1986).

hypothesize that an increase in maintenance and repair may be linked to genetic results arising from dietary restriction (p. 29).

Kirkwood and Holliday's model shows that, as expenditure in ϱ, that is, the fractional investment in maintenance and repair, is increased within its limits of 0 and 1, survivorship increases in a monotonic manner, as is to be expected (Fig. 1.7*a*). The variation of the reproductive rate **m**, however, changes differently in those circumstances (Fig. 1.7*b*). In the early parts of the life span, the time of the onset of **m** is reduced, and its amplitude increased: maturation occurs earlier and more use is made of it as ϱ rises. However, the duration, defined, say by the difference between the age of commencement of reproduction and that at which the rate has dropped to half the maximal (initial) value, increases with ϱ. Other things being equal, the areas under the curves which represent the total number of offspring produced by a pair of parents should be constant. The effect of ϱ on survivorship and reproductive rate can be combined to yield figures for the intrinsic natural rate of population increase, **r**, as a function of the investment made in repair and maintenance (Fig. 1.8). At present, there is no known currency wherein to estimate the costs involved. This is why models depend on

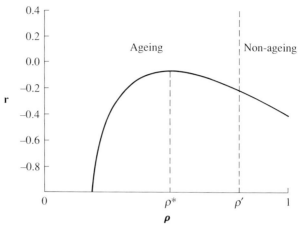

Fig. 1.8 The relation between investment in somatic maintenance and repair ϱ and population increases **r**. It is assumed here that when ϱ > 0.8 the rates of damage and repair are equal. Hence no ageing occurs here and for larger values. However, for smaller ones, e.g. ϱ = 0.5, ageing occurs. After Kirkwood and Holliday (1986).

the introduction of arbitrary numerical values. The particular set chosen by Kirkwood and Holliday show that there is, indeed, an optimal value of ϱ (ϱ*) which serves to maximize **r**, and that it is substantially smaller than the critical value ϱ' beyond which no ageing takes place because the repair facilities can keep in step with the insults to which the individual is subjected.

The above model is based on the Gompertzian mortality function, and an estimate of a putative life span is inherent in its formulation. It is, therefore, possible to estimate the effect of the somatic repair constants of longevity. Using hypothetical values for the basic constants as before, Kirkwood and Holliday find that, consistently with the operation of the above mechanism, one can expect from a reduction in environmental mortality, **e**, a proportionately greater one in the reproductive rate per annum, an almost doubled optimal maintenance and repair constant ϱ*, and an increase in calculated longevity, in nearly inverse relation to the drop in **e**.

Some further bio-economical considerations

It is understandable that, when no one presents a bill for a resource, its supply is assumed to be infinite. In many countries, water is used on the basis of such a tacit assumption, and other natural resources, like timber in England in the Middle Ages and in Brazil today, have been, and are, looked upon in a similar manner. Within well-known limits, solar energy, and, therefore the energy supply on this earth, fall into a similar category.

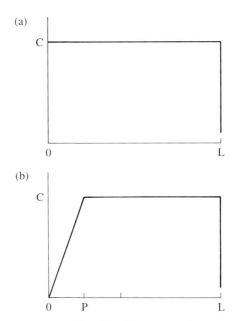

Fig. 1.9a A constant cost (C) of maintenance throughout life-span (OL).
b Economies during the growth phase OP.

However, the supply of energy has to be distinguished from the provision of an organization for its use. It is here that the elements of cost and efficiency appear. The energy used for biological purposes, and formation of amino acids, proteins, macromolecules, tissues, organs, and bodies forms no exception. A progressive increase in organization is involved that corresponds to what the physicist would refer to as a rise in potential energy. The potential energy of physical bodies tends to be minimal consistently with their stability: it is not useful for Swiss postmen to transport mail from one valley to another over the top of a mountain if they can avoid it.

The principle of minimum energy expenditure also applies on the biological level. Suppose there were a type of human race who were created mature, did not age, but died at some age **a(d)**. If the cost of keeping them alive is **C** energy units per year (Fig. 1.9*a*), then each of them would cost the Universe **C.a(d)** (energy unit).years to maintain or keep alive. This cost does not include that of creation, nor does it allow for the discount produced when dust returns to dust and the energy organized in the body is made available for maggots or daisies.

It is easier for mothers to bear smaller individuals, and the initial overall maintenance cost is therefore comparatively small (Fig. 1.9*b*), though this may not necessarily be true for the energy cost per unit mass (growing birds eat a significant fraction, if not a small multiple of their weight per day). For the above-mentioned hypothetical human race to be produced *ab ovo* (Fig. 1.9*b*) involves an increasing rise in cost. We are still considering only maintenance costs; evidently investment has to be made also in growth.

For a given life span L, considerable savings are achieved with a small initial slope: as the notional maintenance cost is reduced in this system from CL to $CL - 0.5C.a(p)$, where $a(p)$ is the age of maturation, economy would seek to maximize $a(p)$. But a large value of $a(p)$ runs counter to another evolutionary interest, namely that of a finite turn-over time of the generations (see above). There is also the consideration implicit in the disposal-soma hypothesis: a non-reproducing individual is a parasite as far as natural resources are concerned. Nevertheless, in homo sapiens the period $a(p)$ is well over 10 per cent of even a hypothetical maximum life span, the reason being human encephalization.

The brain and its potential develop slowly, the and the putative growth curve of the whole organ (Fig. 1.10) is clearly raked, which suggests that, phylogenetically speaking, evolutionary pressures acted during at least two periods for the present product to appear (Thatcher *et al.* 1987).

Given that the age of puberty $a(p)$ is, therefore, a compromise solution to the competing interests of maintenance cost, turn-over frequency, and specific development time, one asks how else costs can be cut. A tentative answer is to be found in this compromise. From an exclusively biological point of view, maximum maintenance costs spent on one generation can be justified only as long as it is necessary for the succeeding one to mature (p. 233). Now the period of reaching puberty is subject to variations, for example on climatic and/or dietetic grounds, but it ranges more or less within the limits of 12–18 years. One would therefore expect the maximum cost of maintenance to be confined to the age-range between 20 and 40 years, allowing for some variability. This has been noted to be approximately the case (p. 85).

Hence the above balance sheet can be further modified (Fig. 1.11). Maximum investment for maintenance having been made between the ages of $a(p)$ and $2a(p)$, the cost of the third phase reduces from a non-ageing value of $C[L - 2a(p)]$ to half this value. The notional maintenance cost for the whole life span is thus reduced from the original $C.L$ to $0.5C.[L + a(p)]$. If maximum investment were confined to a very brief period, the saving in cost would amount to about 50 per cent. The actual saving is $0.5C.[L - a(p)]$ with a fractional cost value of $F = 0.5(1 + [a(p)/L])$.

In practice one would expect to find parabolic rather than trapezoidal age-related variations of physiological functions (see Svanborg 1988) without preujudice to their precise algebraic form. The latter almost always represents a simplification. There is evidence, contested by Economos (1982) on the basis of studies not necessarily applicable to human beings, that a number of important physiological functions follow a linear age-related decline. This is considered in Chapter 5.

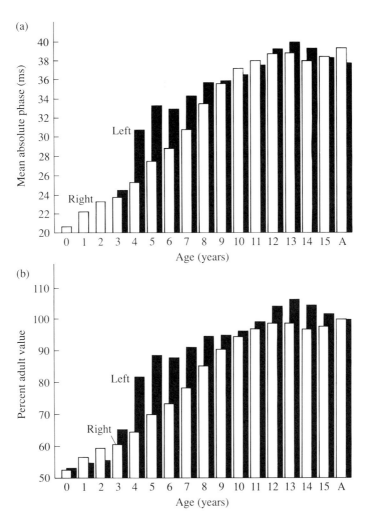

Fig. 1.10 The brain – an example of a non-uniform growth rate. These data (a) were obtained from electro-encephalographic measurements, and represent the development of the mean absolute phase in milliseconds from the left (black blocks) and right (white blocks) frontal occipital hemispheres. The implication is that phase varies with mass; (b) represents the same data expressed as a percentage of the adult (cf. final) values. After Thatcher *et al.* (1987).

The comparison between the physical fitness, presented as maximum oxygen consumption, of the Masai men in Kenya and North American men (Mann *et al.* 1965) provides an interesting illustration of an age-related variation of

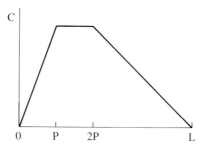

Fig. 1.11 Senescence as an example of bio-economics: (see Fig. 1.9). OP = period of growth (puberty), P-2P = period of growth (puberty) of offspring, OL = life span.

function (Fig. 1.12). Six weeks' physical training somewhat improved the graph of the physiology of the American men but still failed to enable them to match the Masai who were 'untrained'. There is no proven link between physical fitness and rates of survival, but it is not far-fetched to postulate one, even though the older Masai men may be subject to disease processes, which are absent, curable or controlled in the USA. Note the similarity between the apparently trapezoidal shape of the data for the Masai men and Fig. 1.11.

It will be noted that the fractional cost depends only on the ratio of the age of maturity to that of the life span. Although the fractional value **F** increases when **a(p)** is fixed but **a(d)** falls, that of the actual cost is linearly reduced: fatal diseases after the age of 2**a(p)** are biologically highly cost-effective.

It is important to avoid an error, which is not altogether obvious at first sight. The notional value in maintenance is the cost of performance, for the investment is made so that the species may continue successfully. But there are also hidden costs, such as the maintenance of blood vessels, of nervous lines of communication, etc., which appear in the overall balance sheet but are liable to be overlooked. For example, measurements of the visual threshold show that a small number of light quanta suffice to produce a visual sensation. However, many more quanta are needed for this small number to be able to act. For reasons to be discussed in Chapter 4, the number rises with age. The cost of the performance in terms of stimulus intensity has increased. The fact that physiological responses decrease with advancing years is to be seen not as an increase in absolute cost but in relation to a cut-off in investment.

The considerations of cost apply not only to the growth and maintenance of organs but also to the function of the latter. Svanborg (1988) has considered this is a general manner and suggested that the rate of decline can be variable. This is only a way of expressing an uncertainty of the underlying algebraic function. For example, the absorbance of the human crystalline lens appears to rise, that is, the lens appears to darken in a complex manner (Pokorny *et al.* 1987) only

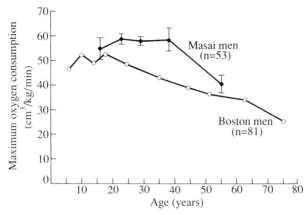

Fig. 1.12 A comparison between the physical fitness of Masai and American men. The data show the age-related variation of the maximum oxygen consumption. After Mann *et al.* (1965).

if it is not realized that the change is exponential. Not all variations need be simple, but a change in rate is no guide.

The general curves in Fig. 1.9 and 1.11 represent gross simplifications designed to introduce the notion of cost. The variation of the size or mass of specific organs, the measure of which is referred to as allometry, is far more complicated. Within wide limits, and subject to the critical remarks made by Hart and Turturro (1985), relations have been found to exist between species body mass and life span, generally on the assumption that mortality is Gompertzian (Chapter 5). Calder III (1982) has shown that, within limits,

$$\ln \mathbf{t(d)} = -0.02 + 0.27\ln \mathbf{M} \qquad (1.1)$$

where $\mathbf{t(d)}$ is the time in which mortality doubles and $\mathbf{M}$ is the body mass in kilograms. It is probable that this, too, represents a simplification for which it will be hard to find a theoretical explanation because the growth of individual organs obeys a variety of different functions. Perkkiö and Keskinen (1985) have assumed a power law for organ mass and time (the Gompertz function being a special case of this), and identified four broad types of human postnatal organ growth (Fig. 1.13). Three of them show the type of delay noted in connection with Fig. 1.10: they are the 'general' type (said to resemble Gompertzian growth above the age of 4 years), the lymphoid, and the genital types. Only the neural type, characterized by the largest initial rate of growth, is describable in terms of solely an amplitude and a rate constant, like in the accumulation of a single radioactive product. The authors stress that the allometric constants are liable to vary with time, which may provide a partial explanation for the variability

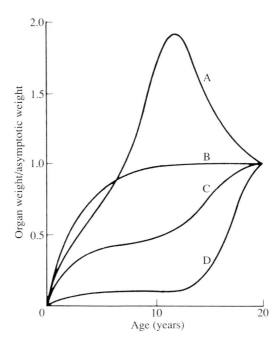

Fig. 1.13 Different types of growth rate. A, lymphoid, as exemplified by the thymus which grows in infancy but declines after puberty; B, neural; C, general (see Fig. 1.11); D, genital. After Perkkiö and Keskinen (1985).

in the allometric relations for body mass and life span set out by Calder III and other authors.

A comparable analysis of the relation between the rate of the development of the crystalline lens and the maximum achievable life span (MAL), illustrates some of the attendant problems. Tréton and Courtois (1989) noted that the lenses of many mammalian species appear to show two principal rates of growth, namely a fast one during early life and a slower one later on. They drew tangents to them and called their point of intersection the lens development stage (LDS). A plot of LDS against MAL yielded a regression with $r = 0.89$. The high r-value is almost certainly the result of the regression being calculated for a non-uniform distribution of the data points. The authors' method of determining rate constants of what appear to be logarithmic growth curves is unusual, and may oversimplify a growth progress which is not necessarily smooth (Brewitt and Clark 1988; Weale 1963). Nevertheless, in some form or other the correlation is likely to be valid and to join others involving brain- and body-weight (see Calder's expression above).

The fallacy of biomarkers

The above doubt as to the justification of arguing from performance to mortality has not worried many people. Driven either by their own scientific curiosity or the equally detached interests of insurance companies, they have spent a great deal of time and money in attempting to establish predictors of debility and death. Although certainty about other people's mortal future would be an actuarial pearl beyond price, so far it has proved beyond reach. Even sophistic-ated batteries of tests of physiological performance measured as a function of calendar age have failed to provide an answer.

From the point of view of studies of the processes of senescence, the value of biomarkers is questionable (Adelman 1987), not to say overrated. Even if one disregards the fact that some of the components may be functionally linked (Weale 1970), as was the case in the battery of biomarkers proposed by Comfort (1969), they suffer from an inherent difficulty which is perhaps due to the concept that death and senescence are causally linked. The difficulty in question is that the batteries represent an exercise in correlation. To be successful, the correlation between performance and mortality has to be maximized. However, the mutual independence of each component of the battery from one another demands that the partial correlations should be as nearly zero as may be. This conflict is unresolved.

Some correlations may be subject to secular changes or, indeed, unsuspected man-made influences. For example, there is a link between dentition and age, even when milk dentition is disregarded: we start adult life with 32 teeth, but, on average, have lost 4 by the time we have reached the seventh decade. Owing to dental practices then prevalent, this average would have been appreciably higher a generation or two ago, and, given the present advances in conservation, it is probably going to be much lower in the forseeable future. While no battery appears to include this variable, many use hearing thresholds. Their value has become debatable since the introduction of modern portable music-players. The high volume used even in socially relatively acceptable instruments causes considerable irreversible rises in auditory thresholds amongst users, who are mainly people in the younger age groups. The resulting presbyacucia will reduce the apparent biological age as long as this variable remains part of batteries of biomarkers.

Another difficulty is that, by being based on averages, biomarkers have little demographic value. For example, if one knew what fraction of a given popu-lation and age-group reached such and such criteria, useful predictions might be made. Svanborg (1988) complains of the difficulties attendant on the inter-pretation of the age-related variation of blood pressure; but dividing the population into four groups with increasing pressures (Weale 1982*a*) shows that there is a high correlation between pressure and mortality only insofar as the group with the highest pressure is concerned.

Moreover, we noted earlier (p. 4) that the definition of health has to obey rather more stringent rules than are commonly observed (see also Smith *et al.* 1988). This would seem to imply that, insofar as these have been ignored, we may lack the standard data whereon correlations between performance and mortality are hypothetically based. But if criteria of health affect one so-called biomarker, it is easy to imagine what chaos is likely to be created when batteries of some twenty tests are subjected to validation procedures.

The most serious objection to the use of biomarkers is, however, that they entail a confusion of categories. It has to be remembered that mortality involves a count of people. Thus mortality pressure can be defined as the number of people of a given age dying during a 12 month period, expressed as a fraction of the number of people (of the same age) that were alive at the beginning of that period. Performance data, however, are expressed as thresholds, for example the strongest possible hand-grip, the weakest visible light intensity, the maximum volume of expired air, etc. Because hand-grip and air volume decrease, and the visual threshold rises, with age, these entities have found their way into test batteries.

It is possible that if performance tests involved the setting of suitable criteria, involving the number of people at various ages who attain them might prove informative. Thus the correlation between blood pressure and age is less than overwhelming. But the correlation of the number of people suffering from the highest range of pressures and mortality is fairly close (Weale 1982*a*; Brant personal communication).

The emphasis on 'suitable criteria' is not a whim but demanded by the exigencies of metrological comparisons. Mortality is not achieved by degrees: it is a criterion, the only parameter for which is the number of people to have attained it. The fact that they can be grouped according to cause, sex, race, etc. is not always relevant since similar sub-divisions can be used in physiological criteria. It is probable that the fraction of people above the age of 90 years to have a very faint, but defined, grip will be large: if finite, the grip value might provide a criterion. Whether the same is true of a criterion visual threshold is questionable (but see pp. 111 and 175) in a safe environment, as it is possible to survive without sight. It would seem that any proposed battery component would have to be analysed from some such point of view. This might enhance its scientific credibility even though its value for gerontological understanding might be left in doubt.

1.3 Resumé

The review of theories of ageing has shown that some successfully fit special cases, as is true, for example, of those underlying the age-related loss of immunity. Again, there are important aspects of cellular theories which allow hypotheses which stem from them to be proposed and tested. But it has proved much harder to advance and to justify an all-embracing theory which would have catholic validity in the sense in which this is true of some physical theories. It is possible, though, that the disposable-soma theory may lay some claim to generality.

It is rooted in the theory of evolution which is an inherent advantage, and based on economics which is a regrettable necessity. It may well have difficulties in making predictions, but it may provide a criterion which any *ad hoc* hypothesis of senescence may have to satisfy to survive. The form, if not also the substance, of its economic aspect is something that can be examined in connection with the life of the eye and its function.

2. The retinal image

2.1 Image homoeostasis

2.1.1 Introduction

In this section the eye in general is discussed, with particular emphasis on the structures that serve to form the retinal image. The term 'homoeostasis' in the heading was not chosen inadvertently. The subjective criterion of an image being sharp — which is quantified in terms of its angular size and contrast — represents a baseline for its resolution. There are reflex mechanisms to maintain either the image intensity or the sensory response it elicits within physiological limits, just as there are devices for the preservation of an optimally focused image of a targeted external object.

A progressively increasing difficulty in the maintenance of homoeostasis of the retinal image is one of the correlates of senescence. The principal ocular structures involved in the formation of the retinal image are the cornea, the iris, and the crystalline lens. Although comparison with a camera invites the idea that the crystalline lens fulfils in the eye the role played by the camera lens in photography, the notion is mistaken. The principal image forming device is the cornea, with the lens acting as a subordinate, but nevertheless very important, assistant.

The reflex ability of the visual system to image objects within a great range of distances from the eyes is known as accommodation, and its continual attenuation with advancing years is called presbyopia (Greek: sight of the elderly). Strictly speaking, the physiological substrate of presbyopia can be shown to originate in childhood; however, the designation is reserved for the presence of actual symptoms arising from it. The need for reading glasses when presbyopia exceeds one's tolerance of the condition explains why it is the best known of all the ocular attributes of senescence.

2.2 A brief survey of the optics of the eye

2.2.1 Lenses

Most people know how thin lenses, such as magnifying glasses, work. When they are used as burning glasses the distant object, the sun, is imaged on a surface. Similarly, photographic lenses (which are complex and not thin) produce images of distant objects on the surface of a film. Glass lenses have two surfaces, each of which takes part in the process of refraction, i.e. the formation of an image. In contrast, the eye works, in effect, with only a single refracting surface, namely the cornea, which acts by virtue of its curvature and by its refractive index ($= 1.376$) being very different from that of air. Although some refraction occurs also at the internal corneal surface, this can be ignored for the purpose of this explanation.

The lens is an important operational refinement to the eye; however, its existence makes no difference to our being able to regard the·eye as using but one refracting surface. Indeed, the so-called reduced eye, invented by Gullstrand almost a century ago to rationalize ocular optics, altogether ignores the lens, but modifies the numerical values of some of the physical attributes of the real cornea so as to take account of lenticular refraction. Naturally the reduced eye cannot deal with accommodation.

If our eyes were provided only with corneae, the images of external objects would not be formed on the retina but behind it, and would be perceived as blurred. The eyes would be severely long-sighted. Such a condition, known as hypermetropia, is remedied by the provision of convex or positive spectacle lenses, which increase the dioptric power of the eyes. Similarly, the presence of a powerful double-convex crystalline lens increases the power of the eye from its aphakic state of hypermetropia to the normal in-focus situation, or emmetropia.

In this state, the eye can form sharp images of objects that are at optical infinity. In practice, infinity means six metres or more. Suppose now that one looks at an object only half a metre away. In this situation the eye is once again hypermetropic: the image of such a near object is formed behind the retina, or it would be so formed, if the retina were transparent and a suitable screen were present behind the eye to receive the image. Once again, the remedy is found in an increase in the ocular dioptric power. But instead of a lens being added, the dioptric power of the crystalline lens is increased as a result of an increase in the curvature mainly of its anterior surface. This is the consequence of the operation of a nervous loop following the route of retina − hypothalamus − intra-ocular musculature, which constitutes the reflex mechanism of accommodation. When the loop fails symptomatic presbyopia is said to have set in.

2.2.2 *The role of the pupil*

The pupil is the optical aperture of the eye; that is, it delineates the cross-section of the beam of light that enters the eye. The particularization of the image − which, in effect, constitutes it − is realized only in the retinal plane; all rays of light traverse the pupil in an unresolved manner. The contrast variation across

the image that permits its ultimate resolution increases in magnitude progressively between the pupillary aperture and the retina in planes perpendicular to the
optic axis of the eye.

The pupillary area is variable owing to the muscular components of the iris.
Its area is controlled by the competitive actions of the radial dilator muscle, a
phylogenetically old structure, as against the circular fibres of the contractile
sphincter, a younger, but much sturdier, muscular partner. The fact that the
pupillary area varies with the illumination received by the eye appears to have
been discovered by Leonardo da Vinci (1513). The name of whoever first
observed that its area also declines with advancing years, a condition known as
senile miosis, has been lost, but Schadow (1882) and Silberkühl (1896) appear
to have been amongst the first people to have measured it. In fact, Schadow was
greatly surprised to find that the diameter does not change monotonically with
age, but reaches a maximum in mid-life. Understandably, stimulus controls
applied at this time were inadequate in terms of our present knowledge, and the
maximum diameter occurs in this first gerontological study of pupillometry
some two decades later than is shown in Fig. 2.1. That first result is almost
certainly partly artefactual.

It has often been suggested that pupillary constriction serves to protect the
retina from excessive illumination, including ultraviolet radiation (see Weale
1986*a*). It would probably be more correct to say that the protection is from
glare rather than functional hazards: facing a sunny day with dilated pupils is
a cause of acute discomfort, if not pain. It would, however, be erroneous to
deduce from these considerations that a beneficent evolutionary pressure has

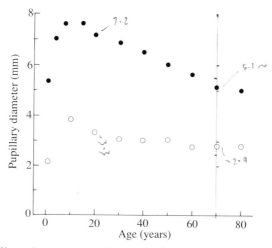

Fig. 2.1 Pupillary diameter as a function of age. The filled circles represent
the state in dark-adaptation, the open ones in light-adaptation. The data are
compiled from a number of authors (see Weale 1982*a*).

acted to protect the elderly from discomfort glare; a possible anatomical reason for senile miosis will be considered later.

The constriction of the pupil in physiologically useful, i.e. photopic, illumination has an important optical corollary, which requires some attention in view of the role with which it has been credited in accommodation and also in presbyopia. In a camera, the aperture is reduced when there is some uncertainty about focusing. A reduced aperture minimizes the effect of the camera lens and turns the apparatus into something resembling a pinhole camera, which is an invention of Leonardo da Vinci's, although the principle is well set out in Roger Bacon's much earlier work (1896). The pinhole camera forms sharp, but rather faint, images of objects at any distance from the camera.

The optical advantage of the pupil constricting consequently enables the eye to image objects in more than one plane perpendicular to the line of sight. Note that, in the young eye, this constriction occurs in a reflex manner whenever there is a stimulus to accommodation. Actually, there is a triad of nervous messages involved in this: the reason is that the convergence of the visual axes which enables an object to be imaged on the two foveae, parts of the retinae where contrast sensitivity is optimal, also leads to pupillary constriction. The response is therefore called the near reflex. Although functional presbyopia impairs the reflex focusing of the crystalline lens it is not accompanied by any impairment of the extra-ocular musculature: our visual axes can be made to converge at close objects provided visual acuity is normal, and hence the near reflex is maintained. This is, however, insufficient to turn the eye into a pinhole instrument, the smallest pupillary diameter being of the order of 2 mm (Fig. 2.1).

Pupillary constriction reduces the area of the ocular aperture: with the cross-sectional area of the beam entering the eye being proportional to the square of the diameter, retinal illumination is similarly reduced. This explains why the reflex is evoked only under photopic conditions when there is a surfeit of light. At low levels of illumination, an approach to pinhole vision would be useless because contrast sensitivity (Chapter 4) is too low to enable the retina and brain to benefit from the optical improvement resulting from pupillary constriction.

2.2.3 The depth of focus

The ability of the ocular optics to produce sharply perceived retinal images of objects in different planes perpendicular to the line of sight is called the depth of focus. The topic is so rarely dealt with analytically in textbooks on ocular or other optics (Gleichen 1921) that, now and then, it is treated *de novo* (Green *et al.* 1980). It is of such importance for our understanding of both accommodation and presbyopia that a simple treatment of the problem is presented here.

Figure 2.2 shows two objects, **A** and **B**, at distances of D_1 and D_2 cm respectively from the pupil (radius **P** cm), located at **C**. The object **A** forms an image **A'** on the retina at a distance R_1 from the pupil, whereas the image **B'** of the object **B** is formed behind the retina at a distance R_2. Multiplied by 100, the reciprocal values of the four distances are expressed in dioptres; for a given optical system, the sum of the object and image dioptres is a constant and a measure of the dioptric power of the image-forming device. If the sizes of the two images are assumed to be equal, then the blur edge of the unfocused image will be represented by **GH**. The limiting ray from the pupil to the image **JB'** crosses the optic axis at **K**, i.e. **N** cm from the pupil. Assume that the object consists of a parallel-bar grating of period **c** cm. It then follows that

$$N/(N - R_1) = P/(c/2 + GH)$$

Further,

$$N/(N - R_2) = 1/(1 - R_2/N) = P/AG.$$

Hence,

$$R_1/N = 1 - (c/2 + GH)/P;$$

and

$$R_2/N = 1 - AG/P$$

so that

$$1/R_1 - 1/R_2 = (1/P)\{[(c/2) + GH]/R_1 - AG/R_2\} \qquad (2.1)$$

Let

$$d_1 = 1/D_1; \; d_2 = 1/D_2;$$

and

$$Q_1 = 1/R_1; \; Q_2 = 1/R_2;$$

$$Q_1 + d_1 = Q_2 + d_2.$$

The former set relates the distance in metres to dioptric power. The last expression states that, in a given optical system, the dioptric sum of the object and image distances is a constant determined by the optics of the system.

It follows that

$$1/R_1 - 1/R_2 = Q_1 - Q_2 = d_2 - d_1 =$$
$$(1/P)\{[(c/2 + GH)/R_1] - AG/R_2\} \qquad (2.2)$$

But, if **GH** is a just noticeable increase over **GD**, **AG** $\sim$ c/2. It follows from eqns (2.1) and (2.2) that

$$d_2 - d_1 = (1/P)(c/2)\{d_2 - d_1 + [GH/R_1(c/2)]\}$$

so that

$$d_2 - d_1 = (GH/R_1)(1/P)(1 - (c/2P)) \qquad (2.3)$$

GH/R₁ is the angular subtense of the blur edge in radians; **c/R₁** is the grating constant in radians with **1/f** cycles per radian, where **f** is the angular frequency. Since **(R/2P)²** is the numerical aperture **NA** of the eye

$$d_2 - d_1 = [GH/P][1/(R_1 - \sqrt{NA}/f)]$$

The depth of focus **d₂ − d₁** is therefore inversely proportional to the pupillary radius **P**. In practice, $\sqrt{NA}/f$ in the last pair of brackets in eqn (2.4) can be neglected. Then

$$d_2 - d_1 = (GH/R_1)(1/P) \qquad (2.5)$$

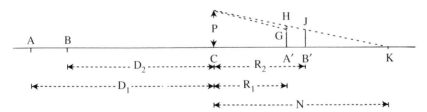

Fig. 2.2 Diagram illustrating the derivation of the expression for the depth of focus (see eqn 2.5) (see text).

Since **GH/R₁** is the angular measure of the just noticeable blur edge, this expression tells us that the magnitude of the blur edge perceived is proportional to the visual resolution of the eye−brain system. It is evident that given poorer visual acuity, blur will be harder to perceive even though the optical system may have produced it (see Chapter 4). Substitution of 1′ for **GH/R₁** and putting **P** = 0.2 cm gives a value of 0.145 D for the depth of focus. Vision is not, however, usually constrained to work under threshold conditions, and a value of between 0.3 and 0.5 D is to be expected. Indeed, Campbell (1957) found the empirical relation of **(d₂ − d₁)** = 0.5/**P**, which is consistent with the above theory if one bears in mind that that author was specifically concerned with the

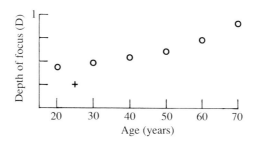

Fig. 2.3 Variation of depth of focus with age. The circles are values based on eqn 2.5, the cross represents a measurement due to Campbell (1957).

detection of blur, and would have used a better criterion for its detection than is implicit in one based on three times the acuity threshold.

If it is assumed that blur is easily detected at a level of one third of one's visual acuity, and the variation with age of the pupillary diameter (Fig. 2.1) and that of the visual acuity (Fig. 5.1b) are substituted in eqn (2.4), the values shown in Fig. 2.3 are obtained. Note that, even well past the age when presbyopia has become acutely symptomatic in the fifth decade, the depth of focus barely exceeds 0.5 D. Consequently, the depth of focus provides a small amount of accommodation, in the sense that resolution remains constant over a dioptric range of about 0.5 D. For example, the emmetropic eye will see objects between 2 m and infinity equally sharply; or, as regards resolution, it does not matter whether an object is 40 or 50 cm away from the eyes. These examples illustrate that, the nearer the object, the narrower the distance over which the depth of focus bestows any benefit. In other words, it is no substitute for the youthful physiological mechanism which permits adjustment between some 10 cm from the eyes to infinity on a reflex basis. It follows from eqn (2.5) that the optical latitude in image formation could replace physiological accommodation only if the pupillary diameter were very small compared with the focal length of the eye. This implies a numerical aperture so small that insufficient light would enter the eye to be able adequately to stimulate the retina. The significance of this result for the interpretation of data on accommodation will be noted below.

2.3 Static refraction

The scientific and commercial interest in presbyopia has led to the neglect of another important question, namely how ocular refraction changes with age. True, there have been some considerable inquiries in the past, amongst which those of Brown (1938) and Slataper (1950) covered large numbers of cases. However, adequate statistical treatment in this field is of relatively recent origin, and the latest studies also suffer from a lack of information.

Effects associated with senescence appear even at the level of techniques of measurement. It is important to note that there are both subjective and objective methods for the determination of the refractive properties of the eye. In subjective ones, the patient has to respond in some way, either by indicating the sharpness or otherwise of a test target, the equal lack of sharpness of two targets, etc. In objective techniques the specialist decides when he or she believes that a given correction should optically abolish any defect that may be present.

Millodot and O'Leary (1978) used retinoscopy for the objective, and the duochrome test for the subjective, tests. Retinoscopy depends on the specialist's assessment of the movement of a light sent into the eye and emerging from it after reflexion, whence its name. The authors found that, in young eyes, retinoscopy records hypermetropia or long-sightedness, whilst the subjective method might indicate emmetropia. The difference between the results of the two methods tended to zero during the sixth decade, after which they reversed their signs: the objective method gave readings relatively myopic to the subjective ones. As the patient is assumed to know best, the authors scrutinized the basis of retinoscopy, but did not resolve the problem beyond suggesting that it is likely to be due to changes in the relative refractive index between the media at the interface of which retinoscopic reflection occurs. A change in the second decimal place of one of the relevant refractive indices would be required, but hard to establish experimentally.

Kragha (1986) failed to confirm Millodot and O'Leary's conclusions. He studied a Nigerian population, and noted that 'the discrepancy between retinoscopy and subjective refraction was extremely small' (about ± 0.1 D in his results). But it has to be noted that the prevalence of refractive errors amongst several African populations is thought to be smaller than almost anywhere else, and that this may be a genuine ethnic difference between the two studies.

Lavery *et al.* (1988a) studied spherical equivalents and astigmatism in a population in the age range of 76 to over 90 years, with the number of subjects of the upper age being understandably few. They confirmed the trend toward hypermetropia, observed by earlier workers, and, again in confirmation of earlier work on keratometry, found an increase in astigmatism against the rule. There was no significant difference between the refractive progress of the two sexes. The study population was selected from a small town in central England, and it might be thought, therefore, that the type of variance one might expect in the presence of, say a considerable East Asiatic ethnic complement, would be absent. The English Midlands are, however, hosts to a large population notably from the Indian sub-continent, and it is a matter for regret that the opportunity was not seized either to tell the reader that the sample consisted largely of native people or, better, whether the data had been analysed by ethnic origin, and no significant variation had been detected. It is unfortunate that the present-day ethos, rightly condemning racism, should have led to wide spread losses of information by the suppression of ethnic details, which, as regards classification, would be a scientific sine qua non in any other field of research.

Ethnic homogeneity is mentioned in a larger study carried out in a rural part of Israel on a population mainly of East European birth or descent (Hyams *et al.* 1977). The age range extended from 40 to over 70 years, i.e. it covered the presbyopic moiety of a local population. There was, again, a trend toward hypermetropia in the higher age groups, but men tended to show more (mild) myopia than did women. The authors suggest that the late hypermetropia may be due to a lenticular flattening, and to 'changes in the relative refractive power of the lens cortex and the nucleus'. All the evidence (p. 66) points to the senescent lens becoming more curved with advancing years (though, on the basis of relatively inadequate evidence, past conventional wisdom proclaimed the view advanced by Hyams *et al.*). The hypothetical relative changes in refraction would have to be based largely on changes in hydration, but the present evidence singles out the human lens as being remarkably stable in this respect (see Fisher and Pettet 1973; Nordmann 1973; but see also Siebinga *et al.* 1991).

The most analytical study to have appeared to date is by Saunders (1986), who compared transverse with longitudinal values. Although the numbers studied are relatively small, and potential refractive differences between the two sexes have not been analysed, his analysis confirms and elaborates Slataper's broad outline (Fig. 2.4). The hypermetropia of infancy and childhood is replaced in many Caucasian eyes by emmetropia, if not mild myopia perhaps as a result of schooling. After the early 30s there is a return to hypermetropia, as we noted above. In the late decades of life a second reversal appears to be taking place: earlier workers have attributed this in their data to the presence of some cataractous eyes, which might have shown the onset of myopia typical of nuclear involvement. This cannot be ruled out, though modern workers usually offer an assurance as regards the absence of pathological conditions in a sample intended to illustrate senescence in healthy eyes (see p. 108).

An alternative hypothesis can be based on the observation that the upper eyelids tend to become loose and perhaps to weaken with age. The resultant ptosis has been estimated only qualitatively (Sanke 1984), but may nevertheless play a role in the refractive reversal. The reason is that, as O'Leary and Millodot (1979) have reported, ptosis can lead to myopia. A local action is involved since unilateral ptosis causes ipsilateral myopia, and the authors draw attention to the fact that ethnic groups with narrow palpebral fissures, such as the Chinese, tend to be myopic. There is nothing universal about this, because the Burmese, who have a similar ocular anatomy, fail to exhibit a comparable degree of myopia.

The early reduction in hypermetropia is almost certainly due to changes in the shape and thickness of the crystalline lens. Figure 2.5 shows that there is good agreement between measurements of the optical power of the crystalline lens and a prediction based on its diameter and thickness (see also Fig. 2.9). The curves

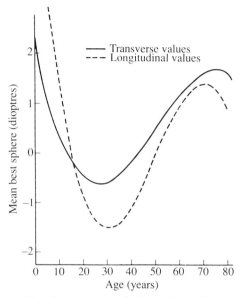

Fig. 2.4 The age-related variation of the spherical equivalent. The latter corresponds to the spherical correction plus one half of the cylindrical correction, if any. After Saunders (1986).

published by Saunders are computations, but there is little doubt that changes in shape can account for them.

The reversal (i.e. the increase in the best sphere) is more of a problem. Changes in refractive index spring to mind, but it can be shown that, unless these are of an altogether unexpected nature and involve changes more drastic than expected on the basis of hydration, nothing more than a few hundredths of a dioptre could be accounted for in those terms. The changes involve, however, about two dioptres. A change of this magnitude is explained most easily in terms of a slight shortening of the eyeball. Several authors have, in fact, reported just this (see Weale 1982a). But Fledelius (1988) makes a valid point when he draws attention to the effect of secular changes in the human make-up (see also Gsell, 1967). There is a positive correlation between body size and ocular diameter; recent generations are taller than their parents; therefore the latter will have smaller eyeballs, which in transverse studies will create the impression of an ocular shrinkage with advancing years.

However, Saunders found the reversal also in a longitudinal study (Fig. 2.4). While there will be a considerable time interval between the young in transverse and longitudinal studies, the difference is minimized in the higher age groups who will be more nearly coeval. The relatively more marked myopia in the longitudinal data could be due, as Saunders noted, to some secular effect:

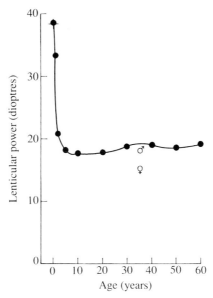

Fig. 2.5 The variation of the optical power of the lens with age. The solid circles represent points calculated from eqns 2.7, 2.8, and 2.9 (see pp. 64–5), the cross is a result due to Luyckx (1966), and the open circles are based on data obtained by Weale (1983).

dietetic changes have been suggested previously. On this basis, a secular change could have affected the older age groups in both samples in Fig. 2.4. But, since the rise has also been noted decades earlier (see Slataper 1950), it is more likely to be due to endogenous causes. The elasticity of the sclera is not yet fully understood, but older sclerae are thinner than young ones (Friedenwald 1952; Vannas and Teir 1960), and this would cause flaccidity even if the elastic properties were unchanged. The fact that intraocular pressure does not seem to vary greatly with age in the normopressive eye (Cagianut 1978; Shiose 1984) does not affect this issue. It would seem, therefore, that a slight deformation of the eyeball results from scleral changes, and that, owing to gravity, the vitreous humour sags and hence shortens the optic axis of the eye. This observation is not confined to Caucasian eyes, as Kamiya (1987) has observed a fractional shortening of the Japanese eyeball, and attributed it to one of the vitreous chamber.

An interesting point that may have become obscured by Saunders' analytical treatment relates to the steady rate or otherwise with which refraction changes occur. In a reappraisal of longitudinal measurements obtained on school-children of both sexes by Sorsby *et al.* (1961) it was shown that the decline in refraction (see Fig. 2.4) appears to proceed intermittently in steps separated by 3–4 years (Weale 1963). Attention was also drawn to Goldmann's measurements (1937) of disjunction stripes in the living crystalline lens, the number of which increased with age, one forming approximately every 4 years. Brückner (1967) observed similar periodic variations in longitudinal measurements of the amplitude of accommodation in observers between the ages of 15 and 25 years, and notes that they are not frequent, but have also been recorded in older observers. In this case it is not clear whether the variations occur in the far point, i.e. static refraction, or the near point, and hence with an accommodative phenomenon – this was not a point studied by Sorsby *et al*. It is, of course, possible that the results are due to chance, but the point seems to be worth investigating. A periodic change occurring every three or four years is unusual, and there is no obvious hypothesis to account for it.

It may be noted that theoretical considerations of emmetropization, i.e. the harmonization of various changes in the ocular components accompanying growth and senescence, can be carried out analytically without any attention to experimental detail. Thus, Carroll (1982) has derived conditions in which the variance of refractive errors is reduced during growth, which is necessary for adult eyes to be emmetropic, given the natural variance of normal development. The errors in infancy are distributed normally, but leptokurtic in adulthood: their distribution is relatively compressed.

2.3.1 *Glancing backward at evolution*

The decline of hypermetropia during the first two decades of life, toward a brief stay of refraction in the neighbourhood of emmetropia (Fig. 2.4), and the return toward hypermetropia over the next two decades or so, recall the notion of a quasi-trapezoidal variation discussed on p. 40. It raises the question of whether there is any special biological expenditure in achieving it. Fisher (1969*b*) was the first to emphasize the role played by lenticular shape in the storage of energy: a flat lens is more capable of being deformed than a rotund one. The lens is at its flattest during the second decade of life (Fig. 2.4). After the third decade the likely flaccidity of the sclera tends to make for a return to hypermetropia. Roughly speaking, therefore, insofar as emmetropia is concerned this is an example of maximum biological investment appearing when it is needed.

2.3.2 *Chromatic aberration*

The chromatic aberration of the eye is related to its optical power and deserves attention because of the adverse effect which it may have on visual performance. Chromatic aberration is due to the fact that, in an optically isotropic medium and in the absence of anomalous refraction, a curved surface will have a shorter focal length for short wavelengths than for long ones. This phenomenon tends to produce coloured fringes which are easy to see in cheap telescopes or opera-glasses. Several authors have studied the question of whether chromatic aberration of the eye varies with age. There is no doubt that it exists, and that it is readily explained in terms of the refractive index of water, presumably because the main optical medium − the vitreous − is aqueous in composition.

Mordi and Adrian (1985), who studied the matter objectively with a refractometer, reported a longitudinal change over a period of 20 years for wavelengths shorter than 520 nm. Bulked data for individual age groups revealed systematic changes from about 550 nm, much as Millodot (1976) had found earlier by a subjective technique. Mordi and Adrian used cycloplegics to paralyse the action of the ciliary muscle, but Millodot did not use any drug. Aphakic subjects were found to have only about two thirds of the normal chromatic aberration, which amounts in the young to 1.5 D between short and long wavelengths, but decreases to one third of this value amongst the oldest observers studied. It is clear that, on the basis of this evidence, ocular media other than the lens bear the burden of this aberration.

Howarth *et al.* (1988) also used a subjective method, involving a Badal optometer which enables one to measure refraction with a constant image size. They did not observe any variation of chromatic aberration with age, and believe that Millodot's stimuli may not have been truly monochromatic. In itself this would not account for the difference he observed between normal and aphakic observers. Their criticism of Mordi and Adrian regarding the small number (eight) of subjects used, when they used only two, hardly seems compelling. It is possible that a covert difference in technique may explain why they did not detect any variation with age. Millodot used a target that consisted of 'a printed text of black letters of high contrast and of four different sizes and characters', designed to facilitate fixation and accommodation. Howarth *et al.*, on the other hand, used a target consisting of two vertical hairs. It is possible that the differences between the two spatial configurations used in the two studies may be the reason for their different results. For, whereas Millodot's observers would be expected to identify the text, those of Howarth *et al.* might have used the criterion of seeing the two hairs. This merely illustrates the difficulties associated with complicated subjective measurements.

A little consideration shows, however, that both the sense and the magnitude of the results reported by Mordi and Adrian and by Millodot can be explained in terms of the variation of ocular refraction discussed on p. 54. We noted from Saunders' curves that, on balance, our eyes become hypermetropic by about 2 D after the age of 30 years. It is after this age that the above authors observed the main change in chromatic aberration. Now if the young eye is myopic for short wavelengths by about 1.5 D in relation to long ones, and if the older eye becomes virtually emmetropic for short wavelengths and myopic for long ones, then a hypothetical shortening of the eyeball, which leads to the hypermetropia referred to on p. 55, would explain these observations on the age variation of chromatic aberration. In other words, both qualitatively and quantitatively, these results are consistent with the notion that the axial length of the eyeball shrinks by a fraction of a millimetre.

2.4 Accommodation

This property of the visual system has received close attention during the last two centuries, in fact, ever since Thomas Young (1801), in imitation of Leonardo da Vinci (1881) but with considerable more insight, immersed his eyes in water, and convinced himself that accommodation resides in the crystalline lens.

There is a tendency for biological measurements which can be made with a semblance of precision to be endowed with too much respect. Both Steinhaus (1932) and Bernstein and Bernstein (1945) were so convinced of the predictive value which premature presbyopia, however determined, held for the early demise of the unfortunate patient that insurance companies were persuaded to use the results for the assessment of premiums for life insurance policies. Their shareholders have, however, probably benefited, for, as Brückner *et al.* (1987) have shown, none in a varied list of causes of death was predicted in any way by any attribute of longitudinal measurements of accommodation which they were able to pinpoint.

2.4.1 *The measurement of accommodation*

Accommodation of the lens is distinguished from the above static refraction, not by the optical power of the eye being labile, but by its reflex ability to form detailed images of objects at different distances. Operationally these vary from infinity − in practice 6 metres or 20 feet − to the near point of vision. The latter is the shortest object distance from the eyes at which the lenses are capable of forming a detailed retinal image. For the emmetropic eye infinity is the so-called far point, clearly optically the greatest distance for which a sharp image is obtained: this is partly a circular argument, because this condition defines emmetropia. In long sight, the far point lies behind, in short sight, in front of, the retina.

If the limiting distances are reciprocally expressed in dioptres, then their difference measures the amplitude of accommodation. This tends to differ with the degree of static refraction, being larger in young high myopes than in coeval emmetropes and hypermetropes (Fledelius 1981; McBrien and Millodot 1986). The peak is reached, however, in mild myopia, the amplitude exceeding 10 D compared with approximately 9.5 D for emmetropes and 8.5 D for hypermetropes.

Consequently, even if an inhomogeneous population is rendered emmetropic with suitable corrections, the above variation introduces an additional variance into statistical measures of the amplitude of accommodation which is better avoided if it is left undetailed. Several authors have reported sex differences in refraction errors (see Krause *et al.* 1982) which may well be reflected in measurements of the accommodative amplitude (Drew 1941). The fact that women may become presbyopic earlier than men is consistent with their having a smaller accommodative amplitude, and with men tending to be more emmetropic than are women (Krause *et al.* 1982). There may be an ethnic factor involved in this: Nigerian women appear to become presbyopic later than men (Adefule 1983) − or, perhaps, they have been taught not to complain.

Just like static refraction, the amplitude of accommodation can be measured in two ways. The older method is subjective and by no means obsolete: the observer tested decides whether or not he or she sees a sharp image when presented with a test object at various distances in turn. If it is assumed that the eye is emmetropic, then the near point, say **n** metres away, provides a measure of the amplitude of accommodation, defined, it will be recalled, as $1/\mathbf{n} - 1/$ (**distance of far point**). The second post equals zero when the far point is at infinity, whence the above result. The value of $1/\mathbf{n}$ decreases systematically, and virtually linearly with age (Fig. 2.6): symptomatic presbyopia sets in when the ordinate value drops below approximately 3 D. This means that the near point has receded further than 0.33 m, the conventional reading distance. In other words, the emmetropic eye requires a reading or 'near' correction at the corresponding age of onset of presbyopia.

Brückner *et al.* (1987) report a number of longitudinal studies on the amplitude of accommodation, which extended over 20 years. Some of them revealed excursions which might be predicted to be larger than the expected error of this type of measurement. They were unsystematic, and apparently unrelated to other organic events (see p. 59). Hofstetter (1965), who studied only two observers over a period of about 7 years, recorded, but made no comment on, similar features.

Presbyopia has also been said to occur when the amplitude of accommodation has dropped, not to 3 D, but to 5 D. There is no physiological or operational reason that would seem to be able to justify such a choice; however, as we shall have occasion to note in another connection, it is a way of persuading people, for whatever reason, that they may need reading glasses sooner rather than later.

There is considerable evidence to suggest that the age of onset of presbyopia, however defined, depends on people's place of abode. Temperature has been suggested as a possible cause (Weale 1963, 1981; Miranda 1979), and though there may be some technical factors contributing to the different results (Kragha 1986) which were almost certainly all obtained by subjective methods, there is a broad consensus in the matter (Bamba 1987; Peters 1987; Weale 1989*a*). It is found, by and large, that the higher the average ambient annual temperature the lower is the age of onset of presbyopia. Roughly speaking, a rise of 1 °C lowers the age by about 8 months.

Objective measurements of refraction can be made either by the technique of retinoscopy or with instruments called refractometers, which can also be used

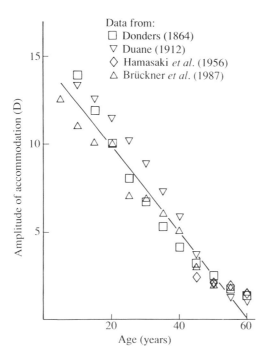

Fig. 2.6 The variation of the amplitude of accommodation with age. After Weale (1990).

in objective measurements of the accommodative amplitude. The latter may suffer from short-comings noted in refraction measurements (see p. 59), but they overcome the problems arising from differences in criteria as to what is meant by the sharpness of an image.

This brings us to a difficulty occasionally faced in daily measurements of refraction, but hardly ever in those of accommodation or its variation with age. Campbell and Green (1965) measured contrast sensitivity (see Chapter 4) as a function of a number of parameters. During the last three or four decades this visual function has been measured with gratings, i.e. periodically repeated patterns consisting of pairs of bars of alternately differing luminance. The latter is kept constant parallel to their length: if it does not vary across their width the gratings are said to be square. If it does, the grating is usually arranged so that the profile is sinusoidal. A light and a neighbouring darker bar constitute the period of the grating. The spacing between pairs is therefore the spatial wavelength. Usually the difference between light and dark is adjusted to threshold, whence its reciprocal is called contrast sensitivity. It is found to decrease with the wavelength of the grating.

When focus was one of the parameters used by Campbell and Green in their study of contrast thresholds, its effect turned out to be relatively unimportant for long spatial wavelengths, i.e. coarse gratings. Ward (1987) studied accommodation with gratings of three periods in turn, namely, 1.67, 5.0, and 15 cycles/degree, i.e. the period of the last had an angular width subtending at the eye a period of only 4 minutes of arc. This is nominally about four times coarser than visual acuity. Ward concluded that there is a variation in the stability with which accommodation can be maintained, and that the 5.0 cycle/degree grating, i.e. one with a period of 12 minutes of arc, is optimal. It follows that attention has to be paid to the visual target used to elicit the process of accommodation.

This is of considerable relevance to an assessment of claims for the method of stigmatoscopy (Hamasaki *et al.* 1956; Marg 1987) which is said to measure accommodation without the data being contaminated by the effects of the depth of focus (pp. 49, 84). As its name implies, this method is based on the observer viewing a point-image and attempting to bring it into focus by exerting his or her accommodative powers. Fourier transforms of point images have a large content of high spatial frequencies, which, as just noted, form less than adequate stimuli for accommodation. Protagonists of the technique have consistently overlooked this point, and this will be discussed further along with explanations of the mechanism of accommodation and presbyopia (p. 84).

It has been noted already in connection with the discussion on the ocular depth of focus (p. 51) that visual acuity decreases with age. In other words, the use of a fixed target, the 'sharpness' of which an observer has to judge when his or her accommodative amplitude is determined, offers physiologically different stimuli to observers of different ages. It is not a sound principle to intermingle more than one variable in a measurement; but this is precisely what happens when the accommodative amplitude, found to vary with age, is also likely to vary with the perception of the target employed to adjudge 'sharpness'.

Furthermore, pupil diameter is also often one of the uncontrolled variables. Ward and Charman (1985) have studied its role in accommodation. They found that, once the pupillary diameter D has reached a minimum value of 1.5 mm, the slope of the stimulus/response curve remains approximately independent of D. Earlier workers have found that, for $D \cong 3$ mm, the classical measure of visual acuity reaches its maximum: optical aberrations, manifested at larger diameters, and diffraction effects, becoming important at smaller ones, seem to come to an operational compromise. In accommodation, however, the pupils especially of the older pre-presbyopes may well constrict to less than 3 mm as a result of the operation of the near reflex. It follows that both the physiological and the optical conditions disadvantage the performance of the older eye in measurements of accommodative amplitude: it remains to be determined to what extent, if any, this affects the numerical values in Fig. 2.6.

The use of objective refractometers may circumvent some of these problems, but may create others. For example, they all depend on an analysis of the retinal image, the contrast of which varies with the fraction of the incident light reaching, and reflected from, the retina. Changes in the transmissivity of the lens (p. 88) and in the pigmentation of the fundus oculi may affect the accuracy of refraction measurements, and so introduce a variation not present in subjective studies. Evidently, the nature of the retinal image plays a role. The optical difficulties inherent in objective measurements preclude the use of a high-frequency (short-wavelength) target to be imaged on the retina; but low frequencies, as we noted above, are less able to pick up differences in focus. It is unlikely that Fig. 2.6 is gravely in error, but the elucidation of some of the above difficulties may lead to an ultimate improvement of the results for the higher age groups relative to those obtained for the younger ones.

This view is reinforced by the fact that very few authors have considered the role of the spectral distribution of the stimulus used to elicit accommodation. The reason is that it is generally thought that the retinal resolving power is optimal in the green or yellow part of the visible spectrum (see Ripps and Weale 1976). Moreover, the photopic spectral sensitivity of the human eye is highest in this region, so that, broadly speaking, 'white' light is considered very suitable for measurements of refraction. However, in view of the existence of chromatic aberration which implies that the eye is myopic for light of short wavelengths, the matter needs some attention. Brückner (1967) and Brückner *et al.* (1987) report measurements on accommodation measured with black Landolt C's on red, green, and white backgrounds in turn. No exception was found to the rule that, amongst the younger age groups, green light registered an accommodative amplitude of between 1 and 2 D more than did red. White tended to give intermediate values. Furthermore, the difference between the two colours systematically diminished after the age of about 30 years (Fig. 2.7).

There is little doubt that these results are explicable in terms of chromatic aberration and its variation with age, as set out above.

2.4.2 *The shape of the human crystalline lens*

The lens is biconvex, the anterior surface having the smaller curvature or the larger radius of cuvature **R**. Approximate values of **R** are 12 mm for the anterior surface, and 6.8 mm for the posterior one. As the difference between the refractive indices of the cortical parts of the lens and the surrounding aqueous and vitreous humours is 0.0707 the power of the anterior surface is approximately 7 D, and that of the posterior surface about 12 D.

In vivo, the thickness of the human lens grows, then declines, and finally grows again, much as is true of rhesus monkey lenses (Denlinger *et al.* 1980). The continual growth throughout life of the equatorial diameter is well documented (see Weale 1982*a*), and the capacity for lens epithelial cells to grow in

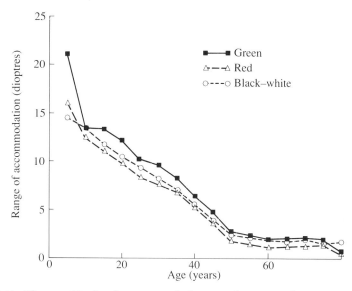

Fig. 2.7   The amplitude of accommodation as a function of age, as measured with targets of three different spectral compositions. After Brückner *et al.* (1987).

tissue culture has been documented even for a 94-year old donor (Bermbach *et al.* 1991).

The rate of lenticular growth and size may be subject to environmental conditions. The eyes of pigs are so similar to human ones that they are often used as a model for the latter. It is, therefore, noteworthy that there is a high correlation between a pig's body weight and lens nitrogen (Kauffman *et al.* 1967), an observation which may be of use in the interpretation of ethnic variations in human lens size. Moreover, there is a marked correlation between the season of a pig's birth and the weight of its lens (Alaku and Steinbach 1982): it would be interesting to know whether this is also true for human lenses, say insofar as concerns their thickness, and whether, therefore, those born at a certain time of the year are at a greater risk of developing glaucoma than are others.

It is sometimes convenient to express the shape of the lens in an algebraic form. Its circularity presents no problem; however, its sagittal profile is complicated by being asymmetrical, as is evident from the above different radii of curvature. To a first approximation each principal section can be represented by an elliptical surface referred to the axes **x**, **y**, and **z**, and the lenticular volume by an ellipsoid of revolution, namely

$$(x^2 + z^2)/R^2 + (y/a)^2 = 1 \qquad (2.6)$$

where **R** is the lenticular radius and **a** is half the sagittal thickness. In the case of the meridional section, the ellipse is simplified to a circle of radius **R**. The above-mentioned asymmetry leads to some uncertainty as to the precise value to be ascribed to the latter even in very accurate work (Fisher 1971), and the lack of symmetry cannot be ignored. The algebraic description is not a matter just of abstruse interest: it is well known that, given such a description for any two-dimensional function, simple differentiation yields a value for the radius of curvature at any point. For an ellipse, there are two principal radii of curvature, and, as regards the crystalline lens, we are interested in the value at the minor axis where **y** = **a**, i.e. at the optic axis of the lens. It is

$$\varrho = -R^2/a \qquad (2.7)$$

Although, as emphasized above, eqn (2.7) is the result of an approximation, some consequences important from the point of view of accommodation and presbyopia stem from it, because the constants of the right-hand side also define **V**, the volume of the lens:

$$V = kR^2a \qquad (2.8)$$

where **k** is a pure numerical constant, namely $4\pi/3$.

It is to be emphasized that eqns (2.7) and (2.8) impose an insurmountable constraint as regards changes in shape which the crystalline lens may undergo as a result of accommodation or as a function of age.

It has been noted (p. 47) that accommodation involves a relaxation of zonular tension, with the result that the capsule moulds the lens matrix into a more nearly spherical shape. A corollary of this must be that the lenticular radius is reduced, and the thickness increased. Almost 70 per cent of the lens is water, and it is unlikely that a physiological change in its shape, such as that entailed during accommodation which can be completed within 0.5 seconds, will be accompanied by one in volume. In other words, eqns (2.7) and (2.8) are not independent of each other. Within certain limits, one can predict a value for one of the three lenticular variables if the other two are known. It follows that changes with age in any of them are likely to affect the accommodative process.

Figure 2.8 illustrates the usefulness of the above concepts. The ordinate scale measures the radius of curvature of the anterior surface of the lens. The straight

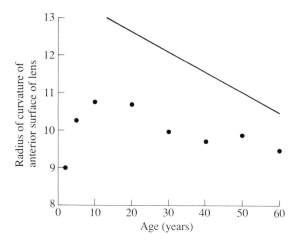

Fig. 2.8 Age-related variation of the radius of curvature of the anterior lenticular surface. The points are values calculated on the basis of eqn 2.7, the regression was obtained by Lowe and Clark (1973).

line is a regression based on the work of Lowe and Clark (1973) who measured the radius of curvature ϱ of the anterior surface of the crystalline lens as function of age. It shows values which are overall lower than those obtained photographically a year later by Brown (1974), whose statistical analysis is open to doubt and to argument. Lowe and Clark allowed for corneal refraction by means of keratometric measurements, and determined the depth of the anterior chamber (AC) ultrasonographically, which minimizes problems due to refraction. The data points are based on the geometry of the lens, and calculated from published values on the lenticular thickness and diameter (see Weale 1982a), and substituted in eqn (2.7). Values calculated for children's lenses are added for the sake of completeness in order to indicate that the radius of curvature as based on lenticular geometry reaches a maximum during the early teens. The data due to Lowe and Clark are too sparse in the younger age-groups to permit the regression to be extrapolated validly to infancy, but it is unlikely that the radius of curvature at birth could be as large as 12 or 13 mm.

The discrepancy between the Lowe and Clark's regression and the calculated values is worthy of comment. Lowe and Clark's results were obtained *in vivo*. There are also numerous studies on the thickness of the lens *in vivo* yielding data which, some remarks made below notwithstanding, permit the use of eqn (2.7). But, so far, the size of the pupil has made *in vivo* measurements of the lenticular equatorial diameter impossible. The equator is always covered by the iris, except in the rare condition of aniridia (see Fincham 1937), and no datum except for excised lenses is available. However, excised lenses are freed from zonular tension, and their diameter would therefore be expected to be smaller than *in vivo* or at any rate *in oculo*. If the diameter is smaller, so will be the radius of curvature (see eqn (2.7)), as seen in Fig. 2.8.

In addition, as noted below, the ability of the capsule to mould the lens diminishes with age; one would therefore expect the discrepancy between measured and predicted values of the radius of curvature to very inversely with age: this is also seen in Fig. 2.5. A small extrapolation suggests that the difference should vanish during the ninth or tenth decade of life. It would seem to follow that eqn (2.7) provides a useful control for the application of corrections for optical effects, such as corneal refraction and photographic variables.

However, a study of the role of the shape of the crystalline lens in theories of accommodation and presbyopia is not confined to considerations of its anterior surface. In fact, it has often been argued (see Fincham 1937) that lenticular accommodation is manifested optically by changes in the power solely of the anterior surface, and that the posterior one can be neglected in this respect. Let us consider the optical power of the lens, and how it varies with age.

If both surfaces are ellipsoids of revolution, then it follows from eqn (2.7) that the ratio of the depths of the ellipsoidal segments, which are divided by the principal meridional plane, is inversely proportional to that of the radii of curvature on the visual axis. It can be shown that this leads to predictions of dioptric values of the radius of curvature of the anterior surface which are not only incompatible with the magnitudes shown in Fig. 2.8, but which also fail to reflect the observed variation with age.

If, however, one makes the assumption that the posterior lenticular segment is described, at any rate, in its axial and paraxial region, not by an ellipsoid, but by a spherical cap of radius equal to the radius of curvature and a width equal to **a** (eqn (2.7)), i.e. half the thickness of the lens, one obtains the function shown with the filled circles in Fig. 2.5. Values for younger lenses (Gordon and Donzis 1985) are shown in Fig. 2.9. Not only does the calculation predict the high neonatal value obtained experimentally by Luyckx (1966), it also agrees with experimentally determined figures for excised adult lenses (Weale 1983). There was no significant difference between results for male and female lenses, and there was no significant variation of the dioptric power with age. The slight rise seen in Fig. 2.5 over the age range between 10 and 60 years is not significant either, but it could become so with the availability of more, and intermediate, values.

It is pertinent to mention that Fisher (1982), who studied the mechanical properties of the lens and its containing capsule as a function of age, found that there is an asymmetry in the elastic properties of the anterior and posterior parts of the capsule, respectively. His explanation of accommodation and presbyopia in terms of the shape and elastic properties of the lens (Fisher 1969*a*, *b*, 1971, 1973*a*, *b*) rests in part on the immobility of the posterior part of the capsule (see also p. 83).

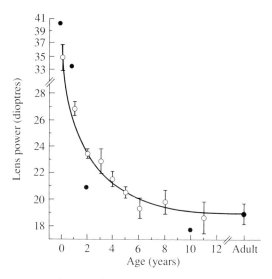

Fig. 2.9 Power of the lens in dioptres as a function of age. Curve and small dots from data due to Gordon and Donzis (1985); large black dots based on eqns 2.7, 2.8, and 2.9. (See also Fig. 2.5.)

2.4.3. *The power of the eye*

How does the power of the lens relate to that of the eye as a whole? Numerous textbooks on optics (see Fincham and Freeman 1977) show that the power **P** of thick lenses, or of systems of lenses, can be expressed in terms of those of the individual surfaces in the first case, and of those of the component lenses in the second.

Thus the power of the eye is made up of that of the cornea $\mathbf{P_C}$ and that of the lens $\mathbf{P_L}$:

$$\mathbf{P} = \mathbf{P_C} + \mathbf{P_L} - \mathbf{d}.\mathbf{P_C}.\mathbf{P_L} \qquad (2.9)$$

where **d** is the reduced distance (i.e. the distance divided by the refractive index) between the so-called principal points of the two systems or surfaces. In the case of the eye, **d** amounts to less than 1 mm.

In other words, the power of the combination is equal to the powers of its two components minus a small, but not entirely negligible correction.

Equation (2.9) leads to an interesting consequence. It predicts that the accommodative requirement of an eye varies inversely with the depth of the anterior chamber.

If the expression is first differentiated with respect to **d**, and then integrated with the appropriate limits,

$$P_L = 1/(1 - P_c.d) \qquad (2.10)$$

since **P** and P_C are constants, the distance of an external object imaged on the retina being fixed by definition.

Obstfeld (1989) has used this simple idea to show that there may be ethnic variations in acommodative effort because there are reports of significant ethnic variations in the depth of the anterior chamber (Clemmesen and Luntz 1976; Clemmesen and Olurin 1985).

Equation (2.10) also has some gerontological significance. There is good evidence to suggest that the anterior chamber contracts with advancing years. This had been measured by optical means a long time ago (see Raeder 1922), and has been confirmed ultrasonographically by Larsen (1971a) and others. There is some confusion in the account of a longitudinal study (Brückner *et al.* 1987): these authors state that 'in the longitudinal analysis . . . no aging trend was found'. But, on the other hand, they note an increase in the depth of the anterior chamber (AC) up to the age of 20 years, with systematic decreases thereafter. The finding that the left AC tends to be deeper than the right one is thought to be significant.

The growth of the lens has also been charted by ultrasonography (Larsen 1971b), as has that of the axial length of the vitreous humour. Basing their conclusion only on optical measurements, Brückner *et al.* (1987) believe that, with occasional exceptions, the length of the eyeball remains constant after the age of 30 years. A similar conclusion is reached by Weekers *et al.* (1973). They combined optical with ultrasonic measurements, and concluded that the reduction in the vitreous chamber is fully accounted for by the growth of the lens. No comment is made on the possibility that this would put the vitreous humour under pressure with problems arising from its incompressibility. Moroever, Weekers *et al.* base their conclusion on this particular issue on measurements on selected eyes, the lengths of which were within narrower than normal limits.

All other authors who have studied this appear to agree that the posterior pole of the crystalline lens virtually stays put. In other words, the contraction of the anterior chamber is due to the lens, partly to its growth and partly to its forward displacement, a point to be considered on p. 83. But, if the anterior chamber, and, therefore, **d** in eqn (2.10), decrease by about 0.1 mm every year after the age of 20 years, the power of the eye increases by about half a dioptre every decade. This does not do away with the need for accommodation as we get older, but makes what is available go a little further. Though marginally advantageous, this statistical result is insignificant from an evolutionary point of view.

2.4.4 *The photography of the human accommodative processes*

One of the problems in this subject, however, relates to the question of measurement. *A priori*, the optical barrier of the cornea, meridional variations in its radii of curvature and their dependence on age (Löpping and Weale 1965) and some uncertainty about the values of refractive indices of the media lead one to prefer measurements directly on excised lenses. But, as noted above, released from zonular tension, the lens assumes an unphysiological shape, which it is difficult to allow for with an accuracy greater than that indicated in Fig. 2.8. Ultrasonography is more reliable than optical *in vivo* measurement when it comes to the determination of distances between the various refracting surfaces, but it is of no use, for example, in the determination of **R**. For these reasons great efforts have been made either to refine optical techniques (Brown 1972, 1974; Koretz *et al.* 1984) or to combine them with ultrasonography (Lowe and Clark 1973). Brown's study provides instructive insight into some of the problems encountered.

This author developed a photographic slit-lamp based on the Scheimpflug principle. The principle itself takes into account the fact that, when an eye is photographed during illumination with a slit-beam, its different parts are at different distances from the camera, the axis of which includes an angle with that of the illuminating beam. Consequently, only a small part of the picture captured by the camera can be in focus. By sacrificing uniformity in scale across the picture to orthogonality of the image plane, the principle improves image quality. Brown elaborated it with a number of optical refinements which include the reproducible alignment of the eye under examination. Brown controlled corneal refraction by means of photographing an artificial eye, and obtained accurate biomicroscopic results on the eyes of four normal individuals aged 11, 19, 29, and 45 years who were expected to accommodate to stimuli between 0 and 10 dioptres.

It must be questioned whether they actually accommodated by the required amount. For example, Obstfeld (1989) has said that an object at a dioptric distance of 2.5 D (40 cm in front of the eyes) requires an accommodative effort of 3.25 D because of the depth of the anterior chamber (see p. 69). On the face of it, the photographic evidence should be sufficient and conclusive. However, if the recorded change in the refraction of the anterior lenticular surface is plotted against the optical stimulus giving rise to it, Brown's data reveal a deficit of several dioptres for stimuli greater than about 5 D, and smaller, but significant deficits for lower accommodations: only the 19-year old managed to match his response to the stimulus up to 4 D. As he dilated his subjects' pupils with phenylephrine, presumably to facilitate photography of the lens, he may have deprived them of an accommodative facility which the pupillary sphincter provides in rhesus monkeys (Crawford *et al.* 1990), and may provide in man (p. 82). However, phenylephrine may have caused a deficit more directly. Alphen *et al.* (1962) applied epinephrine to an eserinized (i.e. contracted) ciliary muscle preparation of a monkey: the subsequent application of 10 μg of epinephrine served to reduce the tension in it.

If the response cannot match the stimulus, one could also argue that there is some accommodative insufficiency, not to mention functional presbyopia. For example, Daum (1983) has shown that accommodative insufficiency appears to be a fairly widespread condition. In over 100 pre-presbyopic persons, he found only 14 whose accommodative amplitude followed the trend shown in Fig. 2.6.

It is perhaps a little regrettable that, with four carefully chosen subjects, Brown had not found it possible to compare subjective and objective responses, thereby leaving open the question of whether the various optical controls were sufficiently rigorous.

This point is emphasized by another of Brown's important results. He was able to show that, during accommodation, the lens advances by a fraction of a millimetre, much as it advances during the course of senescence: but by an extent which, according to Lowe (1970) amounts to only 0.2 mm in 50 years. In Brown's study, the anterior surface and the centre of the lens were found to move forward systematically, but no such movement could be detected for the posterior surface. A forward movement of the lens would not be altogether surprising: it was noted earlier that eyes more primitive than those of mammals possess a type of accommodation that depends on the lens advancing along the optic axis. Such a phylogenetic trace could be preserved in our eyes in a rudimentary manner. There is also good anatomical evidence, based on sections of the ciliary muscle (Stieve 1949) to suggest that the lens moves in this manner. It is, however, easier to detect movement of the anterior lenticular surface than of the posterior surface. A problem that needs resolving is to what extent, if any, Brown's measurements of the advance of the anterior lenticular face during accommodation may be affected by the type of optical effect considered by Obstfeld (1989).

When accommodation takes place, the interior of the lens and the posterior surface are viewed by an external observer through additional powers, which increase with the accommodation of the examined eye. There is an implicit apparent reduction in the distance of the object viewed so that lens surface and centre will appear to approach the camera. While there are also mechanical reasons (Coleman 1970) to support the view that the posterior surface is relatively immobile, the matter is still unresolved. It is possible to show by the application of optical principles appertaining to the analysis of thick lens systems that accommodation would lead to an apparent movement of the lenticular centre of about 0.1 mm/D. A consideration of the additional power through which an external observer has to view the inside of the accommodated lens makes the qualitative aspect of such a conclusion highly plausible.

A considerable amount of work has been done during the last decade or two using slit-lamp photography, and it is appropriate to discussion the suitability of this technique for the provision of quantitatively reliable biometric data. There is no doubt that the method is well suited for the detection and relative topography of lenticular opacities (Hockwin *et al.* 1983). However, its suitability for basic measurement is an open question, in particular as no analysis of its underlying optics seems to have been done.

The problem is presented in Fig. 2.10. In well-controlled measurements a narrow illuminating beam enters the eye under test along the optic axis and continues without deviation through the cornea, aqueous humour and the crystalline lens. The observing beam, which coincides with the axis of the slit-lamp camera, is set at 45 degrees to the illuminating beam. It is clear that, owing to corneal refraction, the rays that will mainly enter the camera originate from a part of the lens that is well removed from the ocular axis; in fact, they will travel approximately along a path including with it an angle of some 30 degrees. Because of the finite size of the pupil, there will be a solid angle of pencils emanating from that lenticular area, as indicated in Fig. 2.10. In this situation the lamp illuminates one part of the lens surface, but the camera is looking at another. The two beams do intersect in the interior of the lens, but confusion is likely to arise if the region of intersection is mentally projected onto the lenticular surface, which gives rise to a vignetted image. Indeed, Niesel *et al.* (1976) decline to give any measurement for the posterior lenticular surface

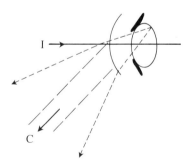

Fig. 2.10 Schematic bird's-eye view of Scheimpflug optics. I, incident pencil of light; C, beam received by the camera. The optic axis is horizontal (solid line). An arbitrary point on the posterior surface of the lens emits pencils, the angular boundary of which is shown by the short-dashed lines. The upper of the pair of long-dashed lines indicates the angle between camera axis and ocular (visual?) axis, the other line indicates that, in theory, the camera can scan the pupillary aperture.

because of the pronounced 'vignetting', which is accentuated especially after the age of 50 years.

This simple analysis has ignored the complications likely to arise when refraction by the lenticular nucleus is also considered. Viewed in a vertical plane, its effect will be more pronounced near the axis than away from it, confounding the quantitative interpretation of the lenticular slit-lamp image.

Imagine next that the situation shown in Fig. 2.10 is adapted to a measurement of accommodation. With the two axes fixed, an increase in curvature of the anterior surface of the lens necessitates that the camera looks at areas nearer the optic axis. This approach to the lenticular pole progresses with the degree of accommodation. In other words, the use of the Scheimpflug principle in studies of accommodation involves the examination of different lenticular regions in turn; this entails the traverse of the different parts of the highly refractile nucleus. Therefore this only serves to increase the difficulty met in trying to interpret apparently definitive results, for example on the changes in curvature of the posterior lenticular surface. The optical problems encountered are illustrated by a comparison of Scheimpflug photographs taken of an eye when accommodation was relaxed, and in action (Harding 1991). Defocusing is shown to have taken place between the two steady states, and it is probable that correcting it would vitiate the basis of such biometric measurements as photography may subserve.

This is highlighted by the notion that the Scheimpflug appearance of the posterior 'surface' can be represented algebraically by a hyperbola (Koretz *et al.* 1984); as the profiles from the posterior lenticular pole must lead symmetrically to the highly curved diametrically opposed equatorial regions the use of a hyperbola is likely to be so restricted as to compel one to ask oneself whether there is not perhaps some distortion involved in this type of imaging.

2.4.5 *An outline of the physiology of accommodation*

Accommodation is not a simple mechanism, and the extent to which it may be multifactorial is still a subject for debate. What is beyond argument is that it operates by virtue of changes in lenticular shape (Helmholtz 1855). This is not an essential requirement; accommodation in the eye of the frog is based on lenticular displacement, as in the camera. In the horse, there is a ramp retina with parts of the retina being progressively further removed from the fixed lens. But the human lenticular shape changes in a reflex manner which has evolved with a sensitivity involving muscular movements of small fractions of a millimetre. The lens is attached to the rest of the eye via the suspensory ligaments, collectively known as the zonule. This is derived embryologically from a precursor of the vitreous humour.

There is little information available on the fate of zonular mechanical properties throughout life. In a histological study of human eyes covering a wide

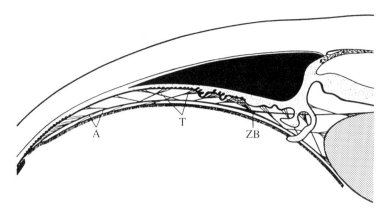

Fig. 2.11 Schematic diagram of the structure of the human zonular complex. A, anchoring ligaments; T, tensile fibrils; ZB, zonular bifurcation. After Rohen and Rentsch (1969).

range, Alexander and Garner (1983) showed that the suspensory ligaments consist throughout life mainly of oxytalan. This is the name given to immature fibres able to resist prolonged acid hydrolysis. In a sense such fibres may be looked on as precursors of elastic ones.

It is unlikely that the suspensory ligaments can stretch very easily. This important point does not seem to have received any attention. Suppose, for the sake of argument, that the ligaments are highly tensile, and stretch easily when accommodation is relaxed as a result of the ciliary muscle fibres contracting to their unstimulated state. The result might be that the ligaments extend without the muscular pull being transmitted to the lenticular attachments of the zonule, and the lens remains in its accommodated state. It would seem to follow that, for the zonular suspension to be efficient in terms of the accommodation of the lens, the ligaments must be relatively rigid, a point perhaps consistent with their oxytalan constitution.

The ligaments form a complicated system of fibrils which has been elucidated during the last two decades or so as a result of painstaking studies done with transmission and scanning electron microscopes.

In an examination of pre-presbyopic and older eyes, Rohen and Rentsch (1969) discovered that, leading from the lenticular insertions, the ligaments form bifurcations (ZB) that are covered by the ciliary processes (Fig. 2.11). This may explain why the ligamental divisions were not discovered for a long time. At the point of bifurcation the system is said to divide functionally into two parts. The continuation of the ligaments forms the anchoring system (A) of the lens. According to Roll *et al.* (1975) part of the fibres (Fig. 2.12) continue between the basal membrane of the pigmented ciliary epithelium of the pars

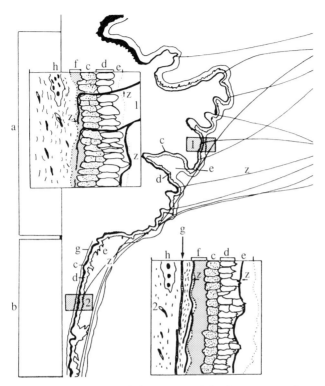

Fig. 2.12 Schematic diagram of the course of the human zonule in the partes plicata (1) and plana (2) of the ciliary body. One part of the ligaments (z) in (1) courses through the external limiting membrane (f), the other traverses all the cellular layers and reaches the external limiting membrane (f). In (2), part of the ligaments appear in the superficial layers of the unpigmented epithelium (d), whereas the other runs separately between the external limiting membrane (f) and the elastic moiety of Bruch's membrane (g). After Roll *et al.* (1975).

plana b (the flat section) and the elastic tissue of Bruch's membrane g. These ligamental bundles continue within the basal membrane in the crypts of both the pigmented (c) and the unpigmented (d) epithelium of the ciliary pars plicata a (the folded section), whereas another set of bundles stretches across the surface of the unpigmented part d of the pars plicata, the ora serrata, and the retina.

It is likely that the superficial system represents Rohen and Rentsch's anchoring fibres (their work being apparently unknown to Roll *et al.* and vice versa), and that the other system (T) is what the earlier authors called tensile fibres. Figure 2.11 shows that they course behind the zonular bifurcation in an anterior sense in the eye. They seem to occupy a key position for a modern understanding of the mechanism of accommodation.

The ciliary muscle, which mediates the response of this mechanism, consists of a composite arrangement of fibres, which run partly in a posterio-anterior direction, and partly radially by turning through a right angle near their anterior aspect. This anatomical arrangement has the consequence that, when an inner-vation arrives at the muscle from the third cranial nerve, the muscle fibres contract, and the muscular complex moves inwards and forwards.

Following the contraction of the ciliary muscle, the tensile zonular fibres are levered forward and hence extended (Fig. 2.11). This reduces the tension on the ligamental (anterior) portion between the bifurcation and the lenticular insertion of the zonular elements. Therefore the balance between the elastic forces of the lenticular matrix and the capsule containing it permits accommodation to occur in the non-presbyopic lens. This is to say that the lens surfaces increase their curvature. But a more nearly spherical shape is equivalent to an increase in optical power: in other words, the eye is in a state accurately to image a near object on the retina. The main optical work appears to be done by the anterior lenticular surface. A number of workers (for example Fincham 1937, Brown 1973) have studied changes in lenticular shape during accommodation, and there is general unanimity on this optical matter.

The pull in the tensile zonular fibres also prompts an increase in the tension in the ligamental part posterior to the zonular bifurcation: this stores up energy which is used to flatten the lens when the innervation of the ciliary muscle has ceased. The tensile fibrils terminate in ciliary crypts (Ober and Rohen 1979, see Roll *et al.* 1975), which is mechanically sound. Were they to terminate on the spongy processes of the ciliary epithelial crests they would be unlikely to exert the tension needed to operate accommodation and its relaxation.

The existence of the above complex zonular system is denied by Davanger (1975). He studied five human eyes of unspecified ages with the scanning electron microscope. His excellent photographs appear to distinguish between suspensory ligaments inserted on the anterior and posterior surfaces of the lens respectively. Whereas those originating on the anterior surface appear to terminate in the anterior ridges of the ciliary processes, the posterior ones seem to lead into the vitreous humour. But even some of the anterior ones could actually be leading through, rather than just to, the ciliary processes. Unlike some of the above authors, Davanger is unconcerned by the relation between his observations and our understanding of accommodative mechanisms, and has not considered the question of the stability of the crystalline lens suspended in accordance with his scheme in a human being on the move, yet desirous to see well.

2.4.6 Aspects of presbyopia

The ciliary system

The mechanical agent in the accommodative process is the ciliary muscle. It lines the anterior part of the inside of the eye, beginning in the anterior aspect near the ocular equator beyond the line at which the retina abuts the ora serrata. Its anterior end is anchored at the scleral spur, just below the corneal limbus. In the Cynomolgus monkey, separation between spur and muscle abolishes accommodation (Flügel *et al.* 1990). At the time of birth, the radii of curvature of the cornea and of the eye are similar. Afterwards, those of the cornea remain unchanged (see Weale 1982*a*), whereas the emmetropic eye grows until just after puberty. Consequently there is a slight increase in the angle between the principal axis of the meridional muscle section and that of the eye. The apparent benefit which this might bestow on accommodative efficiency is, however, constrained by the fact that the cornea also grows slightly. Although smooth, the muscle assumes aspects of striped systems (Flügel *et al.* 1990), and there are regional morphological differences. In rhesus monkeys, the circular section of the fibre system revealed senescent changes at an age which corresponds to the third decade in human terms.

The ciliary system is believed to contribute to presbyopia by a progressive reduction in the mobility of the muscle fibres. According to one authority, this is brought about by the formation of connective links between them after the age of 30 years (Van der Zypen 1975). These are said not only to create friction but also to block an outflow channel for the aqueous humour, and thereby to increase a disposition for glaucoma. However, the idea that senescence of the ciliary muscle is accompanied by the formation of significant amounts of elements generating friction is denied on histological grounds by Lütjen-Drecoll *et al.* (1988) insofar as concerns the rhesus monkey: 'Age-related increase in connective tissue within and adjacent to the muscle seems far too small to immobilize it, with the muscle remaining compact and non-hyalinized'. More-over, impedance cyclography (Swegmark 1969), which involves the application of external electrodes that can record potentials from the eye when the ciliary muscle contracts has failed to show any marked change in the amplitude of the potentials up to the age of 60 years, that is to say well after presbyopia has reached its full extent. However, there was a slowing down in the rise time of the potentials as age advanced.

Morphologically, there is a progressive change in the meridional shape of the human muscle (Stieve 1949). It grows during the first three decades of life, reaching its maximum volume during our 30s. Thereafter it not only shrinks but also changes from a nearly spindle-shaped section to almost a triangular one. The latter shape is similar to the one the muscle adopts in accommodation. Lütjen-Drecoll *et al.* studied the shape of the (rhesus) muscle following the application of atropine and pilocarpine, and conclude that, as it ages, the contraction of the ciliary muscle becomes isometric. This may be due to a reduction in the muscular ability to contract (Lütjen-Drecoll *et al.* 1987). The change would be looked for in the structure of the fibres rather than in impediments between them.

A zonular contribution

Gärtner (1970) studied the ultrastructure of eight zonulae in the age range between 0.75 and 78 years, and confirmed that their structure does not differ from that of vitreous supporting fibrils. Fibroblasts, from which the ligaments are derived, are present also in the oldest pars plana, on which attention was focused, but they tend to be quiescent. There was no variation in the ligamental diameter with age, but the periodicity of transverse striae dropped marginally. In infancy, the cilio-zonular basal membrane was found to be a monolayer, but became converted into a multilayered structure in adulthood and beyond. Degenerative changes, related to those observed for example in skin, were observed in the collagen which glues the fibres into bundles, and this may explain the fragility of older ligaments.

The method whereby suspensory ligaments are inserted at their distal ends has already been discussed. As regards the proximal zonular ends, it is agreed that they are anchored in separate bundles on the posterior and anterior lenticular surfaces respectively. The posterior lens surface apparently playing a subsidiary role in accomodation (p. 83), and therefore in presbyopia, its insertions do not appear to have been studied. However, Farnsworth and Shyne (1979) have examined the distance between the insertions and the lenticular equator as a function of age, and compared it with the circumlental space.

It will be recalled that there is a progressive increase in the equatorial diameter of the lens (p. 66), and, provided there is no appreciable change in the width of the ciliary system, the observed reduction in the circumlental space is explicable in terms of lenticular growth. Farnsworth and Shyne observed that the distance between the proximal zonular insertions on the lens and the ciliary edge abutting the circumlental space remains constant throughout life. This implies that the suspensory ligaments do not stretch (cf. p. 74). If they did, the lens would sag *in situ*: a visual system having to cope with an optic axis determined by the cornea and another due to the lens would have problems with visual resolution which, were they appreciable, would have been detected by now.

The mechanism whereby this is achieved is thought by the authors to rely on zonular shifts. It is not clear what force there might be to produce such shifts. The authors say '. . . it is obvious that the shift of the zonules onto the anterior surface correlates with the changes in elasticity of the capsule (Fisher 1969*b*)'. This is shown in Fig. 2.13 where Farnsworth and Shyne's experimental points are compared with the reciprocal of the curve drawn by Fisher through his

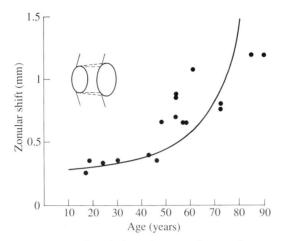

Fig. 2.13 Change in zonular shift with age. This is shown in the inset in relation to the lenticular diameter. The curve represents reciprocal values for Young's modulus of capsular elasticity. After Farnsworth and Shyne (1979).

points for Young's modulus of capsular elasticity: this provides a measure of strain, i.e. the extension of a body stressed by an elastic force. The relatively satisfactory fit suggests that the diameter of insertion, i.e. the distance between diametrically opposed insertions on the anterior surface remains constant throughout the age span studied (see the inset in Fig. 2.13). Owing to the different elasticity of the posterior capsular surface (Fisher 1982), the latter stretches much more than does the anterior surface, and this difference extends into the equatorial region, hence possibly producing the observed result.

It remains to be seen whether Farnsworth and Shyne's suggestion that these shifts are a factor in the aetiology of presbyopia is valid. Figure 2.13 shows that major shifts occur only after presbyopia has appeared. Clearly, any increase in distance between zonular insertion and lenticular equator reduces accommodative efficiency; whether it also reduces the amplitude has yet to be established.

A lenticular contribution

The conventional wisdom is that the main reason for the appearance of presbyopia resides in the lens, as first postulated by Young (1801). For decades it has been thought that the lens scleroses even though no one had measured its mechanical properties to substantiate this argument. Those who have worked with normal crystalline lenses know that lenses similar to glass (i.e. sclerosed) are found in the eyes of fish: these are hard to transect even with a new scalpel. Another reason why sclerosis was postulated is that many animal lenses lose some of their water content, but this is not true of human lenses (Nordmann 1973). Indeed, measurements of the water content of human lenses by means of

Raman spectroscopy (Siebinga *et al.* 1991) show that their nuclear water content increases with age at the rate of 0.11 per cent of lens mass per year. As regards the cortex, an age-related decrease in water content was observed only for the equatorial region of the lens. No change was observed near the anterior or posterior polar regions. The implication of these observations for the optics of the human lens is that a reduction in the refractive index of the nucleus occurs with advancing years.

In a felicitous combination of surgical skill with a competent knowledge of engineering mathematics, Fisher undertook a detailed study of the mechanical properties of the human lens matrix and capsule as a function of age. By clamping the capsule in a steel ring, he was able to subject it to various pressures and to measure the strain which they produced. This yielded values for the capsular modulus of elasticity (Fisher 1969*b*): it was found to decrease in old age to one seventh of its juvenile value; after the age of 40 years the rate of decrease more than doubles.

Young's modulus of the lens matrix was obtained with an ingenious arrangement wherein the isolated lens was spun on a rotor. The centrifugal force mimicked ciliary stresses, and could be calculated from the speed of rotation. Concomitant changes in the shape of the lens were photographed and analysed. In contrast to the capsular trend, Young's modulus of the lens matrix remains approximately constant up to the age of 30 years and then rises to triple its value during the eight decade of life (Fisher 1971). The rotary method has been criticized by van Alphen and Graebel (1991) on the ground that spinning is liable to turn initially clear lenses into opacified ones. They mention in particular 'varicose swellings . . . presumably indicating that the [lenticular] fibres were leaking'. This observation was based on lenses between 56 and 80 years old. Not only is it hard to see how the mechanical properties of such lenses can be significant for our understanding of accommodation and presbyopia, it is also worth recalling that Young's modulus rises quite steeply before the onset of this age range (Fig. 1.2*a*).

The above-mentioned age-related variations in Young's modulus hold approximately both for the equator and the lenticular poles. Since the deformation of the lens-capsule system varies with the ratio of the two elastic values, it follows that the 70-year old lens is more than 20 times harder to mould than is true of the young one. This is presumably the explanation for the outdated notion that presbyopic lenses are sclerosed.

It is worth noting, however, that during the fifth decade, when presbyopia has become symptomatic, the above ratio is only about 2.5 times it juvenile value; in other words, while more resistant to deformation than that of a child, the lens is far from hard. Fisher (1969*a*) has been able to show that the two elasticities are not the only factors to lead to presbyopia: the shape of the lens, as characterized by its equatorial and sagittal diameters, and the energy the capsule is capable of storing also have to be taken into account.

Changes in lenticular shape were discussed also on p. 63. Thus the capsular moulding pressure is higher in the human lens than in the lenses of the cat and the rabbit, because the latter are more curved. Fisher also showed that neonatal capsules store between one third and one half the maximum energy stored during the early 20s, the lenses being almost spherical. In this connection it may be noted that although babies can accommodate to those physiological distances for which they were tested, namely down to 0.75 m (Braddick *et al.* 1979), the precise amplitude of their accommodation does not appear to have been determined, though about half the adult range appears to be present at the age of a few months (Banks 1980). Similarly, being by far the less curved of the two surfaces, the anterior surface of the mature human lens is easier for the capsule to mould, even if the inherent elastic anisometry of the lens is disregarded (Fisher 1982).

Using an approach in which the lens and zonule are in turn subjected, not to radial stresses as was done by Fisher, but to diametrically opposed ones, van Alphen and Graebel (1991) studied the mechanical properties of human lenses. They showed for samples between the ages of 1 day and 50 years that the lens is less easily deformed than the zonule, and that the elasticity of the zonule does not vary with age. Without attempting Fisher's more detailed analysis, they also noted that the principal changes in the shape factor when the lens is stressed occur during the first two decades of life both when the loading is low (1.5 g) and as much as 6 g (which is moving out of the physiological range).

In a somewhat indirect way, Fisher (1977) measured the force of contraction of the ciliary muscle, and the effect this had on the shape, and therefore the optical power, of the human lens. Contrary to the earlier assumption of linearity made by Pau (1951) in connection with bovine lenses (which are unlikely to exhibit any significant accommodation), Fisher found that the amplitude of accommodation varies with the square root of the ciliary force. It may be noted in this connection that Van Alphen and Graebel (1991) found an approximate square root relation between applied force and lenticular deformation.

With power functions calculated for the experimental vaules obtained in the above studies, age being the independent variable, Fisher was able to derive the regression shown by the continuous line in Fig. 2.14. The experimental points were obtained by Duane (1922), Brückner *et al.* (1987), Hamasaki *et al.* (1956), and Donders (1964): the dashed line is the regression through these data. Fisher attributes the difference between the two regressions to the depth of focus apparently contributing to the accommodative amplitude. However, the need for a correction for this factor in Fisher's own data appears to have been overlooked: it increases the discrepancy between the two sets of data. It is, of course, arguable that there may not be a significant difference between the two types of study, given that the comparison is made between two regressions rather than two populations of results.

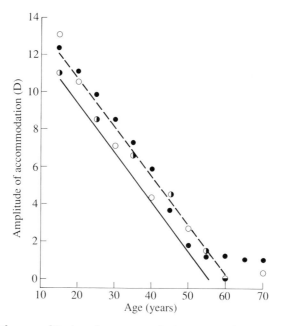

Fig. 2.14 The amplitude of accommodation as a function of age. The continuous line is the regression through the points Fisher determined on the basis of mechanical and morphometric studies of human lenses. The dotted line is the regression through experimental data on the amplitude of accommodation published earlier (see Donders and Duane in Fig. 2.6). After Fisher (1977).

A role of the iridal sphincter

Attention has been drawn to the fact that the ciliary muscle is attached to the scleral spur beneath the corneal limbus. It follows that the root of the iris is in close proximity to the ciliary system. The innervation of accommodation is accompanied by a constriction of the pupil, as is true when the visual axes converge onto a near point. There is a triad of reflexes mediated by the third nerve, and, since it is elicited by the close proximity to the eyes of fixated objects, the resulting miosis (pupillary constriction) is known as the near reflex.

A study of this reflex for a number of age groups (Schäfer and Weale 1970) showed that it occurs also in presbyopes when elicited by ocular convergence. Just as is true of the simple light reflex (Alexandridis 1971), there does not seem to be any physiological stimulus for which the iris ceases to constrict, even though its minimum diameter is about 2 mm under extreme conditions (see Ellis 1981). The question has been raised (Weale 1989*a*) whether the constricting sphincter does not consequently pull on the ciliary region.

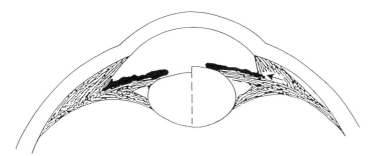

Fig. 2.15 The anterior segment of the human eye when accommodation is relaxed (left), and when it is in force (right). Changes in pupillary diameter accompanying accommodation can exert a pull on the ciliary region, thereby potentially increasing the amount whereby zonular tension is relaxed and hence the lens accommodates. Modified from Stark (1985).

Recent experiments on the macaque monkey (Crawford *et al.* 1990) have illustrated the important role played by the pupillary sphincter in this animal's amplitude of accommodation. The reflex was induced by the ionophoretic application of 40 per cent carbachol, known to elicit a supraphysiological response in this species. Measurements were obtained for the intact eye, and again after it had been iridectomized. The amplitude of accommodation in the intact eye was found to be some 50 per cent greater than in the operated eye, which demonstrates the important role played by the intact pupillary sphincter in this situation.

Figure 2.15 shows that the human muscle can act in a like manner. If one assumes that Hooke's Law holds to a first approximation, that is to say that the stress exerted by a force is proportional to the strain which it causes, then one can postulate that the axipetal movement of the root of the iris is approximately one fifth that of the contraction of its sphincter. But this is measured by the constriction of the pupil. It can be shown that the movement calculated on the basis of Brown's (1973) and other workers' results can probably lead to a significant reduction in zonular tension; consequently pupillary constriction may be pictured as contributing to the amplitude of accommodation.

The results of such an analysis lead to the conclusion that accommodation is a multifactorial event. While it occurs the thickening lens probably moves forward: if this were not the case the incompressible vitreous humour would be subjected to a pressure with nowhere for it to overflow; this argument obviously finds no parallel in connection with the anterior lenticular surface, the volume change caused by the forward movement of which may be taken up by an aqueous humour which disposes over more than one outflow channel. None of this contradicts Coleman's view that the vitreous humour acts in a supporting manner (Coleman 1970). With an accommodative amplitude of 10–11 D at the

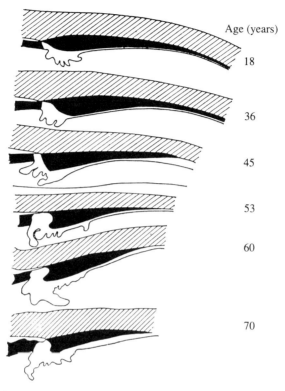

Age (years)

18

36

45

53

60

70

Fig. 2.16   The change in shape of the human ciliary muscle as a function age.
After Stieve (1949).

age of 20 years, this forward movement of the lens and the depth of focus
(Fig. 2.2), would account for a fraction of a dioptre each. But the constriction
of the iridal sphincter could well result in 20–25 per cent of the amplitude of
accommodation; this would leave the major factor of about three quarters to be
explained in terms of changes in lenticular shape, as has been done by Fisher
(see above).

This hypothesis not only offers a contribution to the resolution of the
discrepancy between the two regression lines in Fig. 2.14, but also helps to
explain why the ciliary muscle sets in later life apparently in its accommodated
form (Fig. 2.16). Swegmark's work (1969) shows that the muscle is capable of
action long after the onset of symptomatic presbyopia. It is unlikely that it
contracts every time a presbyope may wish, but fails, to accommodate. Even if
it did, one would have to postulate that the tensile fibres (p. 74) have lost their
function when it comes to the relaxation of accommodation, even though
attention has been drawn to their later fragility (p. 78). But senile miosis, the

progressive constriction of the pupil as we age, provides a ready explanation of a constant pull. Several hypotheses for its development have been advanced, ranging from nervous causes to differential atrophy of the dilator and sphincter respectively and to changes in the iridal stroma and its vessels (see Weale 1982a). It has no obvious evolutionary significance as regards normal pupillary function, but, as discussed later, it may fulfil one insofar as accommodation is concerned.

Another hitherto puzzling observation can be considered at this point. We have noted that the age of onset of presbyopia appears to be under some influence relating to temperature. In most warm countries there is a great deal of sunshine, and in those where measurements have been made pupillary diameters appear to be considerably smaller at all ages than in temperate ones (Weale 1982a). A calculation analogous to that which suggests that the near reflex assists in the relaxation of the zonule leads to the result that in warm countries the naturally smaller pupil may account for as many as 4 D of the accommodative amplitude, which would mean that, in the warm countries, the onset of presbyopia could occur up to 16 years earlier than in temperate ones. This estimate appears to be consistent with observation.

2.4.7 A possible evolutionary pressure

One of the unexplained puzzles of presbyopia is the large amplitude of accommodation observed in childhood. We have suggested that there is no evidence for its existence at or soon after birth, and that the shape of the crystalline lens in early infancy is relatively unsuited for powerful accommodation. There is nevertheless every indication that during the first decade the amplitude far exceeds physiological requirements. There is no known situation which would require a child to accommodate to a distance of 6–8 cm. The argument that monkeys need powerful accommodation (because they spend a great deal of time nit-picking) is clearly inapplicable to the case of a child. How, then, is one to explain this remarkable resource?

Let us return to the notion of bio-economics introduced in Chapter 1 (p. 40) and recall that there is no point in developing a biological mechanism before it is going to benefit its owner. To that extent the putative quasi-trapezoidal shape of the accommodative amplitude – starting from a low value, rising to a peak and then running downhill – makes economic sense. It will, however, be objected to on the grounds that the peak is reached early in life, namely before puberty, and that its magnitude is unaccounted for.

To examine this valid objection one may ask what accommodative amplitude would have been historically useful during that biologically important period when the next generation has to be reared and protected. In the wild, this would be the interval roughly between the individual's puberty and that of its offspring, that is to say, approximately between the 15th and 30th years of his or her life, give or take two or three years. The amplitude needed would be some 4 D so as to ensure good vision between infinity and the distance of manipulation, which is effectively reading distance.

It has been emphasized (Weale 1990) that this value of 4 D cannot be an average; if it were, then half the population might well be disadvantaged by having a smaller accommodative amplitude during those vital years, and suffer the consequences of being visually relatively unfit. With evolution discriminating against them they would be unlikely to be able to provide for their offspring. However, this is not a matter of certainty, and a theoretical way of circumventing the problem is as follows. Assume that, when the amplitude evolved to roughly its present level, the population of the world was about 1 million (McEvedy and Jones 1978). The error of an amplitude measurement obtained for a number of persons is approximately 0.7 D. Statistical tables show, that if the chance of an event occurring is approximately 1 in 10^{10} (which is the order of the present world population), its value would have to be six times greater than the error added to the value postulated. But the latter is, as we saw, 4 D. Hence, to ensure that no more than one person in the whole world shall be disadvantaged by an accommodative amplitude smaller than appears to be necessary for survival, the mean would have to be over 8 D at or just above the age of 30 years. It can be shown that, for the primeval population of about 1 000 000, the value would be about 7.5 D.

Figure 2.6 shows that the observed value agrees with that estimated on the basis of the above argument. It also shows that the decrease varies approximately linearly with age. But this implies that it is governed by two constants, namely its early value or zero intercept, and the slope of the line. The value of the zero intercept is extrapolated, and unlikely to hold, as mentioned on p. 81. It can nevertheless serve to define the regression.

The biological cost of maintaining our ability to accommodate can be expressed tentatively in terms of the area under the regression. Given the above constraint as regards the necessary amplitude of approximately 8 D at around 30 years, it is found to be minimal when the zero intercept is approximately at 16 years and the regression intersects the abscissa at around 60 years. These theoretical values appear to be consistent with the observed data.

One of the advantages of accommodation being a multifactorial phenomenon, depending, as suggested on p. 80 on the four variables of lenticular shape and position, depth of focus, and pupillary action would seem to be that evolution could tune their changes finely enough for the economic result of biological economy to be achieved. As discussed later (p. 227), this is not the only example of this principle to be found in ocular senescence.

2.5 Image degradation

2.5.1 Introduction

Image degradation may appear to be a recondite subject, but it has important practical facets. The question of light losses in the ocular media in general, and in the lens in particular, is important if it involves a variation with age, for provision may have to be made for supplementary illumination for the elderly for tasks easily discharged without such aid by the young. Consideration may also have to be given to the quality, i.e. spectral composition, of such additional illumination. Moreover, in a civilized society, even in one concerned with energy conservation, light is looked on as an amenity: if some types of light, acceptable to the young, prove to be uncomfortable to their elders, then a knowledge of possible reasons may assist in the production of acceptable solutions.

Although the *raison d'être* of the crystalline lens is to support and to refine the image-forming capacity of the cornea, and thereby to maximize the contrast of the retinal image, the make-up of the lens prevents this from being its only function. It can also affect the colour of the retinal image, and, deprived of its pristine clarity, the quality of what is projected onto the retina.

There is a clear distinction between light being absorbed or being scattered. Nevertheless, some experts see an inevitable progression from presbyopia via yellowing of the lens to cataract and visual defects of old age. Of course, in a sense they are statistically correct, in that the probability of those developments occurring increases in correlation with age; but there is nothing inevitable about the sequence, nor has any chain of causes been so far established.

The mechanisms of these modifications have often been overtly linked with the processes of presbyopia; in an attempt to clarify this issue, it may be useful to summarize the physics of image characterization.

2.6 Absorption and diffusion: tea versus egg-flip

The lens absorbs and − sometimes − scatters light. Absorption implies a reduction in transparency: the brightness of the retinal image is reduced. But the brightness of this image can be restored if more light is shed on the object being imaged.

Scatter, on the other hand, means a reduction in translucence: the brightness of the image may or may not be reduced, but its quality is undoubtedly impaired. No amount of increase in light intensity can compensate for this deficit.

An infusion of tea may look dark because tannin strongly absorbs visible radiations; if, however, the layer of tea is thin, a design on the bottom of the teacup is clearly discerned. A repetition of this experiment with egg-flip leads to a different result: with a layer of similar thickness as before, the design is at best diffuse. Though egg-flip also absorbs, it mainly scatters light because of the fragmented proteinous material suspended in it.

These simple analogies may help to illustrate why some authorities have problems in keeping apart lenticular manifestations of senescent processes. The normal lens yellows in a regular manner, as we shall note below. In some people a cataract may develop, which greatly reduces the amount of light reaching the retina. Since the lens then looks dark brown, the cataract is called brunescent. But objective tests show that such cataracts may not impair the image-forming quality of the lens. Although their ability to scatter light may be virtually nil, they effectively abolish the retinal stimulus. Hence the patient's disability.

There are other types of cataract in which the colour of the lens is more or less normal. But the specialist, using an ophthalmoscope or slit-lamp may be unable to see through it because the fragmentation of the normally translucent lenticular structure scatters light, and thereby randomizes the passage of the light rays. Brunescent cataract may therefore be likened to the tea model, while other cataracts behave physically more nearly like egg flip or even shattered glass.

As already noted, the normal lens also absorbs light, whence its physics belongs to the class of tea.

2.7 Lenticular absorption of light

2.7.1 *Basic notions*

Until relatively recently, the direct measurement of light absorption was not possible. The absorbed intensity expressed as a fraction of the intensity incident on the filter was derived indirectly from a measurement of the light-transmitting capacity of filters, including animal and human lenses. The relevant concepts are as follows.

> Let I_i be the intensity of some monochromatic radiation incident on a filter or a lens, and let the intensity which is transmitted be I_t. Then the ratio of the two, namely I_t/I_i is called the transmissivity T. It is convenient for a number of reasons, relating for example to the concentration of colouring materials causing absorption, to use the negative logarithm of this quantity, which is called the optical density D, i.e.
>
> $$D = -\log T \qquad (2.11)$$
>
> It is easily seen that densities are additive; thus, if one measures the intensity of light just as it is about to enter the eye, and the densities of the cornea, aqueous, lens, and vitreous are known, their sum determines by what fraction the original intensity has been reduced.

Equation (2.11) shows that, as the transmissivity grows and more radiation passes through a filter, so its density drops. But the part that is not transmitted (or reflected, usually a negligible fraction) must be absorbed. Expressed as a fraction of the incident intensity it is called the absorptivity $\mathbf{A}$, and needs to be distinguished from the absorbance, which is the part of the density caused by light absorption, but not scatter. It may be noted that, in simple cases, the absorbance is proportional to the concentration of the pigment, to the optical pathlength which it occupies, and to a characteristic constant, the extinction coefficient. This varies with the wavelength, and is determined by the molecular structure of the pigment.

Absorptivity and transmissivity are related as follows:

$$\mathbf{A} = 1 - \mathbf{T} \qquad (2.12)$$

A rise in transmissivity is therefore expressible by a reduction in both the absorptivity and the density of a filter. Note that absorptivities are not additive in the sense in which this is true of optical densities.

At least as regards the visible part of the spectrum, it is found in practice that the principal losses occur in the lens with the virtual exclusion of the capsule (Murata 1987). The other media play a role mainly in the ultraviolet. This used to be considered of comparatively small interest, owing to the fact that the lens offers a strong barrier to the entry of ultraviolet light into the eye, where such radiation may constitute a hazard to the retina. But the use of lens implants, which may be devoid of any material absorbing ultraviolet radiations, has greatly heightened interest in the spectral properties of the other ocular media and how they vary with age. Again, only the lens seems to play a significant role in this respect, and hence receives our attention.

Where technical details of measurement are important, they will be touched upon; in general, it will be assumed that the data discussed are based on eqn (2.11).

2.7.2 *Methods of measurement*

The type of measurement that has been used can be classed as follows:

(1) *in vitro*, when the lens is placed in some form of spectral densitometer, and a print-out is obtained for $\mathbf{D}$;
(2) *in vivo*, when the intensity of the light reflected from the posterior surface of the lens is compared with that reflected from the anterior surface, the ratio providing a measure of $\mathbf{D}$;
(3) *in vivo*, when one eye is aphakic, the other being normal, and spectral visual

thresholds are measured in each: the lensless eye needs less light for the visual thresholds to be reached than does the phakic eye, and the ratio of the two threshold intensities is a measure of **D**;

(4) *in vivo*, when the spectral sensitivity of the dark-adapted (rod-dominated) eye is compared with the absorbance spectrum of rhodopsin, the visual pigment contained in the rods: the ratio of the two can be shown to be equal to **T**;

(5) *in vivo*, when a measurement is made of the fluorescence of the lens exposed to a standard intensity of monochromatic ultraviolet radiation: this method has, so far, yielded only relative values, but is suitable for studies of variations with age, the influence of cataracts, etc.

1. The data obtained by Cooper and Robson (1969) on relatively few human lenses confirmed what had been known quantitatively since the first decade of this century, namely that the lens yellows progressively with advancing years (see Weale 1982*a*). They noted the existence of two large absorption bands, namely one below 300 nm, which is usually associated with proteins, and one at approximately 360 nm. It is this band that bars relatively near ultraviolet radiation from reaching the retina. Cooper and Robson's contribution to the subject lies in the fact that they linked the latter principal absorption band with an eluate they extracted from human lens material. Van Heyningen (1973) identified it as a glucoside of 3-hydroxy-L-kynurenine, which fluoresces under the influence of ultraviolet radiations. Her data show that the substance is concentrated largely in the lenticular nucleus (Weale 1989*b*). The compound provides an example of non-tryptophan fluorescence, a point worth stressing because the concentration of tryptophan itself also increases with age. Non-tryptophan fluorescence emitted by the nucleus is always stronger than any coming from the cortex (Harding 1991).

The absorptive dominance of the nucleus was confirmed experimentally by Mellerio (1987) and by Weale (1988). The former measured the lenticular absorbance in two ways. He first assessed it in intact lenses of various ages. Then he removed the cortex of the lens by manipulation, and measured the absorbance of the remaining nucleus. Figure 2.17 shows that, even at the wavelength of 400 nm, the cortex absorbs on a relatively small scale, independently of age. By contrast, the absorbance of the nucleus rises systematically with age. The results obtained by Mellerio in the region of the 360 nm absorption band reach some 9 density units during the eighth decade of life. It is possible that some of this loss is attributable to the difficult manipulative manoeuvre used in this study.

Weale (1988) confirmed the importance of the nucleus by measuring intact lenses, and subsequently pulping them: the reduction in absorbance of the second measurement was consistent with the idea that this action redistributed the pigment contained in the relatively confined nucleus throughout the whole mass.

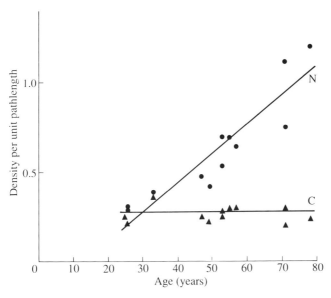

Fig. 2.17 Age-related values for the absorbance of human lenticular nuclei (N) and cortices (C) at a wavelength of 400 nm. After Mellerio (1987).

In a literature review Pokorny *et al.* (1987) suggested that the absorbance spectrum of the lens can be divided into two moieties: one of these is stable after the age of 20 years, whereas the other rises. They also concluded that lenses between the ages of 20 and 60 years follow a law different from those above 60 years, and offered two equations to describe this, the second of them revealing a rate of rise more than three times greater than the first.

This convoluted description can be greatly simplified, once it is realized that the variation of the absorbance **D** of the human lens with age follows an uncomplicated rule.

The absorbance (**D**) of the human lens rises more or less exponentially from birth, following the formula

$$\mathbf{D} = \mathbf{D_0}\, \exp(\beta A) \tag{2.13}$$

where **D$_0$** is the absorbance at birth, **A** is the age in years, and β is a constant coefficient which, like **D$_0$** varies with the wavelength. Although **D$_0$** was determined graphically, it agrees well with direct measurements obtained by Cooper and Robson (1969) on a neonatal lens; this lends confidence in the validity of eqn (2.13).

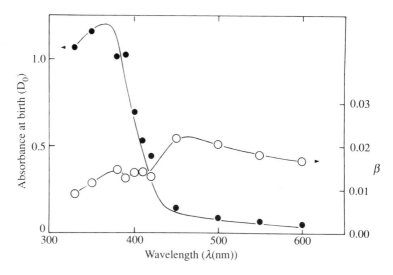

Fig. 2.18 Plots of the values of absorbance at birth (D_0) (filled circles), and coefficient β (empty circles) in eqn 2.13. After Weale (1988).

Figure 2.18 shows plots of both D_0 and β. What they mean is this: we are born with the pigment the spectral absorption characteristics of which are given by D_0; it is probable that this is the aforementioned 3-hydroxy-L-kynurenine. Apparently, immediately after birth there commences an accumulation of another unidentified pigment, with an absorption band at about 470 nm in the short wavelength part of the visible spectrum. However, the concentration of 3-hydroxy-L-kynurenine also appears to increase. The concentration of another powerfully absorbent compound, namely tryptophan (p. 90), also increases with age (Lerman and Borkman 1976). Dillon and Atherton (1990) have reported the formation of a transient pigment also absorbing in the blue part of the spectrum when the lens is exposed to a flash of UVA radiation of wavelength 355 nm. This is also present in daylight and is effectively absorbed by 3-hydroxy-L-kynurenine. Although the pigment produced by fluorescence is transient in the young human eye, a variety of changes in the nucleus may combine to make it progressively less unstable.

The advantage of the above algebraic formulation over others is that the broad run of the absorbance of human lenses in the age range of 0–85 years is easily calculated with acceptable accuracy, but with a proviso which needs a little consideration of a detail relating to measurement technique.

It will be remembered that it is the nucleus of the lens that is now believed to be the principal absorber of radiations in the visible and near ultraviolet parts of the spectrum. But the nucleus, though appreciably smaller than the lens, is also lens-shaped. Moreover, it occupies an approximately symmetrical position within the lens. This implies that more absorption occurs along the sagittal axis of the lens than along any other light path parallel to it.

The matter has recently been analysed when it was found that this excess absorption is not very significant for medium and long wavelengths of the visible spectrum (Weale 1991a). However, for wavelengths of 460 nm and below, the absorption of the lens depends greatly on how much of its cross-section perpendicular to the direction of the incident beam of light is used in image formation. More specifically, *in situ* the lenticular nucleus absorbs on average relatively much more radiation when the ocular pupil is small than when it is large (Fig. 2.18). The discrepancy introduced by pupil size increases greatly with age, and, as discussed in Chapter 4, may help to explain widely divergent results obtained when measurements were made by the method described under (3) above (p. 96).

The results in Fig. 2.19 indicate that, for pupil sizes up to about 4 mm in diameter, the optical density of the lens for short wavelengths may be considered constant, but for larger diameters it effectively drops. When it is recalled that the pupil size is approximately within the former limit in daylight or photopic vision, but that it is dilated in nocturnal or scotopic vision, then it follows that

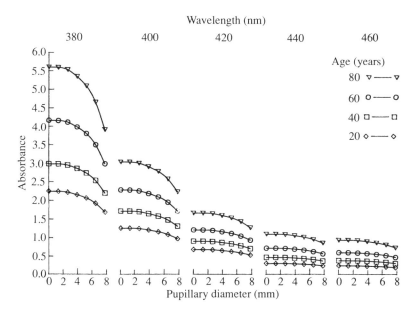

Fig. 2.19 The variation of the absorbance of the human crystalline lens with the lenticular aperture, wavelength, and age (inset). After Weale (1991a).

pupil size or aperture has to be considered in conjunction with lenticular density whenever the functional amount of light reaching the retina has to be determined (see p. 156).

The data in Fig. 2.19 were obtained by calculation from the measurements shown in Fig. 2.18, because the configuration of the beam with which they were obtained was known. While other authors have given us data on lens absorbance and its variation with age, their usefulness is smaller than it might be if the diameter of the measuring beam traversing the experimental lenses in their apparatus had been specified. It may be added that the aperture effect satisfactorily explains the differences found amongst the data obtained by Cooper and Robson (1969), Mellerio (1987), Ruddock (1965), Said and Weale (1959), and Weale (1988).

Equation 2.13 indicates that absorbance increases exponentially with advancing age. When this relation is plotted, the rise appears expectedly slow during the early part of life, but progressively accelerates as time goes on. Before the exponential formulation had been advanced it was not uncommon to see it stated that the absorbance remained approximately constant till the age of 40 years, after which it rose (see Hess 1911; Said and Weale 1959). This may be another example of senescence occurring in a process apparently governed by only two constants which have evolved in such a manner as to preserve an optimal situation after an individual's puberty, without, at the same time, allowing high biological costs to be incurred (see pp. 40, 61, and below).

2. The *in vivo* method for the measurement of lens absorbance depends on a comparison of the intensities of light reflected respectively from the anterior and posterior surfaces of the *in situ* lens (Fig. 2.20). In principle, the pupil of the eye under test is dilated, and illuminated with monochromatic light. As the light reflected from the posterior surface of the lens must have traversed the lens twice in order to emerge from the eye while the light reflected from the anterior surface does not traverse the lens at all, the ratio of the two intensities provides a measure of the light absorbed by the lens.

Said and Weale (1959) used photography to estimate the two intensities. At long wavelengths, their results have stood the test of time, as has the variation with age. However, in the short wavelength part of the spectrum their values are lower than those obtained by other methods (Werner 1982). When one considers the above discussion on the aperture effect, this may not be surprising. As discussed below, Said and Weale did not address effects due to the fluorescence of the lens, but it is likely that this would have been automatically allowed for in their attempt to correct for stray light.

3. It is noteworthy that the method whereby the lenticular transmissivity is determined from measurements of visual thresholds in a pair of eyes one of which is aphakic while the other is normal is, in fact, the oldest of all. It was first used by Hess (1911) who observed, but did not note, an exponential vari-

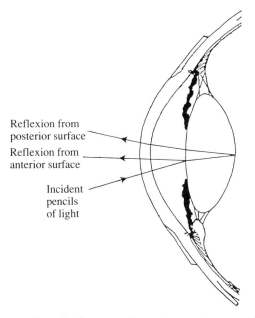

Reflexion from
posterior surface

Reflexion from
anterior surface

Incident
pencils
of light

Fig. 2.20 Lightpaths forming the 3rd and 4th Purkyně images.

ation with age (see eqn 2.13). Its rationale is beautiful in its simplicity, for all it assumes is that the eye, unencumbered by a lens, will be granted a retinal illumination which is larger by a factor equal to the reciprocal of the transmissivity of the lens in the other, phakic eye. The matter is somewhat complicated photometrically if no account is taken of the discrepancy between the sizes of the two retinal images, and if, as was true until about three decades ago, it was thought that the trauma then accompanying cataract operations might permanently change retinal performance, a situation which may not yet be a matter of the past (Owsley and Burton 1992). However, if these matters are kept under control, then the method has something to offer, especially today, when implant operations are carried out in ever younger eyes.

Rather surprisingly, the method has been used in a restricted fashion, and not in the highly instructive manner pioneered by Hess. Thus Werner and Hardenbergh (1983) and Zrenner and Lund (1984), interested in how well lens implants absorb the near ultraviolet, studied the effect of aphakia on the scotopic and photopic spectral sensitivity, and showed that, for wavelengths shorter than about 470 nm, there is a marked rise in the sensitivity of the aphakic eye in relation to the (phakic) standard. Concern was expressed because some implants fail to protect the retina from hazards due to ultraviolet radiation, a point to be considered in Chapter 3.

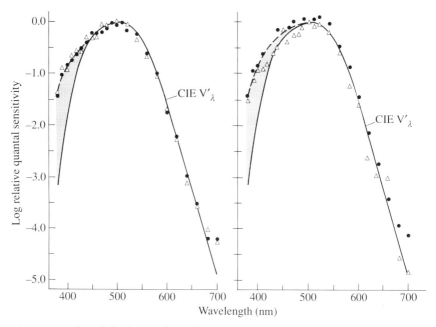

Fig. 2.21 Plot of the log of the relative scotopic sensitivity of an aphakic (●) and a pseudophakic (△) observer versus wavelength. Each of the observers, data for whom are shown left and right respectively, had an implant in one eye and was lensless in the other. The curve CIE V'_λ is the internationally standardized function for scotopic vision. After Werner and Hardenbergh (1983).

The two sensitivity curves in Fig. 2.21 were obtained from a 52-year-old and a 69-year-old observer respectively, the circles representing data for an aphakic eye, the triangles for one bearing an implant. At the shortest wavelength, the differences between the 'aphakic' and the standard sensitivities are somewhat smaller than predicted by Fig. 2.19, but this may be due to the pupil being about 4 mm in diameter. These particular implants therefore failed to mimic the filtering properties of normal lenses, because the V'-curve lies below the sensitivity data measured with eyes containing such implants.

4. This method of assessing preretinal absorbance is related to method (3). It is based on the spectral dependence of a threshold curve on the characteristics of the visual pigment giving rise to it. The best known example is the similarity between the aphakic scotopic sensitivity curve and the absorbance spectrum of rhodopsin, the visual pigment contained in the rods, i.e. the photoreceptors mediating scotopic vision. If, however, the sensitivity curve is distorted because of the presence of, say, a yellow lens, the precise agreement is impaired by an

extent which depends on the absorbance of the lens. The ratio of the sensitivity to the absorbance spectrum of rhodopsin hence provides a measure of lenticular transmissivity. Werner (1982) showed in this manner that the variation with age of the scotopic sensitivity as measured with visually evoked potentials is essentially due to the yellowing of the crystalline lens.

A modification of this principle was used more recently in a study which combined results from normal and cataractous eyes, indicating a continuity between the two populations (Sample *et al.* 1988). However, no diagnosis regarding the type of cataract was offered; the authors' conclusion that average values have to be treated with care in view of the large variances observed is well taken. Their own data exemplify the difficulty of this method which, in their hands, is based on the difference between two threshold measurements. Under good conditions the standard error of such a measurement can easily amount to at least 0.1 log units: other methods for the estimation of the *in situ* absorption of the crystalline lens are likely to be more precise.

5. Such, indeed, is the claim made for the last method to be discussed here. Based on the fluorescence of the lens, it is being used in several laboratories, but has so far provided a description of only a relative change with age of lenticular transmissivity; a spectral analysis is still awaited.

In essence the isolated or *in situ* lens is irradiated with near ultraviolet or other short-wavelength radiation giving rise to fluorescence F in the visible part of the spectrum. F is measured at two points, a value F_1 being obtained from light received from the anterior face of the lens, and F_2 from the posterior face. The ratio F_2/F_1 provides a measure of lenticular transmissivity, and, as discussed below, the value varies systematically with age.

The method is used to distinguish, for example, normal from diabetic lenses, but the theory underlying it has not so far been worked out in detail (see Hemenger *et al.* 1989). This is not altogether surprising because it offers formidable obstacles. One of these relates to the fact that the directions of the exciting and emitted fluorescent beams do not coincide (Fig. 2.22). It is true that, by the time the exciting beam has traversed the lens and reached the point 2, its intensity will be much reduced in relation to its value at point 1. It is also unlikely that the two resultant fluorescent beams traverse similar paths. Indeed, Liang (1990) has shown that the measured amount of fluorescence depends greatly on whether the emitted light is derived from the front surface of the lens or originates at a right angle. Moreover, unlike the exciting beam, emitted beams will not be focused, but stray in all directions. This implies that they simultaneously traverse paths of different absorption, and that the make-up of these paths is likely to differ from the beams emanating nominally from points 1 and 2 respectively.

Their intensities are a function of the two stimulating beams as well as the transmissivity of the lens for the type of fluorescence that is produced (and is rarely simple). These complications were better appreciated in a qualitative manner 60 years ago by Vogt (1931) than by some present-day authors, and they explain why it is hard to relate results obtained by this interesting technique to those obtained by methods (1)–(4) in an unexceptionable manner (see Zeimer and Noth 1984). A simple analysis, based on Fig. 2.22, may help to show both the advantages and the limitations of the method.

Let the intensity of the exciting beam be $I(\lambda_x)$, and strike the lens at the point x_1. A fraction q_1 will give rise to fluorescence. This passes through some lens tissue with a transmissivity $T(\lambda')$. However, more than one fluorogen may be present; this may affect the compositions of the beams emitted at 1 and 2 respectively. Therefore, though the intensity of the exciting beam at point x_2 is $I(\lambda).T(\lambda_1 x_2)$, and that of the emitted beam is by analogy with the first beam $q_2 I(\lambda.)T(\lambda_1 x_2)T(\lambda')_1$, it should not be assumed that the transmitted fractions of the emitted light have similar spectral compositions. This is why they have been distinguished by the numbers 1 and 2. The ratio R of the two emitted intensities is given by

$$R = T(\lambda_1 x_2) \{T(\lambda')/T(\lambda_1 x_1)\}\{q_2/q_1\} \qquad (2.14)$$

The ratio of the qs is unlikely to differ much from unity. To the extent to which the numbered T-values are in the visible part of the spectrum, their ratio may not vary greatly with age. However, $T(\lambda x)$ refers to ultraviolet or short-wavelength radiations, and Fig. 2.18 shows that it greatly varies with age. In other words, method (5) is highly sensitive to age-related changes in lenticular transmission. Note that, even if instrumental arrangements are such that the emitted radiation is measured in the visible part of the spectrum, say in the blue-green, the ratio R is dominated by the transmissivity for the exciting (usually ultraviolet) radiation.

Van Best et al. (1985) have applied the method in vivo (Fig. 2.23), and shown the type of decline to be expected on the basis of eqn 2.14. They obtained higher transmission values than those obtained by other in vivo methods (see Said and Weale 1959), which may be due to an inadequate separation between the filters designed to isolate the exciting from the emitting beams. A large numerical aperture may also contribute to the observation (see Fig. 2.19). However, it can be shown that the variation with age of their data agrees with that derived from Fig. 2.18.

The possible role of lenticular fluorescence modifying absorbance measurements especially in the living eye was examined in vitro (Weale 1985a), but no important effect was observed at short wavelengths.

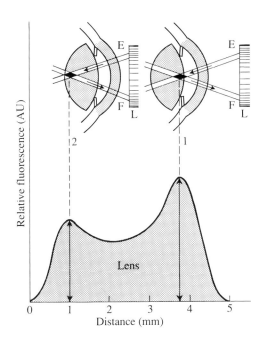

Fig. 2.22 Top: lightpaths involved in the stimulation (**E**) and measurement (**F**) of fluorescence; **L** is the exit-lens of the fluorometer. Bottom: trace of the relative fluorescence of a lens *in situ*, represented in arbitrary units. Note that **E** is generally a pencil of short-wavelength light, which will suffer progressive absorption as it penetrates into the lens. It will therefore give rise to less fluorescence (2) than is observed anteriorly by virtue of being feeble. The emitted rays emanating from posterior parts of the lens are also weaker than those nearer point 1. After Van Best *et al.* (1985).

2.7.3 *Absorption and environment*

Said and Weale (1959) applied method (2), described above, to both British and equally old Egyptian eyes, and found that the latter were slightly yellower than the former. Figure 2.24 shows a plot of the difference between the means of the absorbances for 25–42-year-old lenses for the two ethnic groups. The reason for the difference is unknown. However, one cannot rule out a possible explanation based on the putative presence of diabetes in some of the Egyptian subjects. Using a method based on (4) mentioned on p. 96, Lutze and Bresnick (1991) observed that diabetics in their twenties showed an absorbance for a wavelength of 420 nm higher than normal by 0.2–0.3 density units. This is much larger than the values shown in Fig. 2.23, but the diabetics studied recently had been

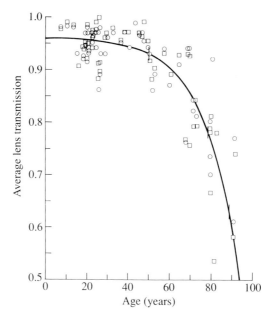

Fig. 2.23 Lenticular transmissivity for blue-green light as measured by method (5). ○, left eye; □, right eye. The curve represents the best fit. After Van Best et al. (1985).

diagnosed as such; Said and Weale had neither considered nor tested this possibility by carrying out the appropriate tests.

The possibility of such a confusing factor in the study of lenticular transmission will henceforth have to be borne in mind, since a number of experimental studies have suggested that exposure of both animal and human lenses to ultraviolet is liable to cause their yellowing (and to promote the formation of a cataract).

For example, Grover and Zigman (1972) irradiated excised human lenses immersed in 0.1 per cent solutions of tryptophan with radiations ranging from 340–380 nm – which form a small but not negligible part of the daylight spectrum – and observed considerable yellowing. The exposure was continued for 48 hours, the intensity being of the order of that of sunlight. If the phenomenon they observed were very relevant to the human condition, we would be expected to suffer from severe brunescent cataracts after a few weeks of summer.

A more direct epidemiological test involved 197 normal-sighted observers in the age range of 18–25 years (Girgus *et al.* 1977). All had grown up in British Columbia, so they should all have experienced similar environmental influences. All of them 'provided extensive self-report data about their habitual use

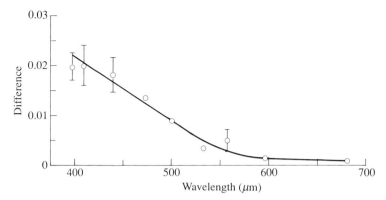

Fig. 2.24 Difference between the *in vivo* optical densities of British and Egyptian lenses of equal ages plotted against wavelength. After Said and Weale (1959).

of both eyeglasses and sunglasses', information which was elicited on the basis of questionnaires. This information formed the independent variable of the test.

The notionally dependent variable was the result of a colour matching procedure dependent on so-called metameric matches. Briefly, white light may be matched visually with a suitable mixture of monochromatic blue-green and reddish purple light, and, alternatively, by one of monochromatic violet and monochromatic yellowish-green lights. The four amounts of light are recorded. The two pairs of matching lights constitute a metameric pair. If the procedure is repeated while one looks through a colour filter at least one of the matches will be disturbed. It is possible to predict the magnitude and direction of the disturbance in terms of the transmissivity of the filter. Girgus *et al.* held that the differential light intensities passing through eyeglasses and sunglasses, used for durations which varied by a factor of approximately 5:1, should have allowed an imprint to be made on the respective crystalline lenses. The differently yellowed lenses, if any, should manifest in terms of systematic disturbances of the metameric matches. None was observed. The authors believed, therefore, to have disproved the photogenic aetiology of lenticular yellowing.

Zigman (1978) rebutted this conclusion on the ground that the sample population was too young to have accumulated sufficient pigment for it to give rise to a significant increase under Girgus *et al.*'s conditions. He is supported in this by the observation that the age-related absorbance rises exponentially (eqn 2.13), and this point will be discussed in Chapter 5. It also has to be said that the use of unverifiable questionnaires has not a great deal to recommend it, nor have the authors tried to relate their results to the very small differences reported by Said and Weale (1959) which have an obvious bearing on their highly important study.

The conundrum is unresolved. Laboratory studies show unambiguous photo-biological effects in isolated human lenses (see Megaw 1984; Dillon 1984; Rao *et al.* 1987), but their relevance to *in vivo* yellowing of the human lens still needs to be established. It may be that excised material is deprived of repair processes available *in situ*; again, the temporal pattern of illumination may play a role; or it may be a subtle effect of ocular temperature, etc. The solution to the problem is important in view of the fact that short-wavelength radiation is also held by some authors to predipose a lens to the development of a cataract. It is, however, unlikely that the mechanism of cataractogenesis, even in sunny countries, is inevitably linked to lenticular yellowing, because, unlike the pathological mani-festation, physiological yellowing is virtually universal. It is also relevant to note that exposure to the sun is linked statistically with cortical and mixed cataracts, and not specifically with brunescent ones (The Italian-American Cataract Study Group 1991).

2.8 Lenticular fluorescence

Fluorescence, already mentioned in connection with the measurement of lenti-cular absorption of light, is not a phenomenon that is just being put to some use for the assessment of the transmissivity of the lens *in vivo*. Whenever a patient's eyes are examined with a slit-lamp, an intense beam of light can be concentrated on the anterior segment of the eye including the lens. It is then noticeable, particularly in older eyes, that there is a greenish tinge in the lens. This is due to the short-wavelength component of the white illuminating light causing the lens to fluoresce.

In such a situation a patient would, if asked, complain of glare, and prove unable to distinguish the discomfort or disability due to this from the subjective results of fluorescence. However, the distinction is simple in principle: glare due to scattered light has a spectral composition either not very different from that of the original light or else it is describable by Rayleigh's four-power law, or a formulation akin to it. In contrast, the spectral distribution of fluorescent light is generally well separated from that of the exciting radiation. It also has to be remembered that everyday life differs from laboratory conditions. In particular, the simplifying assumption that there is only one fluorogen (see Hemenger *et al.* 1989) is almost certainly untrue (Bessems *et al.* 1987), and the continuous spectra of daylight, and also of artificial illuminants, make it likely that the emitted light will cover a broad spectral band.

One therefore faces the question of whether fluorescent light is detectable in levels of illumination more nearly physiological than can be said of a slit-lamp beam. The answer appears to be a circumscribed yes. First, the background against which the fluorescence would be seen has to be considered (Weale 1991*b*), and it would appear that the radiation excited by everyday fluorescent tubes can be visible. The reason is because, secondly, normal daylight illumination suffices for the production of above-threshold quantities of fluorescence; radiation in the band between 360–420 nm can cause lenticular fluorescence, and there is enough present in the daylight spectrum. Its effect may become noticed by careful observers after the age of about 40 years (Weale 1985*a*). It should be noted that this result was obtained for lenses of various ages with both the incident and the fluorescent beams lying along, not at some angle to, their axes. Thus, the situation mimicked what happens from the point of vision and its senescence. Figure 2.25*a* shows that there is a systematic increase of axial fluorescence with age; an approximate rule suggests that at the age of 80 years the fluorescence is twice as great as at half that age. This is confirmed in the results shown in Fig. 2.25*b*, which were obtained *in vivo*, but at an inclination to the visual axis and in a direction roughly opposite to that of the incident, i.e. stimulating, beam (Bleeker *et al.* 1986). Note that both studies show a positive intercept on the abscissa which is, however, statistically non-significant.

Lerman (1988) extended the study of lenticular non-tryptophan fluorescence to two distinct populations. He compared the fluorescence emitted by normal lenses of persons domiciled in Atlanta with others at home in Oregon. Both showed approximately parallel increases with age; the slightly lower values observed for Oregon may be due to a lower exposure to ultraviolet radiations, but Lerman mentioned that several controls other than geographical location are needed to clinch the argument relating to this hypothetical influence of the environment.

Lenticular fluorescence is much enhanced in some types of cataract. For example, Lerman and Borkman (1976) found that, in nuclear cataracts, it can be twice as intense as in equally old normal lenses. The phenomenon may help to account for a symptom said to occur soon after an operation for cataract, namely erythropsia or red vision. It persists for about a week and, though no reliable measurement has been reported on the matter, the sensation of red seems to be a dominant feature. It is plausible that the retina becomes adapted to green fluorescence when the cataract is still there to produce it. Once the lens is removed, retinal stimulation consists of daylight minus green so that the complementary red predominates until the system is re-adapted.

Saraux *et al.* (1984) report a case of transient snow erythropsia, which is long post-operative, and provoked by a protracted exposure of the eyes to intense light in snow-covered mountains. Although the lenticular fluorogens are clearly ruled out as causes, it is possible that a similar mechanism, namely retinal fluorescence (see Chapter 3) may help to explain the sensation.

2.9 Scattering of light

The angular problems associated with the measurement of fluorescence reappear in that of scattering of light. A remarkably ingenious study by Allen and Vos (1967) had shown a long time ago that the slit-lamp provides a useful instrument

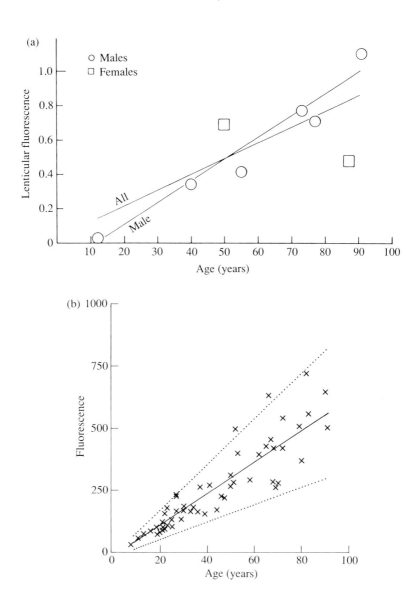

Fig. 2.25 Lenticular fluorescence as a function of age. *a* Excised lenses, fluorescence measured in arbitrary units along the visual axis separately for males and females. After Weale (1985a). *b In vivo* (method (5)) with fluorescence measured in a forward direction and expressed in terms of equivalents of fluorescein concentration. Each point represents the mean for both lenses. After Bleeker *et al.* (1986).

in this field, because it enables one not only to isolate the effects of the cornea from those of the lens but also to identify the several contributions of various lenticular portions. Notwithstanding a considerable variability, the cornea appears remarkably constant throughout life, and shows a rise in scatter only during the ninth decade.

This is in sharp contrast to the lens. Here scatter rises in early life slowly in the anterior part of the cortex and the nucleus, but the rate increases after the age of about 50 years (see Ben-Sira *et al.* 1980). In the posterior part of the cortex, the early initial rise is followed by a plateau. Additional support for the view that it is the lens matrix and not the lens surface that is principally involved in scatter was obtained by Navarro *et al.* (1986) who examined the third Purkyně image with coherent light. It exhibits appreciable roughness (not to be confused with shagreen visible through a slit-lamp microscope); this shows no signficant variation with age during the first six decades of life, and corresponds to only a small percentage of intra-lenticular scatter. The posterior surface of the lens is smooth by comparison.

Allen and Vos also studied a number of visual faculties (see Chapter 4), and reached the conclusion that the hypothesis, that scatter in the anterior eye media as measured by the back scatter from a slit lamp beam might be a major component in the deterioration of visual performance with age, appears to be untenable.

When the efforts that have gone into similar measurements by means of slit-lamp photography at 45° to the visual axis are considered (see Sigelman *et al.* 1974) it is doubly regrettable that Allen and Vos' work has not received wider recognition. This is true also because clinical experience teaches that the links between the slit-lamp appearance of a patient's eye and its performance may be tenuous in the extreme. This was explained in a study of excised human lenses by Bettelheim and Ali (1985) who measured the fraction of polarized light incident along the axis on lenses of various ages. They found that, in general, forward scatter is much stronger than back scatter, that the variation with age varies with the wavelength,, and that the so-called dissymmetry ratio, i.e. the fraction of light scattered at 45° to the axis to that scattered at 135° increases with the size of the scattering loci. As it increases with age, the authors conclude that ageing is accompanied by molecular aggregation.

This work was extended to the living eye when a slit-lamp was used in conjunction with polarized light (Weale 1986c). It was found that a considerable fraction of the apparently scattered light can be extinguished with crossed polarizers. This fraction systematically decreases with age, as would be expected on the basis of the above work; consequently the fraction that cannot be extinguished rises, as shown in Fig. 2.26. All the apparently scattered light is inextinguishable and therefore probably genuinely random once the ordinate value has reached unity. The reason for this is that, at near normal incidence, crossed polarizers would be expected to fail to extinguish random scatter, and

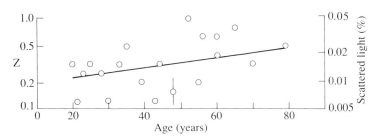

Fig. 2.26 Variation with age of the Log of the ratio of white light scattered by a lens, illuminated by a slit-lamp beam, irremovable by polarization, to the light incident on the eye (z). The right-hand scale gives the percentage of scattered light. After Weale (1986c).

the fact that considerable extinction can be achieved even with *in vivo* eyes over the age of 60 years suggests that some of the so-called stray-light visualized by the slit-lamp is spurious. It may be noted that the fraction of the incident light scattered represents only a small percentage. This agrees with Wooten and Geri's estmate (1987) of 1 per cent obtained by sensory means, and suggests as a result of its lack of change with wavelength that structures substantially larger than the wavelengths of light must be responsible.

The age-related variation of stray light shown in Fig. 2.26 has also been measured with monochromatic light of 470 nm, but for fewer eyes (Weale 1986c). Extrapolating the regression describing it to the age at which polarization probably fails to extinguish any of the apparently scattered light yields a value of 113 years. This value is discussed further on p. 238.

Recent photographic records have also shown that the crystalline lens may apparently diffuse light without being deprived of its ability to form extremely sharp images. Figure 2.27 shows the reflexion of a slit-lamp test pattern from the posterior surface of the lens of a patient whose visual acuity was 1.0. The gap between each pair of points doubles progressively, the smallest gap corresponding to optimal retinal resolving power. The rationale of the method is that if the eye specialist can resolve the pattern in the patient's 4th Purkyně image (which is formed by reflection at the posterior surface of the lens), then the image-forming capacity of the anterior segment must be unimpaired. There is evidently appreciable stray light in the 52-year old lens, but the purely optical resolution remains highly satisfactory even though the patient may understandably complain of glare in some circumstances. The technique has been applied to cataractous eyes, enabling one to quantify the handicap afflicting the patient. The correlation between the objective assessment and the patient's visual acuity stresses the value of the idea also in the clinical context.

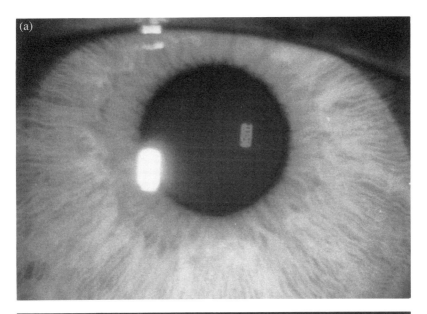

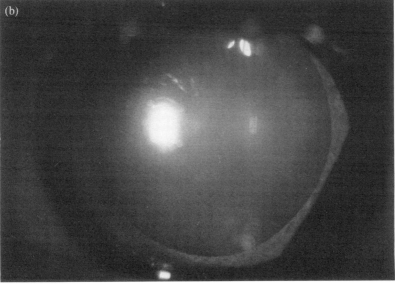

Fig. 2.27 Slit-lamp photographs of human crystalline lenses. Note the faint 4th Purkyně image. It shows the reflexion of a target consisting of six pairs of points, the gaps between them doubling at each step. The closest separation corresponds to an optical quality which would give the patient a resolving power of 2.0. *a* Image in a 26-year old eye which shows hardly any scatter. *b* Image for 52-year old eye: light is scattered by the lens both on the inward and the outward paths, but the six pairs of dots are still resolvable. The patient's visual acuity in this eye was 1.0.

2.10 Cataract

It was noted previously that several authors have discovered a correlation between cataract and life expectancy (p. 10). Its nature is unexplained, and passed off with the comment that the incidence of cataract may be a manifestation of an impaired state of health; in other words, it is not the cataract itself that reduces life expectancy, but that this is the result of some other factor(s), in turn causing the appearance of lenticular opacities.

When these are discovered by the specialist, the patient is usually told that virtually all lenses above the age of 60 years exhibit some opacity. Since not even all the specialists put together are likely to have remotely seen all lenses, a certain amount of extrapolation is taking place which is intended to reassure the patient but impedes an identification of the cause(s) of cataract. Some dozen types of cataract have been classified, and the one with an unknown aetiology is called senile cataract; this is, indeed, how it is defined. It will, no doubt, eventually come to be known as age-related. The progression of the various types of opacity is unpredictable, but may take between 4 and 7 years from a first diagnosis to the state when surgical intervention may be necessary.

Strictly speaking, the clinical expression 'cataract' should be used only when a clinical condition is found to exist. There are those who maintain, on what they see as ethical grounds, that to be classed as a cataract an opacity seen by the specialist should be accompanied by some such symptom as glare, haze, or a reduced visual capacity.

There are several types of age-related cataract. Some, the coronal, appear as a cloudy ring round the edge of the lens. This is never noticed by the individual, and seen by the specialist only if the pupil has been dilated (Fisher 1970). Only if it extends toward the optical centre of the lens is it likely to create symptoms.

Another type, the nuclear cataract, gives rise to haze, but need not at first unduly impair the quality of the retinal image (Kluxen 1985). In some cases, instead of turning cloudy, the nucleus turns a deep yellow or even brown (see p. 88). In this case the handicap, if any, is due primarily not to an impairment of the quality of the retinal image but to its faintness. Some patients can be helped by the provision of intense task-orientated illumination. This increases the brightness of the retinal image without necessarily causing any significant glare.

The posterior subcapsular cataract is optically the least tolerable condition. It is due in all probability to an impairment of the more nearly peripheral fibres of which the lens is made up. They derive from the lenticular epithelium and grow from the equatorial region of the lens. If this is subject to a noxious agent, the fibres suffer damage which is usually irreversible. Hart *et al.* (1979) reported that, during the formation of lenticular fibres, nuclear DNA is liable to accumulate free 3'-OH ends, which are a sign of single-strand breaks, much as have been observed in senescent photoreceptors.

The desire to combat the condition, which is blinding when no surgical intervention can be made available, has led to many studies in search of risk factors, including overtly non-pathological ones (see Hiller *et al.* 1983; Leske and Sperduto 1983). The principal one is age. Another is geography (Miranda 1980), but this may merely be a cover for more specific environmental factors, such as diet (Chatterjee *et al.* 1982) and hygiene (Harding and Rixon 1980). In general, there are more cases in warm climates than in temperate ones, and their incidence occurs earlier in life. This has led to the suggestion that temperature or perhaps long-wavelength ultraviolet radiation is a noxious agent (see Brilliant *et al.* 1983). Bochow *et al.* (1989) have associated it specifically with posterior subcapsular cataract. Myopia has also been impugned (Perkins 1984; Weale 1980), and Kluxen has found an association with nuclear cataract. The latter has been associated typically with smoking (Flaye *et al.* 1989; West *et al.* 1989).

Even approximate statistics relating to cataract operations have to be treated with caution, but Fig. 2.28 gives an indication of general trends. Data points for men and women are kept separate (the later being suffixed), and refer to four different ethnic groups. The data represent the incidence of first cataract operations, i.e. the ratio of patients in a given age group being operated on for a first time divided by the number of similarly aged people in the population from whom the patients were drawn.

Such figures lend themselves to a presentation as Gompertz plots (see Chapter 5), shown in Fig. 2.28. Constants of the regressions are shown in Table 2.1. They are the slope **g**, the intercept **c**, and **a(m)**, the age at which the natural logarithm of the function attains the value of 0 on extrapolation, i.e. when nearly the whole population under consideration is affected. The justification for extrapolating over 20–30 years is arguable; however, in a logarithmic plot, considerable changes in high values produce small ones in their logarithms and this is unlikely to vitiate the subsequent comments on values of **a(m)** on p. 238.

Statictical tests show that there is no significant difference between the several slopes, which tells us that the chance of having a cataract operation (and thereby escaping the chance of becoming blind in one eye) doubles every six years or so probably all over the world. The vertical displacement of the data may be a reflexion of a frequently made remark, namely that there is a geographical factor in the incidence of cataracts (see Miranda 1980). However, in connection with the Pima Indians who live in Arizona and were studied by Schwab *et al.* (1985) (Table 2.1, ref. 1) it is relevant to note that the operations included a noticeable proportion of traumatic cataracts, i.e. not just age-related ones. This would raise

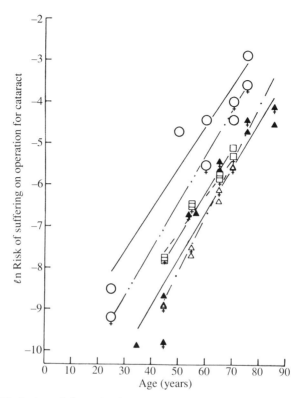

Fig. 2.28 Variation of the risk of suffering an operation for cataract with age. Compare with Table 2.1. Symbols for women are shown with a +. Slopes for line 3(0.132, 0.137) in Table 2.1 have been omitted to minimize confusion. The circles represent data due to Schwab *et al.* (1985) (ref. 1) for Tahiti Indians, the filled triangles refer to a population in and near Oxford studied by Caird *et al.* (1973) (ref. 2), the empty triangles to Israeli patients of European descent while the squares refer to those of Asian origin (Halevy and Landau (1962) (refs. 3,4)).

the points in comparison with the other studies which do not seem to have had to face this problem.

It seems legitimate to average the eight values for **a(m)**, there being no difference between those calculated for men and women respectively. The mean value is 113.17 ± 7.06 years. For the moment it will suffice to say that, by that age, arrived at by extrapolation, virtually everyone will have at least one eye that will have an operable cataract. Since the chance of having an operation appears to double approximately every six years, by the time one has reached the age of 120 years both eyes would be blind in the absence of an operation.

Table 2.1 Gompertz constants of epidemiological studies on cataract

Reference	Slope (**g**)		Intercept (– **c**)		Age constant (**a(m)**)	
	M	F	M	F	M	F
1	0.101	0.114	10.641	12.106	105.35	106.47
2	0.115	0.137	13.539	14.953	117.63	109.31
3	0.132	0.137	14.882	15.054	112.74	110.29
4	0.108	0.093	12.642	11.785	116.73	126.85

A potential biological significance of this figure will become apparent in Chapter 5.

2.11 Resumé

The idea explored in Chapter 1, namely that human performance is likely to be optimal during the third and fourth decades of life, appears to be true.

Age-related changes in the shape of the crystalline lens and the consequential variation of the static refraction of the eye have been found to conspire in the optimization of the image-forming function of the eye during that period. In addition, it was noted that the large juvenile amplitude of accommodation can be understood in terms of the absolute necessity for the eye to be able to form during that period high-contrast images of distant objects as well as of those at 'reading' distance. The fact that the decline of this faculty appears to conform to basic bio-economic principles provides support for those hypotheses of senescence that are rooted in evolutionary pressures rather than in those based on ideas of forward planning.

The next step is to try to discover whether the quality of the nervous pathways also peaks at some time during life. If the answer is in the affirmative, it is also important to find out whether such a peak is in phase with the above period of optimization, and hence when the biological need seems to demand it.

3. Retinal senescence

3.1 Introduction

The retina is an outcrop of the brain, and its senescence might be expected to share features with that of its cerebral parent. Unlike the brain, the eye is exposed to environmental stimuli or hazards, for example, short-wavelength electromagnetic radiations and heat. This difference between the eye and the brain creates difficulties not only for the understanding of retinal senescence, but also makes comparisons with other parts of the body hard to sustain. The reason is that exposure to radiation may produce changes that may be misinterpreted as signs of senescence, not because there is necessarily a change in function, morphology or appearance, but because the resulting signs are cumulative. A film continuously blackens during exposure to light, but no one would suggest that it is ageing; however, were it to be found to blacken when not exposed to light, the ageing metaphor might well be applied. The point is that the mere summation of effects due to the environment needs to be distinguished from progressive changes associable with ageing.

The retina therefore offers a fruitful field of study from the point of view of gerontology in general. But, precisely because it may be subject to more than one cause leading to functional impairment, a brief outline of the relevant features of cerebral senescence may be apposite.

Like those of the brain, the neural cells of the retina are formed very early in life, and, broadly speaking, are not replaced once lost. The number of neurons is one of the determinants of the capacity of the nervous system to process information, and their size may well relate to their metabolic potential (Flood and Coleman 1988). The question of cell death is consequently of paramount importance for an understanding of visual senescence. Also, like the brain, the retina depends for its survival on an intact supply of oxygen (although the period of noxious ischaemia may exceed that needed to produce irreversible damage to the brain); the retina is endowed with two rich vascular systems, namely the retinal and choroidal circulations.

The ambivalent role which this may play is illustrated by reference to senile miosis (p. 48). This is thought to occur because the pupillary dilator atrophies at a considerably greater rate than its antagonist sphincter, and the reason for the differential rate may be due to a more rapid impairment of the vascular supply to the dilator. There are thus secondary, tertiary, etc., causes of senescence, and the above-mentioned environmental difference between retina and brain may not be the only complication in this field. Schulz and Hunziker (1980) note, in an account of a histological study of age-related changes in the human frontal cortex, that vascular modifications in the age-group of 65–74 years precede the neuronal changes which they observed. This is not surprising, as the vascular system of the brain makes an early start on the path of devolution (see p. 123; Leenders *et al*. 1990).

Comparisons with other species are not always helpful: Flood and Coleman emphasize the age-related losses of neurons seen in human brains are not necessarily reflected in those of animals. They do not speculate on the possibility that there may be differential responses to environmental stimuli (p. 11), including effects of diet. They stress areas of disagreement in studies of similar species and cerebral regions, and it is not altogether surprising that modern histological techniques, image identifying methods, and the introduction of computerized morphometry should sometimes fail to corroborate data compiled by simpler methods (Terry *et al*. 1987).

It is also becoming progressively clearer that it is wrong to base speculations regarding ageing processes in one part of the brain − or in the retina (Weale 1975) − on those recorded for others, even within the same species. In a broad sense, there is also evidence to suggest that rectilinear regressions should be treated with more caution in some instances than is, in fact, the case. They may be valid only for relatively restricted parts of the life span, such as the post-reproductive phase. It was also previously noted (p. 42) that the individual does not grow at a constant rate (Thatcher *et al*. 1987), any more than is true of individual organs like the crystalline lens (see Weale 1982*a*). The trapezoidal shape of Fig. 1.11 occurs more than once in studies of the brain, the important feature of myelination in Gennari's line (Lintl and Braak 1983) providing a noteworthy example (Fig. 3.1).

The assumption of uniform ageing, as of postnatal cerebral development, is similarly a gross simplification. More specifically, assessments were made of electro-encephalographic coherence and phase in children whose ages ranged from 2 months to early adulthood (Thatcher *et al*. 1987). While systematic, significant differences were observed between the two hemispheres, it was not possible to assert that one matured faster than the other, because various regions − identified by means of 19 electrodes attached over the head − appeared to be developing at different rates within any one hemisphere (Fig. 1.10).

However, even on a cognitive level, studies on two groups of observers, 21–26 years and 60–73 years of age, respectively, suggest that the two cerebral hemispheres possess different vulnerabilities (Lapidot 1987), which is not surprising in view of the above variation in their rates of development. Ocular tracking was monitored during the elicitation of verbal and visual associations in turn: pursuit movements to the left or right will engage predominantly the left or right hemispheres. If mental overload occurs as a result of simultaneous visual and mental, or visual and aural, demands, the eyes will stop in their

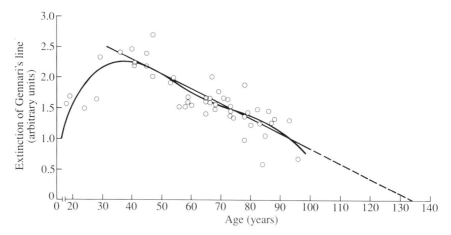

Fig. 3.1   The age-related variation of the myelination of Gennari's line. The curve is a polynomial fitted to all the experimental points. The regression was calculated without the lowest four ages being taken into account. After Lintl and Braak (1983). For extrapolation see Chapter 5.

tracks. Cases of ocular tracking arrest were counted for both parameters and age groups. The older group experienced relatively greater difficulties in their visuo-spatial performance, but this does not necessarily impugn the right hemisphere as a whole.

Asymmetric changes have also been recorded by computerized tomography (Sandor *et al.* 1990), which has the advantage of being non-invasive and, unlike the previous technique, wholly objective. It revealed two regions of marked lateral differences: the intraparietal sulcus showed more regression on the right side of the brain, whereas the central and postcentral sulci were more affected on the left. Nothing of significance was recorded for the visual area 17 (but see below); this may have been due to methodological causes. The authors noted that the main changes were recorded in the central regions of the scans, subtle inaccuracies in the alignment of the head making changes in the frontal and occipital lobes hard to detect.

The variance of results may be inadvertently increased if the possibility that the rate of ageing may differ in the two sexes is overlooked. For example, Friedman *et al.* (1985) recorded evoked potentials in young adolescents engaged in continuous performance tasks, and found that the sex-task interaction on the wave-form was greater than the more modest age-task value. This may have been due to endogenous differences, but superficial ones, such as the size of the head, or perceptual ones involving differences in task strategies, cannot be ruled out.

Yamaura *et al.* (1980), however, used the objective technique of computer tomography on Japanese men and women in the age range of 20–79 years. They called the ratio between brain volume and cranial cavity the cranio-cerebral index (CCI), and defined the brain volume index (BVI) as (100/92) × CCI, because the mean value of the CCI was 92 in the maximal range during the third and fourth decades of life. Both indices showed a decrease after the age of 40 years (Fig. 3.2), that for men being delayed by some 10 years in relation to that for women. There is a parallel with the age-related variation of brain mass (Ito *et al.* 1981), which also peaks during the third and fourth decades (Fig. 3.3). The existence of sex differences was confirmed in an elaboration of that study, when the putative volume of the cerebro-spinal fluid and of the cranial cavity above the level of the cerebellar tentorium were determined. Especially after the age of about 40 years, the rate of change in the indices was greater for women than for men (Takeda and Matsuzawa 1984).

Both groups of authors interpret their data in terms of cerebral atrophy; the idea that dehydration or shrinkage of the tissues may be taking place is not considered. Only when one of the principal investigators, Hatazawa, came to collaborate with teams working in British centres did he seem to appreciate that this is a possible interpretation of the numerous results obtained in his laboratory (see below). Indeed, Leenders *et al.* (1990) specifically state that functional images obtained with positron emission tomography can, but failed to, reveal moderate to gross ventricular enlargement, and hence implicit shrinkage, in older brains.

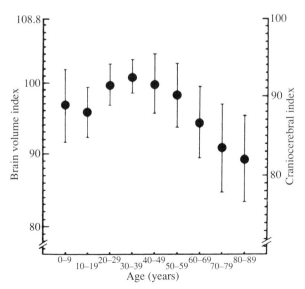

Fig. 3.2 Age-related variations of the mean craniocerebral and brain volume indices. After Yamaura *et al.* (1980).

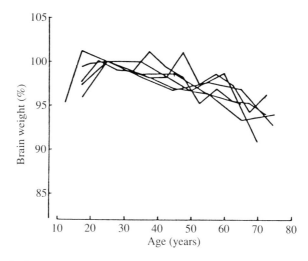

Fig. 3.3   The brain mass at different ages, as a percentage of that of a 20–25 year old. The various lines represent the results of different studies. For details see Ito *et al.* (1981).

   That tissue shrinkage is an alternative interpretation is clear from cell counts done from a midfrontal region (Brodmann areas 9, 10 or 46), a superior temporal part (area 38), and an inferior parietal region (area 39 or 40). Terry *et al.* (1987) distinguished between large ($> 90\ \mu m^2$) neurons and those smaller than this criterion. The number of large neurons was found to correlate well with brain mass, and decreased approximately linearly with age. The smaller neurons, however, became more numerous with advancing years. So far there does not seem to be any reason to believe that neurons are generated in any numbers after infancy, and it is significant that Terry *et al.* found that the increase of the number in small neurons approximately matches the decrease in large ones. It would seem that some kind of pyknosis is occurring, with the larger neurons shrinking in size but not in number. No significant cell loss appears to be taking place in the above cerebral areas, at least during the second half of the life span.

3.1.1 Repair processes during cerebral senescence

These observations lend support to those who believe that a number of repair processes exist in the ageing brain. A variety of mechanisms have been envisaged. For example, Bugiani *et al.* (1978), who did not employ the latest counting method, also studied population densities of large and small cells. The object of their study was the putamen, and the rates of loss were similar in the two cell populations. The authors view this fall-out as a way of balancing extrapyramidal activity, and speculate that, but for its occurrence, a reduced cell population in the substantia nigra coupled with a reduced input from the midbrain to the neostriate region would lead to general parkinsonian symptoms in old persons.

In a study of the brain of the ageing rat, Cotman and Scheff (1979) and Calderini *et al.* (1987) found support for the existence of neurotrophic activity that had earlier been associated with injury. It forms a bilateral response to unilateral cerebral injury, and is much delayed in older animals. According to Cotman and Scheff, this is a pure repair mechanism which appears to ensure that the number of synapses remains approximately constant. Using mice, Coleman and Flood (1986) demonstrated enhanced dendritic growth in old animals following neuronal loss, and, conversely, its absence, also in old animals, when no such loss had occurred. They extend their analysis to a consideration of granule cells in the human dentate gyrus, and calculate that newly formed dendritic material between the ages of 52 and 73 years is four times as great as the estimated loss of such material resulting from neuronal losses. Buell and Coleman (1979) have postulated the existence of two types of neuron, one wherein the dendritic arborizations shrink with advancing years, and another in which they expand. The latter appear to be absent in Alzheimer's disease.

In the light of the views expressed toward the end of Chapter 1 it would be erroneous to look on such processes as results of evolutionary pressures tending to preserve the function of the senescent brain. It may be more appropriate to regard them as inherent in the topomorphology of the tissue, part of its intact nature. The manifest cause of these apparently reparatory events is unknown. There is little doubt, however, that both dendritic growth and its restraint are fundamental to the maintenance of a functioning neuronal network. Without growth there would be no interneuronal communication. Without its restraint, there would result tangles limited not by functional requirements but by volumetric factors.

In the case of angiogenesis, the growth of capillaries in the neighbourhood of major vessels appears to be stopped by the local oxygen tension. It may be speculated that there is a critical concentration, $c(g)$, of nerve growth factor (NGF), below which growth is favoured, whereas inhibition of growth occurs above it. In this manner Nature's abhorrence of a dendritic vacuum would lose its mystery. The two populations postulated by Buell and Coleman may reflect different values of $c(g)$.

Some such hypothesis would deprive so-called compensatory processes in dendritic growth of their status specifically associated with senescence. The growth occurs for reasons of homoeostasis, and not primarily to promote repair.

3.2 Losses in the brain

Terry *et al.* (1987) appreciate that their results are at odds with those of earlier authors, but are at pains to emphasize that this may be due to a great increase in instrumental and methodological sophistication. Although they themselves have not investigated the region of main interest in this inquiry, namely the striate area (17), Haug *et al.* (1984) have done so, and likewise failed to find losses of the magnitude reported earlier in this century. This is in marked contrast to the results of a study in which fixed tissue from area 17 was disrupted by means of sonication (Devaney and Johnson 1980). Since formalin hardens the perikaryon, ultrasound breaks off dendritic processes, leaving the cell body intact and available for counting following a known amount of dilution. Differential fragmentation of cells was controlled, and the authors believe that the loss of cells amounting to some 30 per cent between the ages of 20 and 87 years (Fig. 3.4) from the macular projection onto the striate area may be a low estimate. Haug *et al.* have criticized this work on the grounds that an unrealistic automatic criterion was set for the distinction between glia and neurons. Their own area of interest was centred on the calcarine fissure, which contains projections from the retinal periphery rather than the central area, and this may also be a reason for the difference between the two sets of results (see p. 121).

The extensive data obtained by Haug *et al.* on area 17 for an age range stretching from 18 to 111 years were carefully controlled for age-related shrinkage. Although the area of neurons decreased slightly but significantly with age, neuron density rose, and no theoretical explanation is advanced for this result. The authors stress that each cortical area has its own history of ageing.

Ultimately, the capacity for dying is something with which neuronal cells are created. Embryonic neuronal organization is accompanied by well-orchestrated losses even during the development of the eye-cup (Silver 1978; see p. 20), and Leuba and Garey (1987) have reported this also for the human striate area.

Their study covered an age range from prematurity to 93 years. Blocks from the centre of the upper bank of the right calcarine sulcus were isolated and fixed. The majority of these were reduced for examination with the electron microscope, the rest being mounted in paraffin, which served for comparison with ultra-thin sections stained with methylene blue. No correction for shrinkage appears to have been applied; this may have contributed to the variance of the data, because glutaraldehyde and formaldehyde, the two fixatives used by the authors, appear to cause different amounts of shrinkage.

The youngest samples examined were of a gestational age of 21 weeks and contained over 750×10^6 cells/mm³. By 28 weeks, the density had dropped by 20 per cent. At term, it was reduced to 150 000 cells/mm³, and, in some cases between 0 and 10 days old, there were 90 000 cells/mm³. The nadir was reached between an age of 4 months and young adulthood with a density of 35 000 cells/mm³ or less. Other layers of the striate area showed similar pat-

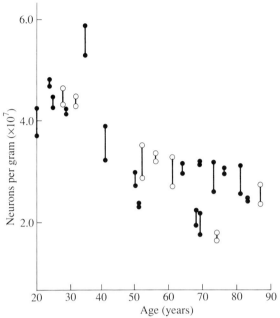

Fig. 3.4 The densities of neurons in the macular projection of area 17. The vertical lines link paired measurements for a given tissue sample. ●, males; ○, females. After Devaney and Johnson (1980).

terns. The decrease is well correlated with the increase and development of dendrites and synapses (see below) as more cortical surface becomes available.

In contrast with Devaney and Johnson's results, which were obtained specifically for projections from the macular region, older adults showed an increase of the order reported by Haug *et al.* (1984), the mean for the oldest group (81−93 years) reaching a value of 44 000 cells/mm^3; this was statistically significant. The authors suggest, as others have done before them, that this is spurious, and due to cerebral shrinkage, known to occur with advancing years.

A complementary study on the development of the density and absolute number of synapses in the visual cortex covered a slightly narower age range, namely 28 weeks of gestation to 71 years. Huttenlocher and de Courten (1987) related their loci of interest to the topography of the visual field: the search for such a link between structure and function is all too frequently overlooked.

In the attempt to quantify synapses, i.e. the gaps between neurons, the problem is even more demanding than that of a cell count, because synapses may stretch across more than one section and therefore be counted more than once. The authors list the stringent precautions they took, which included an analysis of the differential shrinkage of embedded material as a function of age. Both the number of synapses per μm^3 (0.115) and per mm^3 (572×10^6) peaked at the age of 8 months. Thereafter it declined to a plateau between the ages of 11 and 26 years to about two-thirds of those values. The oldest brain studied (71 years) had half-maximal values. Approximately similar courses were followed in all the layers of the striate area.

If it is assumed that the total volume of each cortical layer of area 17 remains constant at 6.16 ± 0.47 mm^3 after the age of 4 months (even though a drop of 10–15 per cent appears to occur after childhood) the results shows that there is an average 41 per cent loss of synapses in all cortical layers. Measurements of the cortical volume and synaptic density enabled the authors to calculate the total numbers of synapses in the striate area. The maximum of 3.5×10^{12} is reached at 8 months, and drops to just over half this value at puberty. It is uncertain whether a further slight fall, recorded for 71 years, is significant.

The authors believe that their results are due to a reduction in synapses, resulting from a reduction in the concentration of dendritic spines (see below) unaccompanied by one of neurons. In other words, it is not neuronal death, but an atrophy, perhaps of arborizations, that may account for the observations. The fact that the number of synapses peaks during the first year of life, long before vision is optimal (Chapter 4), may have little to do with the individual's immediate cognitive needs. It may serve to programme the future monocular and binocular organizations of some of the visuo-perceptual processes. Once they are formed, resources needed for the preservation of synaptic gaps are transferred elsewhere.

Other alterations in the human area 17 have been charted in Gennari's line. It owes its light appearance in histological sections to the presence of myelin, which seems to be reduced in blind persons and in certain cases of senile and presenile dementia. Lintl and Braak (1983) examined post-pubertal brains (18–96 years) by staining sections with a solution taken up in proportion to the concentration of myelin present so that the (relative) absorbance (p. 89) and its age-related variation could be determined spectrometrically (Fig. 3.1).

The authors are cautious as regards the significance of the relatively low values they recorded with the youngest brains, but there can be little doubt that they differ statistically from the rectilinear regression calculated for the other values. It is noteworthy that myelin isolated from human femoral nerves also displays a systematic age-related variation (Spritz *et al.* 1973): it reaches a peak around the age of 50 years. The decline in later life has been associated tentatively with a reduction in conduction velocity which, however, is not very marked (see Chapter 5).

Myelin serves the saltatory conduction of nerve-impulses and is formed very slowly. In the optic nerve, much of myelination is post-natal (Dolman *et al.* 1980; Magoon and Robb 1981), a feature that has misled those developmental scientists who seek to explain the course of visual development only in retinal and cortical terms, and who seem to have overlooked relevant implications of some demyelinating diseases. It will be seen in Chapter 4 that there are perceptual faculties the variation with age of which parallels that of Fig. 3.1.

Moreover, Lintl and Braak's tentative link between demyelination in Gennari's line and the age-related slowing down of visually evoked responses has been confirmed both with structured and flash stimuli. Chalmers *et al.* (1985) observed delays of tens of milliseconds over an age-difference of 60 years, but noted no variation in the amplitude of the potentials. A slightly different result was obtained in another study of the latent period in evoked potentials, which involved the use of both grating and checkerboard stimuli (Bobak *et al.* 1989). Over an age range between 16 and 84 years, the authors also found an increase in the latent period of PI, the first positive wave. But a more detailed analysis showed the variation with age to be parabolic, a slight but systematic decrease up to about the fifth decade being followed by a sharper rise thereafter (Fig. 3.5). The smallest checkerboard pattern caused a greater increase in the latent period than did a grating with similar angular characteristics (2.3 cycles/degree). No such difference was noted for more detailed patterns, i.e. those based on higher spatial frequencies.

Heintel *et al.* (1979) also employed structured stimuli. But, contrary to the results obtained by Chalmers *et al.*, they noted that the second positive peak, P2, showed an early fall in amplitude, which dropped to a minimum during the fourth decade, and then rose slightly. Note that this type of variation with age was also observed by Bobak *et al.*, which suggests that this is not an artefact, although neither group of workers mention adequate stimulus controls.

As regards possible causes of their results, Lintl and Braak cite the finding that lipofuscin, a typical age-pigment, accumulates in many isocortical pyramidal cells (cf p. 146), ultimately displacing granulated endoplasmic reticular material and so impairing function. They conclude with the hypothesis that axonal changes in these cells may explain the observed demyelination.

Haug *et al.*'s observation that there is no dramatic cell loss in the striate area has already been mentioned, and this leaves a comparison between brain and retina that has changed out of all recognition during the last decade or so. Whereas the mere existence of apparently continuous cell loss provided a link between the two, this is no longer so. The brain appears to be relatively stable as regards cell numbers, whereas the retina is not. As discussed below, new pointers discovered during the last decade merely confirm this view.

Relative cellular stability in many of the cerebral regions in later life appears to be maintained by degrees of blood flow and oxygen metabolism which show little, if any, change when computed tomography is used (Itoh *et al.* 1990), but which show well-defined changes as revealed by an ^{15}O steady-state inhalation technique accompanied by positron emission tomography (Leenders *et al.* 1990). It is well known that relatively brief periods of anoxia lead to irreversible damage but, even when attention is confined to the second part of the life span,

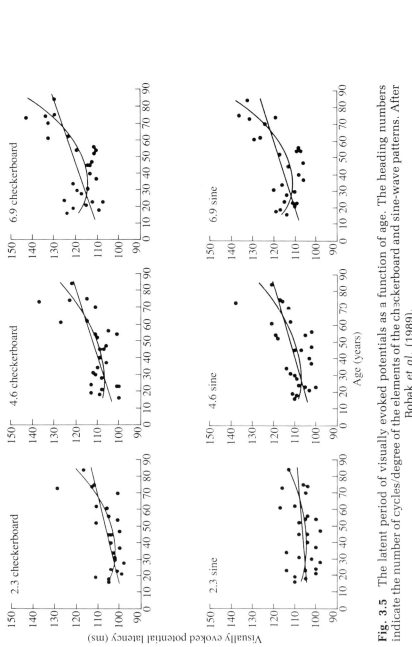

Fig. 3.5 The latent period of visually evoked potentials as a function of age. The heading numbers indicate the number of cycles/degree of the elements of the checkerboard and sine-wave patterns. After Bobak et al. (1989).

mean grey matter blood-flow and oxygen metabolic rate appear to be well maintained (Itoh *et al.* 1990) and independent of tissue shrinkage.

This is not intended to imply that no change in the vascular system can be detected. For example, Lovett Doust (1972) employed rheoencephalography in a study of the cerebral circulation. The age range was far greater than above, and covered 6–70 years. Rheoencephalograms (REGs), recorded with a three-electrode system apposed to the scalp, were accompanied by electrocardiograms. The wave-form of the REG is characterized not only by the angle which its initial rising phase makes with the horizontal (this is a measure of the speed of the dynamic process), but also by the amplitude of the wave. In young persons, there is a peak or double-peak, in older ones there tends to be a plateau. Given that the peak can be identified, a rise time can be calculated. After the fourth decade the rise time increased systematically with age, but the amplitude remained unchanged.

The detailed analysis due to Leenders *et al.* (1990) shows that, between the ages of 20 and 80 years, regional cerebral blood flow (RCBF) drops by about one third, blood volume by almost one half (which may help to explain the aforementioned tissue shrinkage, but contradicts results due to Fujishima and Omae, 1980), oxygen utilization by one fifth, and the oxygen extraction fraction actually rises by some 10 per cent. A somewhat smaller, but still significant, drop of some 12 per cent in RCBF was recorded by Melamed *et al.* (1980). They used the ^{133}Xe inhalation technique, reported that there are detectable regional differences between one hemisphere and another, and concluded that the age-related decline in RCBF progresses continuously from youth through adulthood to old age. As is true of many other studies carried out on a relatively local population, there is at present no means of determining whether a real change with age of the variable is being recorded, or whether it is partly or wholly contaminated by some cumulative environmental factor(s) (see p. 112).

The same technique was used in a study on the age-related variation of cerebral blood-flow in 'cognitively intact' persons by Zemcov *et al.* (1984). It involved an analysis of 32 detectors (16 on each side) of ^{133}Xe washout after inhalation. One of these, number 7, was in close proximity to the striate area. While the majority of the detectors recorded differences between the left and right hemispheres, number 7 and its neighbour number 6 were amongst those to show no important difference although they both indicated a significant reduction in blood-flow.

The morphological basis for the above-mentioned relative stability of cerebral haemodynamics is found in the preservation of the capillary network throughout many decades. In a study of all the cerebral gyri, Hunziker *et al.* (1978) noted that the capillary diameter increased in the pre- and postcentral and the superior temporal gyri. However, the capillary volume, expressed as its projected area, appeared to increase all over the cortex, including the above regions and the occipital pole. The specific area, defined as the ratio of surface to volume of the senescent brains, diminished, which may explain a tendency for the mean inter-capillary distance also to drop. The authors believe that their measurements support the view that the ageing brain exhibits a reduced vascular supply; on the contrary, it appears to benefit from a compensating mechanism, as manifested by a higher capillary density.

It should not be concluded from this that there is a specific evolutionary pressure for the maintenance of the cerebral blood supply in the shape of some delayed angiogenesis. It is more likely that the existing capillary bed is preserved in a shrinking cerebral volume.

In a subsequent study, Hunziker *et al.* (1979) examined all the cortical lobes; their description concentrates on the precentral gyrus of the frontal lobes, measurements for which are harder to compare with results obtained with recent non-invasive techniques than would be true of lateral regions, as noted above (p. 123). However, results for the briefly mentioned, visually significant, occipital pole are given, and follow closely other more detailed information.

The capillary diameter drops from 6.2 μm to 5.7 μm between the late teens and the seventh decade. During the next decade there is a sharp rise to approximately 6.7 μm, and another similarly steep drop follows during the next ten years. Those surviving to the age range of 85–94 years experience yet another gradual rise in capillary diameter to 6 μm. This apparently random zig-zagging mirrors the variation in heart rate: although it would be reasonable to expect it to occur also in the retina, no detailed study appears to have been published on the matter. In spite, or perhaps because, of this variation, only changes between the youngest group and those in the range of 67–74 years were found to be significant: they included increases in capillary diameter, volume fraction, and total length per unit cortical volume.

3.3 Further remarks on retinal vasculature

General features of vascular ageing include an increase in the collagen content and the collagen–elastin ratio of the arteries, commonly, but inaccurately, subsumed by the term of arteriosclerosis (Dobrin 1978). In point of fact this process starts *in utero* (see above). A consequence of this mechanical change in the arterial walls is a rise in systemic arterial pressure in spite of an increase in arterial diameter. The walls thicken and the media becomes wider, with calcium deposits increasing the stiffness of elastin fibres. Stiffening of arteries appears to increase with their distance from the heart.

The retinal and choroidal vessels are not exempt from these changes. Those occurring in the retinal vessels in particular are readily visualized, e.g. by an increased tortuousness. Changes in the capillary bed also occur and can be recorded both entoptically and photographically, for example, by means of fluorescein angiography, a very effective but highly unpleasant procedure. The retinal vasculature seems to be sturdier than the cerebral, and, referring specifically to the capillaries of the choroid, Feeney-Burns *et al.* (1990) observe that their atrophy does not necessarily have lethal consequences for retinal cells.

In a microscopic study of three eyes, aged 58, 64, and 76 year, Lerche (1967) examined a region between the optic disc and the central macular area, determining the relative capillary volume, capillary density, and the mean intercapillary distance, without claiming that the results may have any general validity. For example, from the youngest to the oldest eye, the number of capillaries per 2500 μm^2 in the macular inner nuclear layer dropped from 1.3 to 0.6. There was a marked loss of capillaries in the circummacular regions, and this was linked with a notable thinning of the ganglion cell layer, attributed, in turn, to cell death. The average intercapillary distance changed from 68 to 79 μm between the two older eyes, and there is a qualitative relation between capillary volume and concentrations of succinic and malic dehydrogenases, reported earlier.

These data are partly complemented by others obtained on the brain of macaques, 4, 10, and 20 years of age, i.e. corresponding to human teenage, young middle age and the elderly respectively. The occipital cortex showed a progressive and significant reduction of the capillary area from 37 to 21 μm, and the capillary walls thinning by almost 50 per cent. A similar reduction was noted for the total cross-sectional area of the endothelial cells in occipital areas (Burns *et al.* 1979).

A histological counterpart to these results is to be found in the report that, for example, peripheral retinal capillaries reveal morphological changes at the beginning of the sixth decade (Cogan 1963). The endothelial cells begin to vanish, leaving the mural cells behind. These disappear later so that merely acellular vessels of normal dimensions are preserved for a time. In those cases where the mural cells are the first to vanish more nearly pathological formations like micro-aneurysms tend to appear. At that time of life the cell walls of other, more central, retinal vessels are also liable to become attenuated. The discrepancy in the timing of these events may provide a clue for the age-related constriction of the visual field (p. 190).

A detailed study based on fluorescein angiography is due to Laatikainen and Larinkari (1977) who examined the central avascular retinal regions of over 150 subjects ranging in age from 1 year to over 60 years (Fig. 3.6). Fluorescein was injected intravenously and its appearance in the retinal bloodstream monitored after a timed interval. Its presence was revealed by illumination of the fundus with short-wavelength radiation. This produced green fluorescence which was photographed. The central retinal area (approximately 0.5 mm in diameter) revealed a relative, or even an absolute, scarcity of capillaries, presumably because of the high oxygen tension existing in that region. This is known to inhibit the formation of capillaries and explains why they are absent from the neighbourhood of retinal arteries.

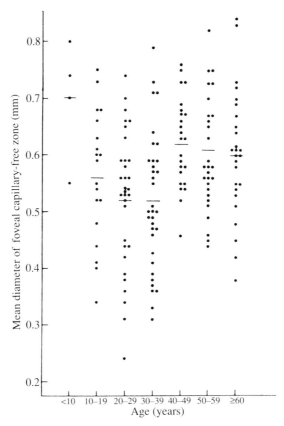

Fig. 3.6 The mean diameter of the apparently capillary-free area as a function of age (decades). The horizontal lines represent the mean in each decade. After Laatikainen and Larinkari (1977).

Estimates of the diameter of the capillary-free area show that it drops from a value of about 0.7 mm in childhood to a minimum of 0.5 mm during the third or fourth decade, i.e. the area is almost halved, but it rises thereafter. The disappearance of the capillaries in later life is probably due less to an increase in foveal oxygen tension than to some of the processes mentioned above.

Wu *et al.* (1985) used a similar technique on Chinese subjects. Their planimetric estimate of the avascular zone was less perfunctory than the above, which was based on the measurements of two perpendicular 'diameters', and they used a higher concentration of fluorescein. Despite this their avascular areas are larger than those obtained for the above Finnish subjects; it would be interesting to know whether this is a real ethnic difference. If anything, the Chinese data show a steepish rise during the second decade of life with a tailing off thereafter.

Hence there are qualitative, in addition to quantitative, differences between the two studies.

Two entoptic methods have been used for assessing the magnitude of the avascular area. In one of them, the sclera is transilluminated, preferably intermittently. This allows the vascular tree to be visualized, and the avascular region to be seen and measured, for example by projection onto a grid. The other method consists in illuminating the retina with light of a short wavelength, and observing the passage of individual blood corpuscles through retinal capillaries close to the fovea. It is possible to measure the smallest area within which no corpuscle is perceived. The latter method formed the basis of measurements on observers below and above the age of 40 years respectively (Yap *et al.* 1987). The mean value for the over-40s was about 20 per cent higher than for the younger group.

There is little doubt that the last three studies may have overestimated the extent of the reduction of the avascular zone. The reason is that both fluorescein angiography and the entoptic method depend for their success on the use of short-wavelength radiation. But this is going to be absorbed more strongly in older eyes than in young ones. Photography, like vision, has a threshold for detection, and the energy needed to produce detectable fluorescence in fluorescein angiography, or to render the blood corpuscles visible in the entoptic method may have been simply too low. It is remarkable that no experiment of this sort has been reported for aphakic eyes. A repetition of these studies seems to be needed.

3.4 Age and the retinal photoreceptors

The external world of radiation and the private domain of nervous messages meet in the retinal layer of photoreceptors. It is here that quantized absorbed electromagnetic energy gives rise to photochemical events in visual pigments contained in the outer segments of rods and cones, and electric potential changes ultimately leading to the brain are initiated.

3.4.1 *Receptor populations*

Disadvantageous age-related changes might be expected to be observed in photoreceptors. Hart *et al.* (1979) report that studies based on alkaline sucrose gradient sedimentation of retinal photoreceptors of dogs (i.e. largely rods) showed that, in these cells, the single-strand molecular weight of DNA decreases with age.

In fact, age-related morphological changes in rods and cones have often been described (see Marshall *et al.* 1979), but the latest review to mention photoreceptors in the context of ageing relies on work done on ageing monkeys rather than people (Curcio and Hendrickson 1991).

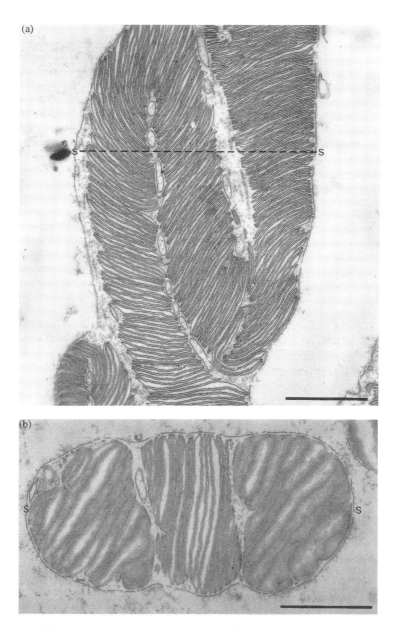

Fig. 3.7 Electron micrograph of a convoluted (senescent) human rod.
a Section parallel to the receptor axis; **b** Section at right angles to it. Scale
bar = 10^{-6} m. Courtesy Marshall *et al.* (1979).

As reported earlier, hypertrophy of the outer segments tends to be observed in rods, and it is attributed to a reduction of the phagocytic activity of the retinal pigment epithelium. Tangential sections reveal under the light microscope the development of nodules along the outer segments (Fig. 3.7). Electron microscopic examination revealed that these enlargements were due to folds or knots, probably arising from a lengthening of the outer limb owing to the actual absence of phagocytosis (Marshall *et al.* 1979).

The cone inner limbs of more than half of eyes over 30 years old were found to contain lipofuscin (Fig. 3.8). The granules were 20−80 nm in diameter, much larger than those observed in the inner, and occasionally the outer, segments of rods (Iwasaki and Inomata 1988). Bazan *et al.* (1990) have demonstrated that the lipid of these granules differs from that of the photoreceptors. But, whereas the latter show an age-related reduction in phosphatidylcholine, no significant change in the components of the lipofuscin fractions could be detected.

Curcio *et al.* (1990) report considerable rod losses in 61−82-year-old retinae. The main losses (30 per cent) occurred in the part of the retina below the fovea. The remaining rods were of increased diameter, and, where the rod loss was maximal, there were also larger cones and larger cone coverage. This suggests that rods are shorter-lived than cones. In particular the peak density of foveal cones overlapped the three-fold range seen earlier in young eyes, and the authors find that the smallness of cone losses is insufficient to account for the observed reduction in visual acuity with age (p. 228).

Although Gartner and Henkind (1981) claim to have observed (unquantified) losses of photoreceptors in the macular region, Figs 5b and 6b in their publication show that, at the ages of 41 and 62 years respectively, cone numbers seem to be well preserved.

This not only agrees with the above observations, but also tallies partly with those of Dorey *et al.* (1989) whose detailed histological and statistical analysis enables them to state that 'although the regression line fitted to the data indicated an annual decrease of 1−2 per cent in the photoreceptor number in the macular and paramacular regions, none of the regions was found to exhibit a significant age-related loss of photoreceptors'. This observation is, however, subject to the reservation that 'the number of photoreceptors remaining in the macula of blacks was inversely related to age'.

The relative sturdiness of the cone receptors may not, however, last much beyond the age of 70 or 80 years. Feeney-Burns *et al.* (1990) compared the population densities of both photoreceptors and of pigment epithelial cells (see p. 131) in human eyes between the age of 90 and 101 years with those found in younger specimens. This raises the question of, and may help to define, pathological changes: they may become the norm, and hence the physiology, of old age. The foveal region exhibited losses in photoreceptors amounting to roughly 40 per cent just during the tenth decade, the variance being appreciable. This may be compared with an approximate 3 per cent loss during the sixth

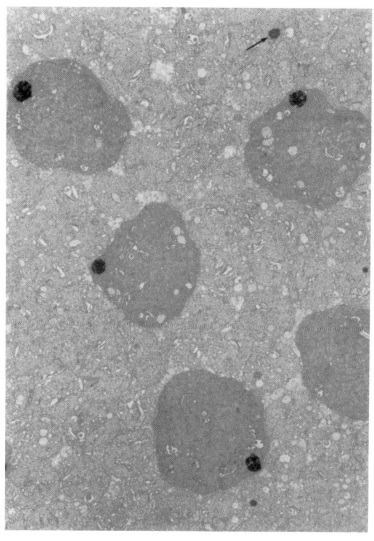

Fig. 3.8 Electron micrograph of a section at right angles to the photo-receptors. The small black spots show lipofuscin in the outer segments of rods, the large ones in those of cones. Magnification × 5400. From Iwasaki and Inomata (1988).

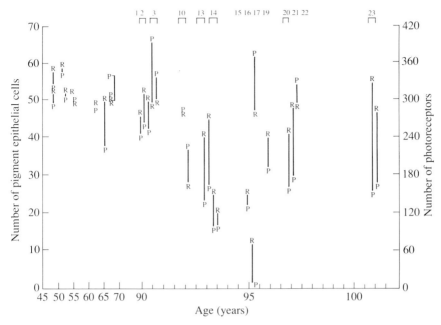

Fig. 3.9 Numbers of pigment epithelial cells (P and left-hand scale) and photoreceptors (R and right-hand scale) in 0.6 mm of sectioned foveae. The number of donors is given at the top. Note that the scales indicate a 6:1 ratio of P:R for retinae less than 90-years old, whereas there is a marked variation at higher ages, see p. 7. After Feeney-Burns *et al.* (1990).

decade (Fig. 3.9). No evidence was found to suggest that the length of the foveal cone outer segments was any shorter in old than in middle-life retinae.

It may be that factors other than population density change with age, and may affect function more severely than might be expected simply on the basis of numbers. Thus Curcio (1986) has raised the possibility that receptor distribution may play a powerful role not only as regards the wide variability observed from one retina to another, but also insofar as the cone mosaic may become dis-ordered. It has not escaped her attention (Curcio *et al.* 1987) that this might be due in part to processing of postmortem material. But the notion of receptor pattern preservation for continuing function is important, and the diminution of its role in senescence, if any, needs to be established.

3.4.2 *The concentration of visual pigments*

The above morphological results are not easily reconciled with studies of the photochemical contents of the photoreceptors. For example, Plantner *et al.*

(1988) found no variation with age in rhodopsin content in a study based on a radioimmunoassay of the pigment and its opsin in human retinae covering an age range from 18 to 82 years, i.e. overlapping the spread in the study in which Curcio *et al.* reported massive losses of rods. Though Marshall *et al.* have not quoted any figure, their qualitative description is consistent with the immunological study, for they report a lengthening of rod outer segments which may partly counteract such losses as may have occurred. Data based on excised parts of human retinae (van Kujik *et al.* 1991) also fail to reveal any systematic variation of the optical density of rhodopsin as a function with age, a situation foreshadowed in earlier and comparatively rudimentary reflectometric studies of the living human retina (see Weale 1982*a*).

In contrast with rhodopsin, cone-pigments have been studied only *in vivo*, two different methods being employed. The first of these was fundus reflectometry, a technique based on ophthalmoscopy; the other, to be discussed below, involves colour matching.

Two fundamental modifications of the well-established technique of ophthalmoscopy used for examining the fundus of the eye were introduced so that qualitative inspection might be replaced by quantitative assessment. In the first place the white light of the ophthalmoscope was replaced with monochromatic radiations, and secondly the specialist's eye gave way to an objective device capable of measuring, or at least comparing, intensities of radiation coming from the illuminated fundus oculi (see Ripps and Snapper 1974). In view of the importance of the results obtained with this technique for our views on retinal senescence, some technical detail may not be out of place.

In principle, a feeble monochromatic pencil of light enters the eye under examination, traverses its media and the dark-adapted retina, is reflected at the choroid, and, on retracing its path, emerges from the eye when its intensity is recorded (Fig. 3.10). Pencils made up of radiations that are absorbed readily by a visual pigment emerge weaker than those that are not absorbed. If the pigment is now bleached with an intense beam of light (Fig. 3.10) and the aforementioned weak pencils are re-admitted into the eye so that the absorption characteristics of the retina may be probed again, little change will be found for those radiations which were originally poorly absorbed. But those that were absorbed strongly, and therefore gave a low intensity reading, will now be much enhanced since the absorbing material has been bleached. A comparison of pairs of intensities for a given type of radiation before and after bleaching therefore provides a measure of the change in absorbance, and hence of concentration, due to the much stronger bleaching radiation. In order to be able to determine what would be expected to result from changes due to age it helps to view the situation in algebraic terms (Weale 1989*b*).

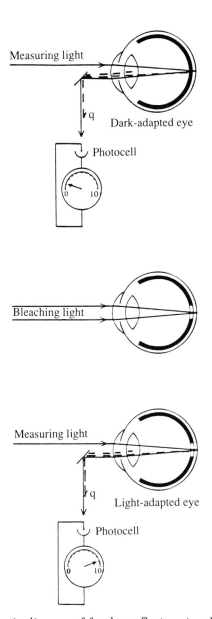

Fig. 3.10 Schematic diagram of fundus reflectometry. For details see text.

If the retina could be considered simply as a pigment contained in the eye, the determination of the above-mentioned change in pigment concentration resulting from a bleaching exposure would be relatively easy. The possible presence of stray light complicates matters. It can take the form of (a) light scattered for example by the lens, or (b) such as has traversed the retina without passing through any photosensitive material. This can occur on the inward or outward journey or on both. It can be shown that if the putative transmissivity of the retina for some monochromatic radiation is $T(r,t)$ if the measurement is made t seconds after an event, and a fraction p of the measuring pencil has traversed pigment while the remaining fraction q has missed it, the measured transmissivity is given by

$$T(m,t) = p.T(r,t)^2 + q \qquad (3.1)$$

The reason for the square is that the light that does traverse pigment is assumed to do so both before and after reflection at the fundus. In case (a) above, $p = R(1-s)^2$ and $q = s$, where R is the reflectivity of the fundus, and s the fraction of the incident light scattered by the lens. In case (b), $p = Rf$, and $q = R(1-f)$, where f is the fraction of the cross-sectional area of the measuring pencil which traverses pigment. In the following, $N = q/p$.

For the fully bleached state b,

$$T(m,b) = p.T(r,b)^2 + q \qquad (3.2)$$

and for the fully dark-adapted state when the pigment concentration is assumed to have reached its maximum following regeneration of the pigment in the dark

$$T(m,d) = p.T(r,d)^2 + q \qquad (3.3)$$

The maximum measured change is given by the ratio of the $T(m,d)/T(m,b)$, say

$$F(d,b) = [T(r,d)^2 + N]/[T(r,b)^2 + N] \qquad (3.4)$$

The change in pigment concentration is proportional to $-\log F(d,b)$. As $T(r,d) < T(r,b)$, N affects the numerator more than the denominator. The measured value of $F(d,b)$ therefore decreases with an increase in N. In other words, measured changes are minimal changes. The burden of this argument is that if $F(d,b)$ is found to decrease with age, this can be due to a real loss in pigment concentration, provided the above effect of stray light has been ruled out. It is true that retinal lacunae, due perhaps to receptor losses, could be a manifestation of ageing, and this shows that it is hard to distinguish a reduction in pigment concentration from one in receptor population.

The rate of regeneration of a pigment after it has been bleached can also be measured by the above technique. If the measurements are made at various times **t** of dark-adaptation following a bleach, then the above fraction takes the form

$$F(t,d) = [T(r,t)^2 + N]/[T(r,d)^2 + N] \qquad (3.5)$$

Here the denominator is more affected by **N** than is the numerator; hence **F(t,d)** is smaller than it would be if **N** were negligible. The corresponding rise in absorbance is, however, larger; this means that the pigment appears to regenerate faster when **N** is significant.

Kilbride *et al.* (1986) and Keunen *et al.* (1987) studied data based on eqn (3.4), for an age range lying beween the teens and 80 years. Keunen *et al.*'s study is particularly interesting because they used aphakic and pseudophakic eyes in order to minimize stray-light effects usually associated with light scattered by the crystalline lens. Like Kilbride *et al.*, they showed that the maximally achievable absorbance change systematically drops with age. Whereas Kilbride *et al.* observed a linear decrease, the results of observations by Keunen *et al.* were constant up to the fifth decade, and started dropping only thereafter (Fig. 3.11a). Although interesting from the point of view of the discussion in Chapter 1 (pp. 36–40), this fact is less important in view of individual variances than that Keunen *et al.*'s data are systematically higher than Kilbride *et al.*'s; this lends support to the view that the former workers had achieved a high measure of control over stray light (see eqn 3.4).

Keunen *et al.* also studied the rate of regeneration of the foveal pigments after the cones had been denuded of them by photolysis. Here again, the values for the time constant do not change up to the fifth decade, but do so afterwards, in this case showing a rise (Fig. 3.11b). This is contrary to the prediction based on eqn 3.5: the presence of stray light leads one to expect a shortening of the time constant (i.e. pigments appear to regenerate faster). Since their results disagree with theory, Keunen *et al.* conclude that cone losses must account for the discrepancy.

But we noted that a simple consideration of the effects of stray light fails to distinguish between scattered light and light passing through, but not being absorbed by, the retina. It is likely, therefore, that the age-related drop in absorbance (Fig. 3.11a) is to be attributed either to cone losses or to a general reduction in pigment concentration, whereas Fig. 3.11b, showing a rise in time constant instead of an expected drop, may have to be explained in terms of a change in regeneration dynamics. These could arise from changes in the activity of the pigment epithelium, Bruch's membrane, and/or a host of other changes overtaking the retina and choroid in middle life (p. 141).

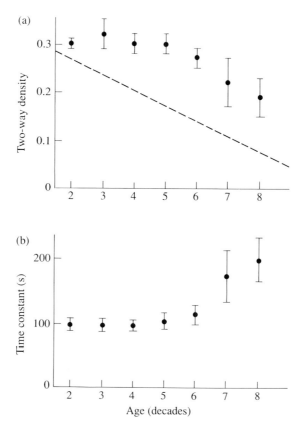

Fig. 3.11 (a) Reflectometric density change $-\log F(d,b)$, see eqn 3.4, as a function of age. (b) Time constant (s) of the regeneration in darkness of the bleached pigment. After Keunen *et al.* (1987).

The possibility of a continued intactness of the receptor population, as demanded for example by the results due to Curcio *et al.* (1990), can be reconciled with the above results on a progressive reduction in absorbance if the latter is due to one in pigment concentration, Keunen *et al.* having practically ruled out any effect due to stray light. However, if there is a reduction in pigment concentration then the ability of the pigment to absorb light is correspondingly lowered, and, in turn, the visual threshold might be expected to be raised. This will be considered in Chapter 4, but it is appropriate to mention here the second method referred to above, namely one used in a sensory study based on colour matches which inform on the absorbance of retinal pigments.

In essence, only those test wavelengths are used which require but two matching stimuli; in practice this means the straight-line part (p. 221) of the chromaticity diagram is involved, with the test wavelength at 590 nm, and the matching stimuli at 546 and 650 nm. The rationale of the method is based on the fact that bleaching with various intensities leads to predictable changes in the relative concentrations of the two principal foveal pigments involved in the matching procedure.

Elsner *et al.* (1988) used the method to study age-related changes in colour matches at moderate light intensities, which provide a baseline; matches at very high intensities, which are related to pigment density; and intensity measurements $I(0)$ yielding the half-way stage, which is a measure of the photosensitivity of the pigment. It may be noted that the latter is independent of retinal lacunae and of pigment concentration. Ages ranged from 13 to 69 years, and the test-field was 4 ° in diameter, which probably explains the relatively low mean computed absorbance (0.27), and the sparse variation. The absorbance reached a shallow maximum at around 30 years, but was too variable to permit any comparison with reflectometric data. $I(0)$ did not vary significantly with age and, at a mean value of 4.37 logtd, was of the same order as values determined by fundus reflectometry (Weale 1959). The ratio of red/green required for the match declined systematically with age; lenticular yellow has not been ruled out as a possible cause. A reduction in pigment concentration is neither demonstrated convincingly nor ruled out.

No systematic *in vivo* study on the relationship between the rod pigment and age appears to have been carried out.

3.5 The macular pigment

The macular pigment, which covers the central part of the ocular fundus, consists of at least two compounds, namely zeaxanthin and lutein (Bone *et al.* 1988). Their ratio decreases systematically with retinal eccentricity, which suggests a close link with the relative distributions of cones and rods.

The optical density of this photically inert pigment, as based on sensory studies, has been estimated at about 0.5 for the maximally absorbed wavelength (about 460 nm), but at only two-thirds of this value when measured reflectometrically. Kilbride *et al.* (1989) attribute this result to lenticular scatter of light (see eqn 3.4): a control experiment on subjects with lens implants has not been published.

The pigment is thought to fulfil three roles (see Werner *et al.* 1987). As a carotenoid it may facilitate the transfer of oxygen in a retinal area not supplied with a rich retinal vascular system (p. 126). In view of its absorption spectrum, it has been seen as a useful filter serving to reduce the untoward effects of chromatic aberration (p. 57) in a retinal region which might be sensitive to them. And, thirdly, it may form a protection against potential retinal damage from short-wavelength radiations. Despite powerful advocacy (Haegerstrom-Portnoy 1988), the experimental evidence for the last is open to argument (see p. 155).

However, a difficulty for all these hypotheses is the great variability in the occurrence and distribution of the pigment. The only systematic correlate apparently detected so far is red hair (Bone and Sparrock 1971). Otherwise its density and, indeed, presence are highly variable (Ruddock 1963), and may vary even between fellow eyes (Bone *et al.* 1988). The putative protective function of the macular pigment could be tested by those who believe to have identified modifications in retinal morphology, appearance or function resulting from measured amounts of radiation: a negative correlation with pigment density would powerfully support that hypothesis.

Although, therefore, the function of the pigment has not so far been pinpointed, it is now agreed without exception that its absorbance does not vary with age (Kilbride *et al.* 1989; Werner *et al.* 1987) except for the first two years of life when zeaxanthin appears to be relatively sparse (Bone *et al.* 1988).

3.6 Other retinal cells

As will be discussed in Chapter 4, there are functional parallels to the progressive loss of rods and the relatively stable number of cones mentioned on p. 127. Second and higher order neurons are concerned not with the detection of radiation, which is the role of the photoreceptors, but with the partial analysis of the information that is carried out. The processing is only partial because, as studies of the brain during the last 40 years or so have shown, some of the data-processing takes place in the brain. Though clearly not in their infancy, these studies have not reached the stage where it would be profitable to speculate on the gerontological significance of this or that visually active cerebral area. It may be recalled, however, that the latest information on cell populations, for example, in the striate area does not suggest that there are marked histological changes in those regions.

3.6.1 *The outer nuclear layer*

This would not be true of the inner neural retina. Gartner and Henkind (1981) found in a light microscopic study that the displacement of nuclei from the outer nuclear layer into the outer plexiform layer occurs largely after the age of 30 years. It is arguable that the phenomenon is progressive: this could be the case during the first five decades. After this a jump occurs, to a plateau which is maintained to the end of the age range studied. Mainly the nuclei of rods appear to be involved in these migrations, which may in fact occur also in reverse through the internal limiting membrane and into the bacillary layer.

When it occurs, nuclear displacement is almost exclusively extra-foveal. Degenerative changes in rods were noted to occur after the age of 40 years.

The authors speculate that the migrations are the result of traction, perhaps due to a shrinkage of axonal or other fibres. This is in stark contrast to the view expressed later, and in apparent ignorance of this work, by Vrabec (1986) who believes that the displacements are 'the result of some sort of morphogenetic accident'. If this is true, and the nuclear positions are, as it were, inborn errors of location, then the above age-related changes, the statistical significance of which cannot be in reasonable doubt, are hard to understand.

3.6.2 *Ganglion cells and optic nerve fibres*

The fact that patients suffering from Alzheimer's disease (AD) have a poor visual performance prompted Drucker and Curcio (1990) to compare cell counts of normal and AD ganglion cells in 66−86 year-old central retinae. The results for the normal (385 K−527 K) overlapped the low end of the range for normal younger eyes (428 K−803 K), and there was no additional loss in the AD retinae (476 K−618 K). It follows that the visual deficit in AD is to be found probably at a more central level. In view of the large convergence of extra-foveal receptors onto ganglion cells it is impossible to decide from these data whether the manifest losses in ganglion cells are in any way related to those noted by Curcio *et al.* (1990) for rods, with those linked to foveal cones being spared, or whether the losses in ganglion cells are general.

As optic nerve fibres are the centrifugal axons of ganglion cells, one would expect close links between the two as regards age-related changes. The macroanatomy of the optic nerve has received repeated attention. Dolman *et al.* (1980) studied the thickness of the nerves, the presence of myelin and connective tissue, of corpora amylacea, and of lipofuscin from birth to an age of 96 years in normal and pathological specimens. 2.8 mm^2 at birth, the cross-section of the nerves doubled by the age of 3−4 years. It rose to 6.25 mm^2 in childhood, and reached its final value of 6.75 mm^2 in the late teens. The density of the axons was found to decrease after the age of 60 years; as no mention is made of a correction for the time elapsing between death and fixation of the tissue (Balazsi *et al.* 1984), this figure may be of limited significance. A similar stricture applies to the results reported by Vrabec (1977). Axonal atrophy was observed in several optic nerve heads ranging in age from 46−80 years, but the variance was considerable.

Corpora amylacea, accepted as a sign also of ageing brains, appear frequently in older lamina cribrosa, but occur also elsewhere in the nerves, notably near their periphery. As foreign bodies, they may exert pressure on individual nerve fibres which could interfere with the conduction of impulses; indeed, in large bunches they can cause visual field losses. Lipofuscin is notable by its absence though found in the brain, in photoreceptors, and in the retinal pigment epithelium (p. 153).

Fibre counts by Balazsi *et al.* (1984) revealed a loss related to **T**, the post mortem time to fixation. When outliers with **T** > 20 hours were eliminated the variation with age became non-significant: but there is an estimated loss of over 5000 axons per year, with an initial value of 1.648 M, which is higher than data reported by other authors (see Johnson *et al.* 1987). The latter authors, too, reported a decrease in axon counts which failed to reach statistical significance. Computerized image analysis led essentially to similar results (Mikelberg *et al.* 1989), allowance being made for **T**. However, the counts were made across a cross-section divided into central and peripheral zones, each being subdivided into eight sectors. The smallest axonal diameters were found on the naso-superior side, the coarsest in the temporal inferior sectors which correspond to the axons of the papillo-macular bundle. The subdivision of the cross-section of the nerve did not affect the conclusion that no significant age-related loss of axons is observed.

The question of age-related losses is unresolved; however, most laboratories report a decline which, with attention confined to their results, is non-significant. The estimate of 5000 fibres lost (Mikelberg *et al.* 1989; Balazsi *et al.* 1984) is modest at about 0.5 per cent. It may or may not commence at birth, and the fact that there are different axonal concentrations in different sectors makes it difficult to predict the functional consequences of the losses. It may be noted, howevever, that this percentage is very compatible with the ganglion cell losses reported above.

To the extent to which axonal losses may occur, Hernandez *et al.* (1989) suggest that the interfibrillar space in the optic disk is filled with macro-molecular aggregates consisting of elastin and collagen. The extent to which a supposedly normal course of events may be departed from may indicate a predisposition to glaucoma.

On the other hand, the relative stability of the optic nerve head has been captured on a macroscopic scale photographically (Lotmar *et al.* 1978). By examining stereoscopically longitudinally obtained photographs of the optic disk, they failed to find any significant change over a period of 8 years in 70 per cent of their subjects. There was no correlation with age, but with one exception, the age range lay below 55 years. A similar constancy in appearance for a period of 11 years was reported also by Robert *et al.* (1985).

3.7 Bruch's membrane

Originally pictured as consisting of two layers, namely the elastic and the cuticular lamina, Bruch's membrane lines the choroid. It is now thought to consist of five layers:

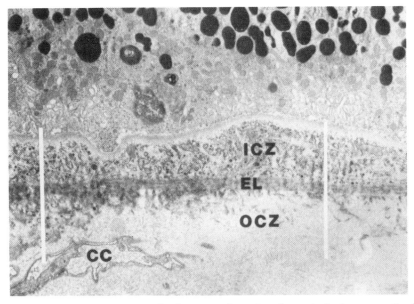

Fig. 3.12 Electron micrograph of a vertical section through the human retinal pigment epithelium. ICZ, inner collagenous layer; EL, elastic layer; OCZ, outer collagenous layer; CC, choriocapillaris. Courtesy Feeney-Burns and Ellersieck (1985).

(I)   the outer basement lamina of the choriocapillaris;

(II) the outer collagenous layer which consists of collagenous fibres reaching to intercapillary spaces of the choriocapillaris;

(III) the elastic layer, readily identified in electron microphotographs (Fig. 3.12), and occupying approximately the central region of Bruch's membrane;

(IV) the inner collagenous layer, similar to, but more homogeneous than, layer No. 2;

(V)   the inner basement lamina, which is part of the retinal pigment epithelium.

The age-related changes in these layers differ and are detailed below.

Nine categories, based on the sequence of age-related changes, were identified by Feeney-Burns and Ellersieck (1985) in a representative study. They included:

(1) the normal unchanged five layers;

(2) short-segment long-spacing collagen in the outer collagenous zone (II);

(3) debris in the inner collagenous zone (IV);

(4) debris in both (II) and (IV);

(5) mineralization;

(6) drusen (which are whitish inclusions visible in the living eye with the ophthalmoscope);

(7) products of secretion located between the retinal pigment epithelium and the inner basement membrane (V);

(8) a combination of categories (4) and (7);

(9) atypical changes involving excess collagen or cells, and an absent elastic layer (III).

Scoring was based on the analysis of 15 contiguous pigment epithelial cells, with alternative methods of assessment being applied to each. Figure 3.13 shows that, from birth to the age of 20 years, non-macular cells preserved a normal Bruch's membrane. The abnormal results for the macular region in this group may be due to post mortem changes. The central age range (21−60 years) showed only two cases of normality. The other eyes fell into category (4) above. In the extramacular zone, there were cases of categories (3), (5), and (6). The last group (61−100 years) contained no normal macular Bruch's membrane, and debris was not confined to category (3); in fact, the main feature was category (4). Category (5) was infrequent, but (6) and (8) dominated in the oldest eyes. The extra-macular distribution showed a wide variance, with category (4) being dominant. Category (8) was not seen before the seventh decade, increasing in frequency with the years.

The authors conclude that the retinal pigment epithelium is the principal source of debris, and suggest that its fragments are released by apoptosis or shedding of aliquots of cytoplasm. From the point of view of the ideas discussed in Chapter 1 it is significant that no debris appears before the age of 50 years: evidently there is a mechanism, perhaps removal of debris by the choroid, which is equal to the task up to middle age. Where the disposal fails, drusen may be formed. These fall into two groups, depending on whether they are hyaline in nature (when they are comparatively harmless), or soft (when they are the forerunners of age-related macular degeneration). The latter lie on the internal side of Bruch's membrane.

A morphometric elaboration of the above findings showed that there are variations in thickness at different ages in different parts of the eye, which is divided for this purpose into the macular (M), equatorial (E), and peripheral (P) regions (Newsome *et al.* 1987). For example, in Bruch's membrane as a whole, (P)

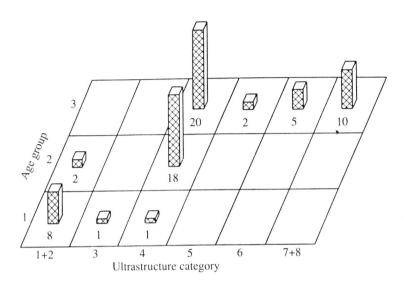

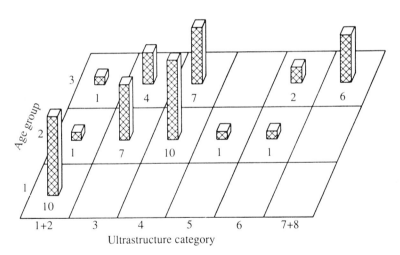

Fig. 3.13 Three-dimensional block chart of the age-related variation of ultra-structurally detected frequencies of categories of cell in Bruch's membrane as detailed in the text. Age groups: 1 = 1 to 20 years; 2 = 21 to 60 years; 3 = 61 to 100 years. Top: macula; bottom: non-macular region. After Feeney-Burns and Ellersieck (1985).

increases from 1.71 μm at age < 10 years to 6.40 μm during the eight decade, whereas (M) barely doubles from 1.64 μm. On the other hand, layer V and the choriocapillaris undergo no change at all. The macular changes tend to lag behind peripheral ones, and became significant only after the age of 45 years (see above). The detailed causes of the volumetric changes are unknown, but it is clear that they are not oedematous.

However, an analysis of layers II and IV in maculae, ranging in age from 1 month to 86 years, concentrated on coated membrane-bound inclusions (CMBI) and their fragments (Killingsworth 1987). Morphometry of their average thickness, together with an analysis of their location, helped to show that they are absent during the first decade of life. They first appear during the second or, more probably, third decade. Their size in layer IV remains almost constant, but increases progressively in layer II, mainly after the sixth decade (Fig. 3.14). Mineralized deposits were rare, and found in layer IV, being derived perhaps from collagen. Killingsworth believes that CMBIs are derived from the retinal pigment epithelium, and that they are bound by plasma membrane, and he views them as normal, rather than pathological, manifestations of their senescent parent tissue.

It may be noted that the noxious potential of inclusions need not involve active toxicity. The mere fact that they are present, either occupying space that might belong to useful material, or perhaps barring or slowing down the passage of substances in transit, may suffice to promote situations which might not arise in their absence.

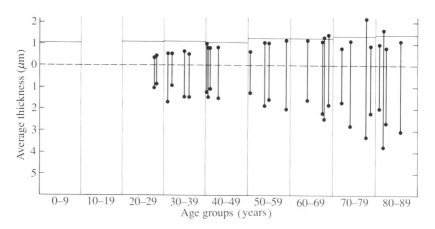

Fig. 3.14   The mean thickness (μm) of deposits and its standard deviation as a function of age. Zero refers to the elastic layer. The distance between this and the mean position of the inner collagenous layer is indicated by the horizontal lines. No figure was obtained for the second decade. After Killingsworth (1987).

3.8 The retinal pigment epithelium (RPE)

Although Gartner and Henkind (1981) stress that they could not observe any changes in Bruch's membrane and the retinal pigment epithelium in non-pathological eyes, Dorey *et al.* (1989) and, of course, Feeney-Burns *et al.* (1990), who had examined some of the oldest eyes ever, found appreciable changes in the cell population of the RPE, as had most of those who had studied this important topic.

A brief glance at a seminal paper published more than 20 years ago (Friedman and Ts'o 1968) shows what advances have taken place since then. Obtained on the basis of only a light microscopic analysis (although the electron microscope had been used for retinal research during the preceding 15 years), the authors drew attention to the differences in shape between macular and peripheral cells of the RPE. In the young, the macular cells are flat and broad, the peripheral ones more compact and rounded. This gradient is reversed in later years, little change being noticed in the intermediate equatorial region. The authors reported on an analogous change in pigmentation: in the young the periphery appeared more pigmented than the central area, the reverse applying in old age. We know now (Feeney-Burns *et al.* 1984) that this observation is partly due to the earlier authors' failure to distinguish between melanin and lipofuscin. These observations virtually paralleled those made biomicroscopically. However, other techniques were needed if the physiological and clinical significance of the RPE was to be understood.

Because the RPE is interposed between the choroid and the neural retina — in itself it represents the vegetative part of this tissue — it is looked upon as a blood-retinal barrier. It controls a two-way traffic. Metabolites needed by the retina traverse it, and it acts as a store of retinol (vitamin A1). Its cellular processes also serve to clean up the daily retinal debris formed by the breaking-up of the photoreceptors, the cones during the night, and the rods during the next morning. However, this discussion is concerned not with a detailed listing of its functions which are, in any case, not fully understood, but with certain aspects of its senescence.

3.8.1 *The pigments of the RPE*

The pigmentation of the RPE — from which it derives its name — has formed the subject of intense and highly sophisticated studies during the last decade or two. At first sight this may seem a little puzzling. The two principally identified pigments, namely lipofuscin and melanin, appear to be inert, yet their concentrations show well-marked changes with age, and have, therefore, commanded considerable gerontological interest. The clinical explanation for this is the increase in prevalence of age-related macular degeneration (AMD), a blinding condition affecting mainly Caucasian populations of the world.

Pigmentation almost of any sort is associated frequently with senescence and often also with pathological conditions, for example, in the skin. It also has the merit of sometimes being quantifiable. It has, however, some very puzzling features, as discussed below.

Lipofuscin in general

This is the age-pigment *par excellence*. It is fairly ubiquitous, having been detected in neurons, the adrenal cortex, the myocardium, and other tissues, including the RPE (see Weale 1989*b*). It is usually detected by its fluorescence, though pigments containing it have also been identified by visual inspection. Sohal and Wolfe (1986) go so far as to say that the 'accretion of lipofuscin is the only consistent age-related morphological alteration detected thus far'. This appears to have been negated in a recent study of RPE cells in tissue culture. When such cells are fed daily with isolated bovine rod outer segments, auto-fluorescent granules were found to accumulate within them within a fortnight. (Boulton *et al.* 1989). The number increased with that of rod doses until the experiment was terminated after three months. One cannot be certain that the accumulated substance is, in fact, lipofuscin, because vitamin E, an antioxidant known to slow down the accumulation of the pigment, failed to do so in these experiments.

However, the pigment is not a single substance; like a chameleon, it tends to reflect its environment: we noted that its constitution may differ even within the retina (Bazan *et al.* 1990). Its mature form exhibits some relatively widespread characteristics, and Sohal and Wolfe defined it as 'a membrane-bound lysosomal organelle, which contains lipoidal moieties, exhibits yellow to brown coloration, emits yellow to greenish autofluorescence under ultraviolet light, and accumulates progressively in the cytoplasm with age under normal physiological conditions'. 'Brown' is not really a scientific designation, but absorption spectra of intact lipofuscin granules have been measured (Boulton *et al.* 1990). They exhibit a limited spectral variation of the absorbance, given, so far, only in arbitrary units (Fig. 3.15). The pigment is absent from fetal cells.

These authors have also measured its fluorescence (Fig. 3.16). The excitation spectra extend for young retinae and also for those over 50 years old from the ultraviolet B to the blue-green part of the spectrum, with a peak at approximately 480 nm. The emission spectra are almost invariant with age, the oldest group revealing a fluorogen emitting at approximately 480 nm in addition to an original one peaking at 580–590 nm. This would suggest that the subjective appearance of yellowish fluorescence in young and middle-aged lipofuscin granules is replaced by a yellowish-green in older ones; in point of fact, Wing *et al.* (1978) and Weiter *et al.* (1986) report the opposite. Sohal and Wolfe (1986) believe that yellow fluorescence is characteristic of the *in vitro* situation, and the fact that the recent work shows blue fluorescence in addition to yellow-green, and especially so in older RPE cells is surely noteworthy.

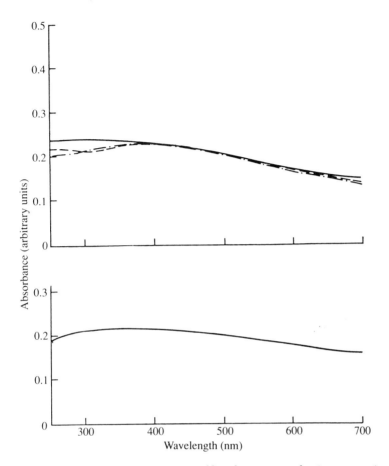

Fig. 3.15 Absorbance (arbitrary units) of lipofuscin granules in suspension as a function of wavelength. Top, L1; bottom L2. Note that the distinction between these types is based on their fluorescence emission spectra (Fig. 3.16). Top: —— = 5–29 years; ------ = 30–49 years; -.-.- = > 50 years. After Boulton *et al.* (1990).

It is not known whether these phenomena occur also *in vivo*. If they do, then it would be doubly unfortunate that the results are not expressed in absolute units. For not only is it impossible to estimate the quantum efficiency of the process, but its significance, if any, for measurements of retinal sensitivity (p. 227) also cannot be assessed.

The genesis of the pigment has received attention, and the present view is that it is formed as a result of the auto-phagocytosis of cytoplasmic material. This is almost certainly true of the RPE, because partly phagocytosed parts of photo-

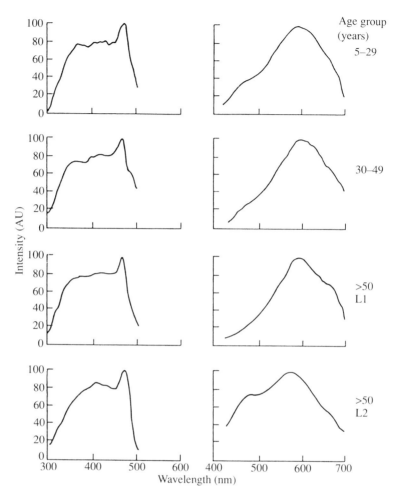

Fig. 3.16 Spectra for fluorescence excitation (left) and emission (right) of intact L1 and L2 lipofuscin granules. Excitation and emission relate to wavelengths of 364 nm and 570 nm, respectively. All intensity scales are expressed in relative units. After Boulton *et al.* (1990).

receptor outer limbs can often be seen in ultramicroscopic sections of RPE cells. The above experiment on the genesis of fluorogenic granules in tissue culture supports this. Sohal and Wolfe describe the process of formation in some detail, and believe that oxidative molecular damage, resulting from free radicals derived from free oxygen is important. Hence the above-mentioned role of vitamin E.

The pigment has been seen as a sign of stress (Aloj Totaro *et al.* 1986), and linked to diet (Mann and Yates 1982), notably in the presence of vitamin E (Katz *et al.* 1984). Sohal and Wolfe's unreserved espousal of lipofuscin as an age-pigment may well be due to their neglect of the literature on the RPE, for this may cast it in the role more nearly that of a calendar than that of a biomarker. But before we consider this, brief attention has to focus on melanin, the other pigment, already mentioned.

Melanin

As its name implies, melanin is black. Analytically, this is misleading since, given a sufficient concentration, any pigment may give the subjective sensation of blackness. Melanin is found in both the RPE and frequently in the choroid, where it appears to fulfil the function of reducing light scatter within the eye. (It is also found in other parts of the body and the eye, such as hair, skin, the iris, etc.). It is sometimes classed with age-pigments, although the correlation with age is negative: as is well known from the example of hair, melanin tends to vanish with time.

In addition to having studied the spectrometry of lipofuscin, Boulton *et al.* (1990) examined that of melanin (Fig. 3.17). During early childhood there appears to be in progress a transformation leading to the reduction and ultimate elimination of an absorption band at or below 270 nm. Melanin also fluoresces, but the variation with age of both its excitation and its emission spectra (Fig. 3.18) is much more complicated than that of lipofuscin. It is clear that the above

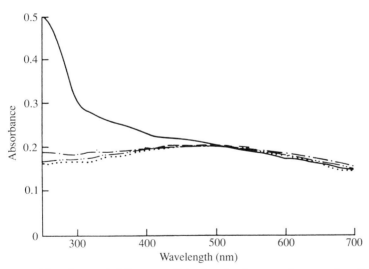

Fig. 3.17 Absorbance (arbitrary units) of melanin granules as a function of wavelength. ——— = fetal; -.-.- = 5–29 years; –··–··– = 30–49 years; ⋯⋯ = > 50 years. After Boulton *et al.* (1990).

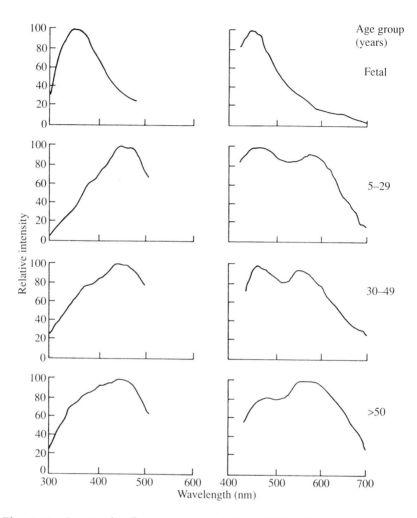

Fig. 3.18 Spectra for fluorescence excitation (left) and emission (right) of melanin granules. Conditions as for Fig. 3.16. After Boulton *et al.* (1990).

stricture regarding the universality of the word 'blackness' is borne out by the difference between the fetal and later excitation spectra respectively (which all relate to black material), when one recalls that excitation is contingent on the absorption of radiation. If different substances look alike, then colour cannot be a useful distinguishing characteristic. There is good reason to believe that different substances are involved, but that they are linked conceptually by their high absorbances.

The distribution of the pigments in the RPE

Neither of the pigments is distributed uniformly throughout the RPE, and the amounts of both follow different age-related courses (Wing *et al.* 1978; Feeney-Burns *et al.* 1984; Schmidt and Peisch 1986; Weiter *et al.* 1986). Their concentrations vary approximately inversely with each other, both temporally and spatially. Figure 3.19 shows this for measurements at apical or basal spots, each point representing a given site; no distinction is made between RPE from Caucasian or negroid eyes (Weiter *et al.* 1986). The reason is that melanin differs for a given age with ethnic group only in its choroidal, but not in its epithelial concentration. The independence of epithelial pigmentation from that of the iris was demonstrated for all ages by Schmidt and Peisch.

The above-mentioned age-related decrease of melanin is accompanied by an increase in lipofuscin, but this is only true in outline. The decrease in melanin appears to be monotonic, whereas the accumulation of lipofuscin is biphasic

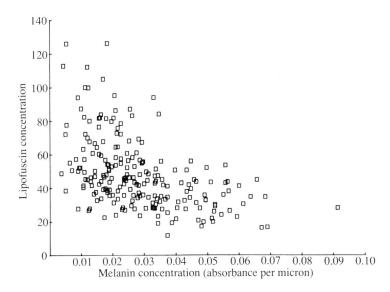

Fig. 3.19   The concentration of lipofuscin (expressed in terms of fluorescence) as a function of that of melanin (in terms of optical density). The points were obtained from five sites per eye (the fovea, two equatorial regions, and two parafoveal areas) and eyes of different age groups. Melanin concentration was derived from apical and basal transmissivities converted into extinction coefficients, and expressed as absorbance per micron. Lipofuscin concentration was measured on the same sections and at the same cell spots as for melanin, and derived from data on fluorescence. After Weiter *et al.* (1986).

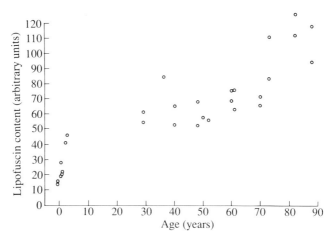

Fig. 3.20 Lipofuscin content of the whole retinal pigment epithelium as a function of age. After Wing *et al.* (1978).

(Fig. 3.20). Moreover, Feeney-Burns *et al.* (1984) showed that there are differences in the rates of increase and decrease of the two pigments respectively in the retinal periphery, which makes it unlikely that there is some form of interconvertibility between the two.

Lipofuscin   The data of Wing *et al.* (1978) show that there is a rapid accumulation of lipofuscin during the first two decades of life. According to Weiter *et al.* (1986), its rate of accumulation is greater in Caucasian than in negroid eyes. The spurt is followed by a quiescent plateau of some 30 years' duration, after which the rise is resumed, albeit at a slower rate than at the start. These results, obtained by auto-fluorescence, were confirmed in detail by Feeney-Burns *et al.* (1984) with cell counts. The results raise the question of how a substance that accumulates at its greatest rate in infancy, childhood, and early adulthood can come by the epithet of 'age-pigment'.

The inverse relationship between melanin and lipofuscin extends, as we noted, also to their spatial distribution. The latter peaks approximately in the central part of the retina (Fig. 3.21), tailing off toward the periphery. Conversely, melanin is sparse in the centre (Fig. 3.22), but increases nearer the equator. Note that both sets of authors observed an indentation in the peak of lipofuscin; this is mirrored by a peak in the trough of melanin.

Both Wing *et al.* (1978) and Weiter *et al.* (1986) suggest that the accumulation of lipofuscin has a photic origin. In support of this they quote that its spatial distribution is paralleled by that of the rods. However, this drops to zero in the region of the central dip of lipofuscin (Figs 3.21 and 3.22) and the probes used in the measurement of its concentration were small enough to detect a zero if

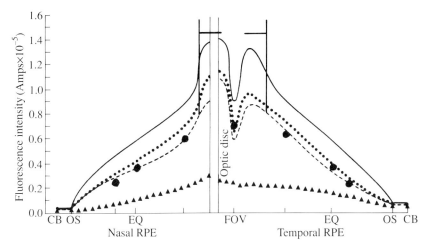

Fig. 3.21 The distribution of lipofuscin (fluorescence) as a function of retinal position. CB: ciliary body; OS: ora serrata; EQ: equator; FOV: fovea. Curves in increasing order of height are for 0, 1, 30, 60 and 88 years. After Wing *et al.* (1978). The spots indicate the distribution of light passing through the normal pupil aperture and the lenticular nucleus. The two vertical lines indicate the angular part of the retina (α) illuminated on the assumption outlined in Fig. 3.26 (see Fig. 3.24). After Weale (1989b).

it exists. The authors postulate the long-term effects of light, acting presumably directly on the RPE, may produce free radicals which, in turn, may generate lipofuscin granules.

The explanation of the temporal changes is confined to the rapid early rise (Fig. 3.20), and leans ingeniously on the age-related yellowing of the crystalline lens discussed on p. 92. In particular, Weiter *et al.* believe that the build-up of lipofuscin is due to irradiation by a wave-band in the range of 295−400 nm. The accumulation stops because the young crystalline lens absorbs more and more of this wave-band thereby progressively reducing actinic radiation actually reaching the RPE. The dip in the lipofuscin peak is similarly due to the presence of the macular pigment (but see above for a possible role played by rods).

To what extent can this attractively simple qualitative hypothesis be quantified? There is, for example, no evidence that the macular pigment absorbs appreciably at the short wavelengths tentatively held to be responsible for lipofuscin accumulation. Again, radiation cannot act on the RPE unless the latter absorbs it, and the above authors have not quoted any absorption spectrum that could represent the requisite mechanism. Although the arbitrary units of the absorption spectra of lipofuscin obtained by Boulton *et al.* do not help much in this respect, there does not appear to be any significantly heavier absorption at

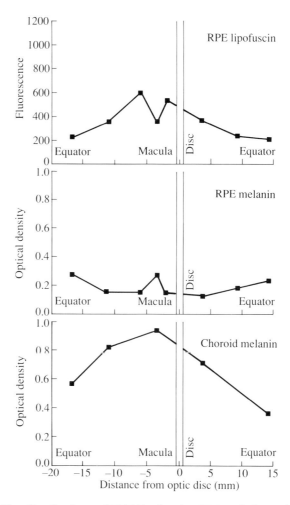

Fig. 3.22 The distributions of RPE lipofuscin, RPE and choroidal melanin at various distances (mm) from the optic disc (average for all ages studied). For units of measurement see Fig. 3.19. After Weiter *et al.* (1986).

short than at long wavelengths (Fig. 3.15). Furthermore, Lerman and Borkman's data for lens absorption referred to by Weiter *et al.* were obtained under unspecified conditions (see p. 94) which render their applicability uncertain.

The necessary radiometric requirements underlying even a tentative comparison between the above experimental data and their hypothetical photic origin were recently set out (Weale 1989*b*). It is necessary to adopt a working model

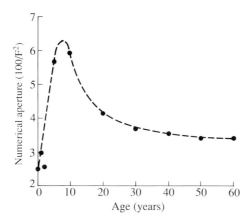

Fig. 3.23 The variation of the numerical aperture of the human light-adapted eye as a function of age. Note how a relatively large pupil and small eyeball conspire to produce a peak in early life.

for daylight, the individual radiations of which are modified on their transit to the RPE. On the physiological side, it is not sufficient to consider only the spectrometric properties of the lens. It has been noted (Fig. 2.1) that the pupillary diameter undergoes systematic age-related changes which need to be taken into account. Even this involves some simplification, because the light-gathering power of the eye is not controlled only by the pupillary area but rather by the ocular aperture, which depends also on the focal length of the eye. Note that its variation with age, as calculated from published age-related values for the daylight pupillary area and the power of the eye, reaches a maximum in childhood (Fig. 3.23).

Finally, some assumption has to be made as regards the efficacy of any hypothetical mechanism which would absorb some postulated band of radiation. If the latter is held to range from UVC to UVA (see above), then such a mech-anism has to be shown to absorb in that range. Weale considered the visual pigments contained in photo-receptors, the 'blue light hazard' (Sliney 1983), retinene (one of the products of bleaching the rod pigment rhodopsin) and retinol (vitamin A1) in turn. For every decade, a calculation was made of the relative amount of the daylight incident on the cornea which reached the retina and was then absorbed by one of the four above substances. The relevant cumulants are shown in Fig. 3.24, where they are compared with postnatal increases in the data due to Wing *et al.* (1978) and Feeney-Burns *et al.* (1984). The curve for cones, which would lie to the right of that for rods, is not shown; note that an increasing effect of lens absorbance moves curves to the left. Consequently the overall photopic sensitivity is affected less than is the curve calculated just for rods.

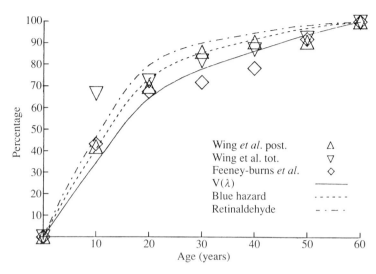

Fig. 3.24 A comparison between the experimental data of Wing *et al.* (1978) and Feeney-Burns *et al.* (1984), and cumulants based on the age-related variation of retinal illumination. POST refers to the posterior pole of the retina, TOT to the total retina. The three parametric curves assume absorption mechanisms of radiation involving the cones, the complex mediating the 'blue' hazard, and retinaldehyde respectively. After Weale (1991a).

The cumulants offer a tentative description of the experimental data on the basis that radiation is indeed responsible for the accumulation of lipofuscin. But they do this only for the first phase, and it is clear that one cannot distinguish in favour of any one of the above mechanisms rather than another.

For more than a decade, the second phase of lipofuscin accumulation was all but ignored. In 1989, two explanations were put forward to account for it. Dorey *et al.* (1989) compared numbers of photoreceptor cells with those of the over-lying RPE cells. Whereas, as noted earlier (p. 129), the former remained approximately constant in Caucasian, but not in negroid, retinae, the latter fell systematically in the macular, paramacular, and equatorial regions by under 50 per cent throughout life. The RPE of Caucasians again fared better than did that of negroes. In general, the number of photoreceptors to survive was found to vary inversely with the concentration of lipofuscin, even though the coefficient of correlation appears to be boosted by two relatively isolated points (Fig. 3.25).

The authors stress that the greatest lipofuscin accumulation was observed in the regions most sparsely occupied by photoreceptors, even though the latter did not vary with age. The RPE in some retinae would have more lipofuscin than would be expected on the basis of their age; this correlated with a low

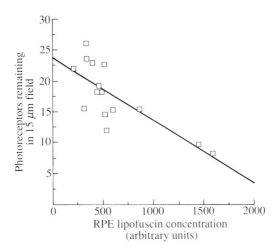

Fig. 3.25 The number of photoreceptors seen in a 15 μm field as a function of the concentration of the lipofuscin concentration in the retinal pigment epithelium. Each point is the mean of six independent observations in the macular area of one eye. After Dorey *et al.* (1989).

photoreceptor count. They conclude that the accumulation of lipofuscin leads to the loss of photoreceptors, and not vice versa, and see support for this in the observation of Katz *et al.* (1986) who found that there was less lipofuscin in dystrophic retinae of rats than in normal ones.

This leads to the authors' explanation of phase 2 in the amount of lipofuscin. Having shown that RPE cells decrease significantly, they introduce the idea of the phagocytic load. This is measured by the ratio of photoreceptor cells to those of the RPE that serve them phagocytically. It is evident that this load increases with age; the fewer RPE cells to survive, the larger the number of photo-receptors that will foist their debris onto them. This will increase the amount of lipofuscin granules per surviving RPE cell. It is, however, not proven that it will also lead to a greater total amount of lipofuscin, which one is led to expect on the basis of Figs 3.20 and 3.22, and which would be needed to explain the resumed accumulation of lipofuscin. After all, Dorey *et al.* do not claim that the RPE cell losses are confined to the over-50s; indeed, their negative linear regression starts at birth.

A problem attendant on Dorey *et al.*'s hypothesis relates to their under-standing of Katz *et al.*'s work on the retinae of dystrophic rats. These authors do not seem to imply that the retinae are abnormal because they lack lipofuscin, and that one would have to deduce from this that the tissues should be dys-trophic. On the contrary, their arguments underline the fact that the lack of functional photoreceptors, and the consequential absence of phagocytosis, lead to a sparseness of lipofuscin. This is supported by observations that vitamin A and lipofuscin concentration are related (Katz *et al.* 1987). The RPE of rats fed a high vitamin A diet was found to contain more lipofuscin than was true of those receiving a low one.

The authors found that 'When retinas lacking photoreceptors due either to light damage or to a genetic defect were studied, it was discovered that RPE lipofuscin deposition was substantially reduced . . . It thus appeared likely that components of the photoreceptor outer segments were being converted into RPE lipofuscin fluorophores. Strong support for this hypothesis came from studies on the RCS [Royal College of Surgeons] rat. In this rat strain, the ability of the RPE to take up shed outer segment components is severely impaired, so that these components accumulate above the apical surface of the RPE. A lipofuscin-like autofluorescence was found to develop in this material, providing the most direct evidence available that components of the outer segments can be directly converted into RPE lipofuscin fluorophores'.

These observations are reconcilable with those of Dorey *et al.* with an additional hypothesis, namely that lipofuscin, once formed, stays put. The inverse relation between photoreceptors and lipofuscin mentioned by these authors could be due, not to lipofuscin causing loss, but resulting from it: where many photoreceptors survive, little undisposed of debris will have been formed, and, conversely, where there is a lot of lipofuscin, not many photoreceptors will remain.

The other hypothesis attempting to account for the late rise in lipofuscin accumulation is based on the notion that, like the early phase, the late one may be linked to radiation. It may well be asked how this may occur when, as we saw, the yellowing lens effectively plugs the pupil and prevents the entry of actinic light, as postulated by Weiter *et al.* (1986). It will be recalled that, in addition to the lenticular nucleus becoming progressively yellower, the ageing lens continues to grow. However, this means that the colourless cortex increases, thereby unplugging the pupil (Weale 1989*b*). Figure 3.26 shows that a cylindrical corridor is formed parallel to the ocular axis; its height ultimately causes the circumferential area through which slanting rays may enter the eye to become equivalent to an additional pupil, to wit one that is not obstructed by a filter absorbing short-wavelength (UVA) radiations.

Rays A and B indicate the limiting angles of the pencils of light that may enter the eye, and strike the RPE. A fraction is reflected. With the progressive loss of melanin (Fig. 3.27) this is going to increase. Although the inside of the eye is not a mirror, even diffuse reflexion becomes more nearly specular as the angle of incidence increases. The rays C and D show the extent of the posterior pole covered by this secondary illumination; C' is shown for the sake of symmetry. Hence the total extent so illuminated is described by the angle α which equals roughly 60 degrees. But this is the angle α indicated in Fig. 3.21. This suggests that the general pattern of accumulation is given by the inverted cup shape shown

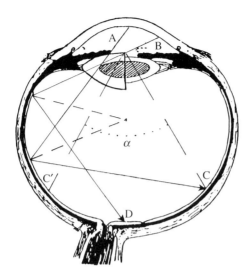

Fig. 3.26 A hypothetical scheme showing how the posterior pole of the eye may be illuminated by short-wavelength radiations which pass through the lenticular cortex without traversing the absorbant nucleus. After Weale (1989b).

in Fig. 3.21 by the black dots; it is due to the transnuclear illumination of the fundus. The excrescence may be due to illumination which misses the nucleus; this can happen also in earlier life as a result of oblique rays traversing only short paths in the nucleus.

Some problems remain unexplained. If phagocytosis following upon irradiation leads to the production of lipofuscin, it is surprising that measurable amounts appear to be present at birth (Wing *et al.* 1978; Feeney-Burns *et al.* 1984). Moreover, the granules occupy only a miniscule fraction of the volume of an organelle (Fig. 3.8) except in old tissue (Flood *et al.* 1984). These authors draw attention to the fact that no mitosis occurs in the RPE postnatally; yet their studies of cells in tissue culture demonstrated not only an age-related delay in proliferation both in macular and in peripheral material, but also an age-related delay in the onset of proliferation in primary cultures. This hysteresis is absent from subcultures. Flood *et al.* postulate that the senescence of the epithelial cells is attained via the action of a clock which − they claim − is lipofuscin. As cells in culture do not augment their lipofuscin content, but reduce it division by division, dilution of the pigment may be a way of rejuvenating them. Flood *et al.* do not address the problem of its biphasic accumulation, but it could be that the plateau reached during the third decade of life is a half-hearted evolutionary attempt in that sense.

It is, however, possible that none of the above hypotheses is valid and that it is not light but some systemic factor that causes the biphasic rise. Even diet may be involved. Remember that when lipofuscin was first mentioned (p. 11), attention was drawn to two relevant studies. Koistinaho *et al.* (1986) had shown that it accumulates biphasically in a variety of human nervous components, apparently without any contact, direct or indirect, with radiation. Furthermore, Mann and Yates (1982) surmised that an ethnic difference in cerebral amounts of the pigment might well be due to marked dietary differences. If this is generally valid, neither the first nor the second phase in the accumulation of RPE lipofuscin may represent anything more than events taking place in the body as a whole. It is also to be remembered that both studies, reporting the two phases and their rates, are based on tissues obtained in the USA, and probably reared and developed under the influence of dietary influences which have, in other respects, not been ideal.

However, there is a crucial test which suggests that light may, after all, play a role. Sohal and Wolfe (1986) quote observations according to which unilateral blindness causes an asymmetry in the amount of lipofuscin accumulated in the human lateral geniculate nuclei. The nucleus contralateral to the blind eye appears to contain less of the pigment than the ipsilateral one. Since the human visual system shows only partial decussation of the optic nerve fibres accurate localization of the pigment and a careful radiometric protocol (see p. 154) seem crucial. Alternatively the study needs repeating on a species in which decussation is complete.

The matter of lipofuscin has been given extended attention here not only because it is said to be an age-pigment, but also because its presence in the RPE appears to create problems of its own. Control measurements on RPE obtained from American negroes solve little if it cannot be shown that their diet differs overall from that of their Caucasian compatriots.

Melanin   Like lipofuscin, melanin can exist in different forms. For example, the absorption spectrum of melanin derived from norepinephrine has a maximum at 310 nm, whereas that derived from the RPE, like that obtained from dopa, peaks at 260 nm (Fig. 3.17). Schmidt and Peisch (1986) carried out an analysis of solubilized melanin obtained from eyes ranging in age from 14 to 97 years, and separated according to its derivation from macular, mid-peripheral, and far peripheral cells of the RPE. No post-mortem reduction in its concentration was observed over 24 hours. In marked contrast to what happens with lipofuscin (p. 153), melanin in the central retinal region showed no significant variation with age (Fig. 3.27). However, a systematic decline was observed outside this area.

It is generally accepted that the presence of melanin in the choroid is an evolutionary adaptation for the protection of the fundus against a surfeit of radiation. From this point of view, the presence of the pigment in the RPE may

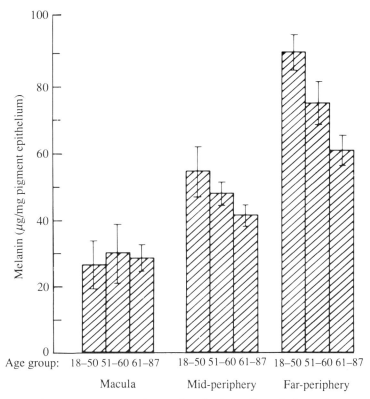

Fig. 3.27 Average concentrations of melanin collected from three regions of the retinal pigment epitheliums for three age groups (n = 5, 4, and 7 respectively). After Schmidt and Peisch (1986).

seem superfluous. But Ulshafer *et al.* (1990) have suggested that it may act as a scavenger of heavy metal ions. It will be recalled (p. 29) that these may be involved in DNA, RNA, and protein synthesis (Eichhorn 1979). Transported through the bloodstream, some of them may bind to functional groups of proteins and act as toxins in sufficient concentration. The RPE acts as a blood—retinal barrier (p. 145), and its melanin may fulfil a role as a sink for such hazards.

Weiter *et al.* (1986) have observed that, whereas Caucasian and negroid RPEs contain similar amounts of melanin, age for age, there is a 1:2 difference in the choroidal quantities. They explain this on the basis of embryological derivation. The choroid is derived from the neural crest and, like hair and the anterior part of the iris, shows marked interethnic variations. The RPE is, however, derived from the neuro-epithelium which provides melanin for parts of the central nervous system not generally in need of protection from environmental radiation; its concentration is, therefore, relatively constant.

3.9 Non-visual effects of visible radiation

3.9.1 *Blood flow and light*

Attention was drawn earlier to the possibility of confusion between age-related effects and cumulative results due to the environment (p. 112), the accumulation of lipofuscin (p. 160) providing a typical example. The situation is complicated not only by our ignorance of the many issues involved, but also by the fact that the results of acute phenomena in the medium and long term cannot as yet be assessed.

The effect of light on the retinal blood flow is a case in point. The laser Doppler technique was used for the purpose. It involves the imaging of discrete retinal vessels, and an analysis of the light scattered by blood flowing through them. A frequency-modulated light signal before incidence on the vessels will be modulated by an amount that is a function of the speed of blood flow since it has been shown that the major vessels dilate by only 2−3 per cent after dark adaptation; consequently it is the speed of the flow, and not its volume, that is the determining factor. Once well-controlled conditions are established, it is possible to demonstrate the synchrony of a retinal arterial signal, as expressed by the maximum Doppler frequency shift, with the separately recorded cardiac cycle (Feke *et al.* 1983).

In each of three subjects (aged 22, 28, and 33 years) the first 30 seconds of dark adaptation were followed by a well-marked rise of some 40 per cent in retinal blood flow. The use of different light intensities made it also possible to demonstrate a close correlation between blood flow, and oxygen consumption and photoreceptor response.

Since the elderly eye admits to its retina at most one third of the light admitted by the younger eye, it is likely that the change in blood flow due to the above effect is reduced in the elderly by some 10 per cent. On its own, such an effect may be unimportant; whether it helps to tip the balance in some adverse manner in conjunction with other reduced performances is unknown.

3.9.2 *Photic hazards*

There is no reason to consider here such well-known traumata as retinal burns resulting from solar irradiation: they have no specifically age-related interest, except that one has to guard against them all one's life. However, the so-called 'blue light' hazard is in a different category since it results from weaker intensities, notwithstanding the link between it and solar retinal burns (Ham *et al.* 1979).

Rhesus monkeys were studied with well-calibrated stimuli of two types, namely laser lines in the range of 441.6–514.5 nm and 610–1064 nm, respectively. Both the macular and extra-macular regions were stimulated with variable intensities so that objectively determined thresholds for identifiable changes could be established both for the RPE and the neural retina. It was found that the short-wavelength group of stimuli caused relatively mild reparable lesions both in the RPE and the photoreceptors. Melanosomes were phago-cytosed by macrophages that had invaded the RPE, presumably from the reticulo-endothelial system. The outer limbs of the photoreceptors later revealed some disorientation of the constituent lamellae. However, after some 30 days repair was complete. This so-called photochemical damage had an action spectrum similar to the absorption spectrum of melanin (Fig. 3.17).

By contrast, the result of irradiation with the long-wavelength laser lines was irreversible thermal damage. The authors deduce from temperature measure-ments that solar retinitis cannot be wholly due to classical burns because the rise in temperature (approximately 3 °C) is too low to achieve them; and that there must be a significant element of the above-mentioned photochemical damage.

These studies have not established whether there are cumulative responses to subthreshold stimuli (but see p. 183). In any case, both *ad hoc* studies and statistical gerontological investigations may be vitiated by a subject's un-recorded photic history. For example, children who had been infants in inten-sive care for treatment of neonatal jaundice, and therefore exposed to light intensities amounting to several thousand lux, may suffer from several modifi-cations of normal visual functions (Abramov *et al*. 1985). They involve cones, with increased thresholds appearing in a marked way for short-wave-length stimuli. There is also a loss in contrast sensitivity, notably for high spatial frequencies. This is somewhat puzzling because the latter are mediated essentially by cones responding to long wavelengths. This apparent incon-sistency apart, and granting that the retinal illumination studied was high, the results suggest that retinal modifications due to ambient radiation may well start to occur at an early age.

It may be recalled in this connection that synthetic (dopa) melanin can be bleached by visible light (Sealy *et al*. 1984). Melanin produces free radicals even in the dark. Irradiation with a wavelength of 544 nm reversibly increases the steady-state free radical concentration. The effect is greatly augmented in the presence of Rose Bengal (RB) which has an absorption peak at 544 nm, and an absorbance at this wavelength 7.5 times greater than that of melanin. The two compounds are unlikely to be bound to each other, yet RB is an effective sensitizer of the production of free radicals, its potency increasing at shorter wavelengths.

An increase in oxygen consumption by melanin was also demonstrated in these conditions. In aerated solutions, RB was destroyed and melanin bleached. Moreover, the production of free radicals became irreversible.

The retinal parallel with this scenario may be only superficial but is none-theless compelling. Melanin in the pigment epithelium may be sensitized by the proximal visual pigments which absorb light in much the same spectral region as does RB. The concentration of the pigment is known to diminish with advancing years (or cumulative exposures to light), and there is no denying that the retina would perish in the absence of oxygen. Sealy *et al.* may have unwittingly spelled out a transformatiion of retinal tissues, the age-related attributes of which may be a mere accident.

Repair processes which depend on DNA synthesis may likewise be modified by exposure to ultraviolet radiation (Fig. 1.6), even if it masquerades as sunlight (Parsons and Hayward 1985), and the pigmentation of human cells containing melanin provides protection which has been detailed by Musk and Parsons (1987). Previous attempts to demonstrate it had failed because of low melanin concentrations and the use of only UVC. Melanin was found to protect its host cells both from sunlight and UVB. While the penetration of the latter to the retina is much attenuated by lenticular absorption in the elderly, this constraint may not operate in the young eye so that the ground may be prepared in some cases for future complications.

That the link between the latter and irradiation is still highly speculative transpires from Andley's review (1987). Although a variety of possible mech-anisms potentially causing retinal lesions is considered, at the time of writing the conclusion was that 'the photochemical mechanism(s) by which light absorption leads to observable lesions in the retina and loss of visual sensitivity are not known at present, evidently reflecting the complexity of the system'. Again, Andley says that the recovery of the capacity of photoreceptors for renewal of their structural and metabolic attributes following photic damage is not established. Clinical reports seem to suggest that this is incorrect. Grey (1978) quotes several instances showing that a mild solar retinitis might be followed by an impairment of visual performance, notably insofar as concerned visual acuity, but virtually full recovery has also been reported more than once (p. 163).

3.10 Age-related macular complications

This is not primarily a clinical text, and there is no pretence that the following observations on age-related macular degeneration, to use a global term, should do any more than draw attention to its existence. It is a moot point whether the progression from retinal senescence to retinal atrophy is inexorable. If, as some of the evidence to be presented suggests, it is not, then its presence in some populations, such as Caucasians, still does not rule out quasi-physiological or even environmental causes. Indeed, the burden of epidemiological enquiry during the last two decades rests on a search of risk factors.

It is fortunate that one of the earlier studies (Sarks 1976) is a model of its kind. Rare, in that it combines clinical observations with subsequent histological analyses, it is based on a sufficiently large number of cases to permit one to form a credible picture of the progression of this frustrating condition. Essentially, there are six approximately consecutive groups (in an Australian population). The earliest, extending over the first six decades of life, is free from any sign in the RPE. The second, coincident with the next decade, is liable to show patchy basal linear deposits in the RPE, some hyalinization in Bruch's membrane and/or the choriocapillaris, and a few cases with disturbed pigmentation in the RPE. In Group III, there is a decreased visual acuity, the basal linear deposit, while still thin, is no longer patchy, and hyalinization and loss of pigmentation increase. This course continues in Group IV, but in Groups V and VI (80–89, 90+years) visual loss is complete, the basal linear deposit is liable to form part of a scar, and geographical atrophy is frequently followed by disciform degeneration.

The study was imitated by Hoshino and Mizuno in 1982 on a somewhat smaller Japanese population, a paper on the same material being subsequently published in English (Hoshino *et al.* 1984). Rather remarkably, the condition appears to be less virulent than in Australia, and seems to start later in life, which is doubly remarkable in that the Japanese have the longer life expectancy (see Weale 1985*b*). However, as iris pigmentation is one of the established risk factors (Hyman *et al.* 1983), it may be recalled that the prevalence of blue irides is probably greater amongst Australians than the Japanese.

The relevance of pigmentation, either in its photic role or in the biochemical protection afforded by melanin (p. 160), has not been discussed by Hoshino *et al.*, which is all the more remarkable since they mention the study by Gregor and Joffe (1978) on black Africans. These workers observed that the incidence of age-related macular changes was amongst that indigenous population less than half of the value noted for an age-matched Caucasian sample studied in London. Disciform degeneration, associated with stage VI in Sarks' classification, was virtually non-existent amongst the Africans, much as it is rare amongst the Japanese. Although Gregor and Joffe do not rule out some effect due to sampling, for example arising from a certain amount of self-selection in the African population, it is unlikely that the vast difference between Africans and Caucasians is an artefact.

This opinion is reinforced by the results of a retrospective analysis of patients who had visited any one of 34 Baltimore ophthalmologists in the late 1970s (Hyman *et al.* 1983). A number of significant risk factors were established. There appears to be some familial influence; cardiovascular complications, exposure to non-specific chemical reagents and smoking cigarettes (males only) correlated positively. However, the most interesting correlate in the present context related to iris colour. Only for brown eyes was the odds ratio (95 per cent confidence limits) equal to 1.0. Both for 'medium' pigmented and for (light) blue irides the odds ratio was 3.6 and 3.5 respectively. Wu (1987) failed to find any link between iris colour and maculopathy in over 1000 patients examined in different parts in China, but gave no indication of any distribution of iris colour in his sample.

The relation between age-related macular degeneration and ocular pigmentation was elaborated by Weiter *et al.* (1985). They found a significant correlation between iris colour and fundal pigmentation, and between iris and hair colour and the presence of age-related macular degeneration. However, their tentative link between macular degeneration and putative light damage is unsupported by a retrospective epidemiological study on over 1200 watermen resident on the East coast of the USA (West *et al.* 1989*b*). The subjects' ocular condition was related to their cumulative exposure to UVA and UVB radiation, and also to work history and dermatological findings as established by personal interview and clinical inspection.

The results showed that there was no statistically significant link between age-related macular changes and exposure either to UVA or to UVB. However, a more recent analysis (Muñoz *et al.* 1990), also based on a study of watermen working on the Chesapeake Bay, showed that a statistically significant correlation ($p = 0.04$) was found to exist between reported exposure to both blue (400–500 nm) and white (400–800 nm) daylight under certain conditions. In the first place, it held if only the more severe age-related macular conditions were taken into account; these would include the presence of disciform scars, i.e. correspond to the final degree of Sarks' classification. Secondly, the crucial period of exposure was confined to the last 20 years of a patient's history. It is therefore noteworthy that the time of great risk parallels a period when the retina might be thought to be relatively well protected by an absorbing lens at least from short-wavelength radiations, but the authors state, of course, that their observation holds for both the above spectral ranges.

West *et al.* (1989*a*) also showed that smoking was associated with a decreased risk of age-related macular changes. As nicotine is held to play a protective role both in Parkinson's and in Alzheimer's diseases, it does not follow thus from their observation that smoking should be advocated: if it were shown conclusively to be beneficial to any or all of these conditions it would probably be possible to devise a topical application which does not involve tarring of the lungs.

It has been suggested more than once that the high prevalence of cataract amongst pigmented populations may protect them from the alleged photic aetiology of age-related macular dystrophies (for example Jain *et al.* 1984). It is therefore important to note that West *et al.* found an association between ultraviolet light and cortical cataract, and that nuclear opacities were, in their sample population, significantly correlated with macular complications.

However, a closer analysis due to Sperduto *et al.* (1981), also of the data collected during the Framingham Study, shows the relation between maculopathy and cataract to be complex. The relative risk of the occurrence of a maculopathy is reduced in the presence of nuclear sclerosis at $p < 0.05$ for ages 65–85 years in right eyes, and for all ages in left eyes. However, the risk is increased in the presence of cortical opacities in the age group of 51–74 years in left eyes, but only for 52–64 years in right eyes. These results are hence consistent with the suggestion that some types of cataract could afford protection for the retina, but other rationales cannot be excluded in view of the results of studies obtained in rats.

The retinae of these animals have been known for almost three decades to be extremely sensitive to light which, insofar as concerns the human eye, falls within the physiological domain. They are liable to suffer permanent dystrophic changes, for example after a few hours' exposure to ordinary fluorescent light. However, two conditions unexpectedly offer protection from such damage. On the one hand, there is hyperthermia (Barbe *et al.* 1988), and on the other, complete water deprivation for three to seven days (O'Steen *et al.* 1990). Neither of these conditions is uncommon in India and Africa, where the prevalence of age-related maculopathies is relatively low. It does not follow from this that human retinae are, after all, sensitive to light, and the above robust experimental procedures merely mimic what circumstances ordain. The reason is that, in the rats, heat shock protein was found to be synthesized in the former study, and that the secretion of arginine vasopressin accompanied dehydration in the latter: this is an important osmoregulatory hormone, and its concentration in the human retina may be worth exploring.

It is possible that, in looking at iris colour, a number of authors may have overlooked a more significant variable. A remarkable study on the transillumination of the iris (Abrams 1964) shows that the tissue is frequently perforated. This is revealed by perpendicular slit-lamp transillumination when the beam reflected by the fundus illuminates the rear of the iris tissue, and reveals trabeculae as red spots or slits, provided the examination is carried out in a darkened room rather than in a contemporary clinic. Abrams divided irides into five groups depending on the degree of iridal perforation; none of them was considered to be pathological. What is significant is that genuinely brown irides never showed any trabecula. Several or many were readily seen in lighter, hazel, and blue irides.

In view of the above evidence, based on epidemiology, that macular dystrophies are unlikely to be photic in origin, it would be futile to argue that a perforated iris protects the retina less well than is true of fully opaque tissue. But what may be the case is that the paucity or absence of melanin causes either tissue fragility, or perhaps an increased permeability to phagocytic agents which disrupt the iris on the one hand and the RPE on the other. It seems desirable to extend the above correlative studies between iris pigmentation and age-related macular degeneration to the quantified transillumination of the iris. This will be achieved probably most readily by a photographic procedure.

3.11 Resumé

In this chapter the line between physiological and pathological senescence has become blurred. Not only are there indications that, as is true of the lens, senescence begins in the teens if not in childhood, but for example the vascular changes noted in connection with cerebral ageing, may, if translated to the retina, cause visual problems. The relation to the outline of theories of ageing in Chapter 1 has also subtly changed. Several of the age-related variations of cerebral attributes exhibit the type of parabolic shape which one can associate with a peak performance after maturity, and possibly co-extensive with the historic period of reproductive prowess. But this does not appear to hold at retinal level. If not monotonic, the rate of accumulation of lipofuscin does not change its sign: it stays positive. Similarly, that of melanin remains negative, as appears to be true of the concentration of the visual pigments. It may be asked whether bio-economics follow a restrictive practice, or whether, as noted in connection with the amplitude of accommodation, there is more than one way of saving biological cash.

4. Senescent vision

4.1 Introduction

The main emphasis in this chapter is on an attempt to assess how the advancing years affect an individual's visual performance. This may take many forms. It can involve merely the awareness of the presence of a visual stimulus. It may be concerned with the differentiation of one stimulus from another, for example, by intensity, spatial location, temporal extension, spectral composition, etc. Many of these variables can now be assessed also by objective means. However, this book is concerned with the senescence of vision rather than that of physiological responses, which is why this chapter is devoted to subjective investigations. Much of it is based on the information given in previous chapters, as it is important to try to establish to what extent, if any, age-related changes in sensory performance are explicable on the basis of relatively simple physical and physiological concepts. More than that, many past misunderstandings of processes of senescence can be attributed to the omission of this fundamental analytical step. No one is likely to avoid such mishaps altogether, but perhaps it is an advance to be aware of the danger.

In this connection it may be helpful to link observations to some basic model. In default of a theoretical framework, an empirical formulation may not come amiss. Quantitative sensory tests involving stimulus as a variable are usually characterized by two features: there is a threshold which has to be exceeded for a response to be recorded at the lower end of the intensity range, and ultimately there is a limiting response which cannot be exceeded no matter how much the stimulus is increased. At this point the response is said to saturate. In general, two constants may suffice in this connection also when a constant other than saturation is considered, as is illustrated below.

Responses can be measured in objective experiments, for example, in terms of the amount of some substance released as a result of stimulation, or when a current is passed in a nerve fibre, etc. But in subjective studies, conventionally measurements are made of a set of stimuli leading to a constant response or to some criterion change in response.

It is of interest to try to apply such a model to senescence, in particular to determine to what extent, if any, it can be used for a distinction between the above mentioned physical or peripheral factors and other more central ones. Since subjective responses are verbal or quasi-verbal they subsume cognitive mechanisms: if these are affected by processes of ageing in larger measure than is true of the peripheral ones, then one asks whether the model can isolate them even though they have no known metric.

The empirical relation between a just noticeable incremental stimulus $\Delta\mathbf{I}$ and the stimulus $\mathbf{I}$ in excess of the relevant threshold to be used here can be derived, for example, from the logistic function, namely

$$\mathbf{R}/\mathbf{R(max)} = 1/[1 + (\mathbf{K}/\mathbf{I})^\mathbf{p}] \tag{4.1}$$

where $\mathbf{K}$ and $\mathbf{p}$ are constants. $\mathbf{R}$ is the response, not amenable to measurement in sensory (subjective) experiments, and $\mathbf{R(max)}$ its putative maximum value. When $\mathbf{R}$ is differentiated with respect to $\mathbf{I}$ and finite differences are substituted for infinitesimally small ones,

$$\Delta\mathbf{R} = (\Delta\mathbf{I})[(\mathbf{p}.\mathbf{R(max)})/\mathbf{I}](\mathbf{K}/\mathbf{I})^\mathbf{p}/[1 + (\mathbf{K}/\mathbf{I})^\mathbf{p}]^2 \tag{4.2}$$

The conventional assumption is that for a differential threshold $\Delta\mathbf{R}$ is constant. Hence

$$1/\Delta\mathbf{I} = [(\mathbf{p}.\mathbf{R(max)}/\Delta\mathbf{R}.\mathbf{I})].(\mathbf{K}/\mathbf{I})^\mathbf{p}/[1 + (\mathbf{K}/\mathbf{I})^\mathbf{p}]^2 \tag{4.3}$$

When $\mathbf{I}$ is very large

$$\Delta\mathbf{I} = [(\Delta\mathbf{R}\mathbf{I})/(\mathbf{p}\mathbf{R(max)}](\mathbf{I}/\mathbf{K})^\mathbf{p} \tag{4.4}$$

But when $\mathbf{I}$ is very small

$$\Delta\mathbf{I} = [\Delta\mathbf{R}/(\mathbf{p}\mathbf{R(max)})].\mathbf{K}.(\mathbf{K}/\mathbf{I})^{(1 - \mathbf{p})} \tag{4.5}$$

If $\mathbf{p} \cong 1$, eqn 4.4 shows that the incremental threshold $\Delta\mathbf{I}$ increases with the square of the stimulus strength: the differential threshold becomes very large indeed, and the response $\mathbf{R}$ is said to saturate. On the other hand, with $\mathbf{p} \cong 1$, eqn 4.5 shows that $\Delta\mathbf{I}$ tends to be constant for very small values of $\mathbf{I}$. Both this feature and the tendency for $\Delta\mathbf{I}$ to rise to very high values when the stimulus intensity is high have been repeatedly verified (Barlow 1957; Hess *et al.* 1990).

The function (eqn 4.1) which is shown in Fig. 4.1 can be modified in various ways, and is introduced here merely to indicate hypothetical changes resulting from a system which ages. For example, it is akin to other psychometric functions discussed by Harvey (1986).

In Fig. 4.1(a) the maximum response $\mathbf{R(max)}$ may diminish with age. In other words, $\mathbf{R(max)}$ acts as a scaling factor for the ordinate. Conversely, the maximum response may remain invariant, but a progressively greater stimulus may have to be applied for its maintenance. In this case, $\mathbf{K}$ acts as a scaling factor for the abscissa (Fig. 4.1(b)) and has the dimensions of a stimulus characterizing some physical or physiological properties of the eye: $\mathbf{K}$ acts as a scaling factor for the abscissa. Aylward *et al.* (1990) have used these ideas in an illustrative manner in a study of the age-related variation of the human electro-retinogram. While this offers a measurable response in the amplitude of

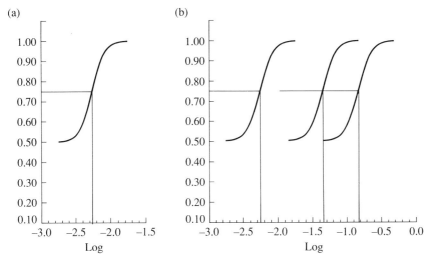

Fig. 4.1 (a) The logistic curve (eqn 4.1) describing a stimulus/response relation above chance responses, i.e. 50:50. The stimulus is given on a log scale. Age-related changes in **R(max)** leave the shape of the curve unaltered. (b) Age-related changes in the stimulus as caused by physical factors lead to a displacement of the curves. Data obtained for higher ages move progressively to the right.

its b-wave and is therefore less open to speculation than are subjective phenomena, it offers a helpful insight into the variation of peripheral parameters, which are likely to affect central responses.

It may tentatively be postulated that age-related changes in the scaling factor of the stimulus describe peripheral variables (see Aylward *et al.* 1990), whereas analogous changes in **R(max)** address non-peripheral ones. Note that, as **I** is expressed in terms of a scaling intensity **K**, it is independent of the absorption of the ocular media, provided both have the same spectral composition. Since **ΔI** is expressed as an incremental intensity, this exemption does not apply to it: it needs to be expressed in terms of quanta absorbed by the photoreceptors if age-related factors in the media and the rods and cones are not to be allowed to mask the results. Then, if the light incident on the retina is absorbed by a class of photoreceptor occupying a fraction **f** of the area illuminated, **T** is the transmissivity of the media, and the retinal absorption coefficient is α, **ΔI(ret)** = Tfα**ΔI(i)**, where **(ret)** and **(i)** refer to radiation arriving at the retina and cornea respectively. As any of the first three factors may change with age (pp. 91, 127, 136), it is material to allow for this if age-related changes in **K** are to be identified when the spectral distributions of stimulus **I** and incremental stimulus **ΔI** are different.

It has been noted above that **R** has no metric, but that its constancy may be useful. The variation, if any, of the other constants in eqn 4.1 can be examined by varying the intensity **I** of a stimulus, for example a background, and by determining the least perceptible value Δ**I** for some incremental stimulus. In the region where Δ**I** rises in proportion to **I** the well-known Weber−Fechner Law may be said to hold, but eqn 4.1 does not predict it in terms of any approximation: it appears simply in the shape of a tangent to the curve at one unique value of **I**. When eqns 4.4 and 4.5 are expressed logarithmically (the right hand side being plotted against log**I**), then **p** can be determined from the slope of the experimental results. The intercepts of both equations are equal so that a measure of **R(max)**, and its variation with age, if any, can be obtained. A relative displacement of the experimental data along the horizontal axis for different age groups means that the scaling constant of the stimulus is changed: as mentioned above, the implication would be a change in a peripheral part of the visual path.

It is surprising that the potential of some such approach for gerontological studies does not seem to have been so far recognized (but see Sloane *et al.* 1988*b*). The above concepts will be related to contrast sensitivity in section 4.7 (p. 204).

4.2 Absolute visual thresholds

Representing a limiting value of eqn 4.1, the measurement of the smallest amount of radiation that can be perceived offers an instructive, if often discussed, example. A number of requirements have to be met for this threshold quantity to be minimal, namely 5−7 quanta absorbed in rods (Hecht *et al.* 1942) and also cones (Vimal *et al.* 1989; see Arden and Weale 1954). Technical means of optimizing the observing conditions are described in detail in textbooks dealing with the physiology of vision (see Davson 1978). The majority of relevant details can be omitted here, with the exception of one, namely the control of the level of visual adaptation.

Adequate dark adaptation is an essential requirement in the measurement of the absolute visual threshold. In practice it has to proceed for about 45 minutes. If the visual threshold is measured in the course of dark adaptation, one obtains the so-called dark adaptation curve, the shape of which depends on the light exposure of the retina preceding the onset of dark adaptation.

The classical gerontological study on this topic is due to Domey and McFarland (1961). The authors and their colleagues studied 241 observers (approximately 30 in each decade) between the ages of 16 and 89 years, having exposed the right eye to a luminance of 1600 mLamberts (mL) for three minutes. The radiation was passed through a violet filter, with a transmission maximum of 405 nm, and, contrary to the view expressed by Pulos (1989), the pupillary diameter was fixed with an artificial aperture at 3 mm. Plotted for

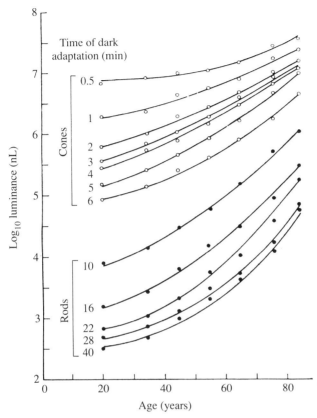

Fig. 4.2 The absolute threshold luminance levels in nanoLamberts (nL) plotted in relation to the age of the observers. The parameter is the time of dark adaptation following exposure to a luminance of 1600 mL. Open circles, cones; closed circles, rods. After Domey and MacFarland (1961).

increasing ages, the dark adaptation curves are displaced vertically upward (Fig. 4.2).

It will be recalled that the early portion of such bipartite functions is attributed to the dark adaptation of the cone mechanism, while the later is held to represent the drop in threshold of the rod mechanism. The family of curves in Fig. 4.2 shows that the age-related rise in rod thresholds is the greater of the two.

The original paper(s) made it clear that the authors were unaware of the fact that the human lens yellows with age, and that this might affect the interpretation of the results. However, it also raises some doubt about their experimental technique, an important technical point which also seems to have escaped other research workers.

The pre-adaptation exposure of 1600 mL represented a fixed physical, but a potentially variable physiological, quantity. The reason for this opinion is as follows. As the results were subsequently to demonstrate, the final absolute thresholds of the elderly were almost 250 times higher than those of the youngest group. Even the putative final cone threshold, as detailed after 5 min of dark adaptation, turned out to be more than 30 times higher for the oldest than for the youngest observers. But this implies that the physiological effect of 1600 mL on the young eyes may have been equivalent only to between 6 and 60 mL for the oldest eyes studied, with progressively higher values applying to the intervening age groups.

It would seem to follow that, whatever the explanation of the age-related changes, young and old were treated differently: the pre-adaptation regime had a much greater effect on the young than on the elderly. If this study is repeated, the level of adaptation will have to be geared to the observers' sensitivity, rather than to the ability of the light source to deliver. To achieve this, thresholds will have to be recorded for a level of adaptation, for example, comparable with the above; but the definitive runs will have to be preceded by a level of adaptation which is a fixed multiple of the threshold. Note that a satisfactory solution is likely to be found only if the cone and rod portions are treated separately, for it has been noticed that the disadvantage of the young in comparison with the elderly is more pronounced in connection with the rod than the cone mechanism.

The original data show that the second youngest group (20–29 years) has a lower threshold than the youngest with $P < 0.01$. If confirmed, this would be further evidence in favour of the view that the progression of senescence in the visual system is not monotonic, but that some sort of reversal occurs before the thresholds start to rise. Figure 4.3 compares the situation after allowance has been made for lenticular absorption: note that the rod threshold, measured after 40 min dark adaptation, tends to remain constant during the first six decades tested, once allowance is made for the increase in lenticular absorbance. However, the cone threshold, as measured after 2 min of dark adaptation, actually decreases after middle life.

It is not easy to imagine an age-related development of the visual system which would entail the considerable reduction in the threshold of the cone mechanism(s) at the highest age groups, once a correction is applied for the senescence of the light-absorbing crystalline lens. It is more likely, therefore, that the solution of this conundrum is to be found in an experimental artefact.

We have noted that radiation betweeen 360 and 420 nm can make the lens fluoresce. The stimulus used by Domey and MacFarland (1961), namely 405 nm, falls within this band. High stimulus intensities had to be used to evoke a visual sensation, particularly when it came to the cone responses of the elderly. It is here that the apparent drop in threshold is observed. Very probably these observers were responding not to the original stimulus but to the greenish

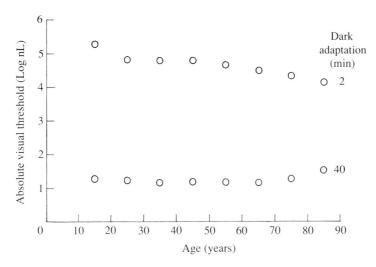

Fig. 4.3 The absolute visual threshold in log nL as a function of age. Dark adaptation of 2 minutes (top), and 40 minutes (bottom). Note that the threshold of the cones tends to fall, that of the rods to rise with advancing years.

fluorescence which it produced in the lens. This would be seen but not measured, and hence would appear as a reduction in the threshold measurement.

This problem, which is unlikely to be important when cone mechanisms are not involved, has to be guarded against whenever short wavelength stimuli are used. It is somewhat ironic that they were used originally to minimize any possible interference between rod and cone mechanisms. Indeed, Hecht and his colleagues, active around the time of the Second World War, used such stimuli specifically to stimulate only rods, or so they thought. Since then new opportunities have been created to study this important problem: younger and younger aphakic but fully functional eyes have grown in number, offering a field yet to be fully explored (see below).

One of the earliest workers to have availed themselves of this chance compared the scotopic thresholds of phakic and aphakic observers using red (619 nm), violet (380 nm), and white stimuli (Gunkel and Gouras 1963). Four other spectral stimuli served to provide an estimate of the scotopic spectral sensitivity function. The ages of the aphakic observers ranged from 31 to 83 years. It was held that a comparison between the extended age ranges of phakic and aphakic observers rendered a detailed control of the pupillary diameter unnecessary. The variation of the log of the threshold with age was approximately linear for all the parameters studied. Table 4.1 compares values for the above stimuli and two sets of observer. The spectral sensitivity data obtained by the authors for the phakic group make it probable that the red

Table 4.1 Comparison of slopes (rise in log threshold p.a.) for phakic and aphakic observers, measured with stimuli of 380 nm and 619 nm respectively

Wavelength (nm)	Rise in log threshold p.a.	
	Phakic observers	Aphakic observers
380	0.025	0.007
619	0.006	0.002

stimulus was being applied to the rods, although some 'cone intrusion' cannot be altogether ruled out.

Again, contrary to the opinion expressed by Pulos (1989), the 619 nm slope for the aphakic observers does not differ significantly from zero even though it has a small positive value ($p = 0.49$). The slope for 380 nm differs significantly from zero for the phakic group but not for the aphakic one ($p = 0.075$). These data therefore seem quite compatible with those shown in Fig. 4.2. It should be noted that the stricture regarding the control of adaptation mentioned above is less necessary in this case because no pre-adapting exposure was used. Nevertheless, even the exposure merely to room lights, mentioned by Gunkel and Gouras, may have had some differential effect on the various ages and have acted differently on phakic and aphakic observers respectively, also on account of differences in pupillary diameter.

In the light of the above, it is questionable what importance can be attached to the data of Sucs (1974); a study of dark adaptation with clinical instruments showed that the logarithm of the logarithm of the absolute threshold slightly rises with age. No allowance was made for senile miosis (p. 48); the use of a white stimulus rendered a consideration of lenticular changes unimportant. Sucs also reported a decrease in the 'speed of dark adaptation' (although his Table IX lists a positive correlation), but it is possible that this is merely a consequence of his use of logarithms of logarithms.

More recently, Pulos (1989) studied scotopic thresholds across an age spectrum ranging from 19 to 61 years. The particular merit of this study is that the retina was sampled at six loci in the horizontal meridian lying between 2.5 and 30 °. Allowance was made for the absorption of the macular pigment which is not negligible even though it plays, at 2.5 °, a role smaller than in the fovea. Corrections for lens absorbance were based on method (4) (see p. 90), and senile miosis was allowed for on the basis of published data (see p. 48). Linear regressions fitted to the data for each of the six retinal locations showed no significant slope for any of the three wavelength ranges used (460, 490, and 580 nm). The author concludes that 'evidence for ageing of the rod system appears to be more elusive than that for its anatomical substrate'.

A parallel study, involving a number of retinal locations within the macular area, was done on a wider range extending from the second to the eighth decade (Jacobs *et al.* 1987). The threshold values were obtained with white light, and presumably covered both rods and cones. They closely follow the age-related variation of the pupillary diameter (Fig. 2.1); this is to be expected in the absence of any control of that variable.

4.3 Incremental thresholds, with special reference to short-wavelength stimuli

The investigation by Haegerstrom-Portnoy (1988), mentioned earlier in the discussion on the function of the macular pigment (p. 138), specifically addressed the question of whether visual properties change owing to senescence or owing to cumulative effects due to visible radiation (see p. 112). Two age groups took part: the average age of one group was 21 years, and that of the other 64 years. The isolation of the responses due to S cones, i.e. those mediating the activity of a short-wavelength mechanism, was achieved by the projection of the 450 nm variable test-target on a fixed broad-band yellow adapting field, 80 cd/m^2 (cd = candela) in luminance. Natural pupils were used. As shown in Fig. 4.4, measurements were done at five retinal locations.

The sensitivity of the older group is significantly lower for the short-wavelength target but not for 578 nm, which was used as a control wavelength. The author concludes that lens absorption cannot explain the results, since it affects the whole of the retinal area examined equally. Moreover, the relatively lower loss in sensitivity near the retinal centre should be attributed to the protective role of the macular pigment, i.e. it is probably due to cumulative retinal damage in the rest of the retina. Since this does not manifest at the longer wavelength of 578 nm, S-cones are, according to the author, particularly vulnerable.

The validity of this conclusion is unfortunately not without doubt, because lack of pupillary control may have led to different retinal illuminations in the two age groups, and their effects could have been wavelength- or receptor-specific.

An analogous study explored the variation with age of short-wavelength mechanisms across a central field 30 ° in radius; the age range covered 20 to 75 years (Johnson *et al.* 1988). The field was examined with an automatic (Humphrey) field analyser which tests incremental thresholds in 76 loci within the central field. As above, the S-cone mechanism(s) were isolated with the test field being superposed on a yellow background. The test field contained only radiations with wavelengths < 500 nm. In addition, the isolation of the short-wavelength mechanism was achieved by the Stiles method with determinations of the threshold for the test-target when the intensity of the yellow background was varied. It may be recalled that generally in this method a background

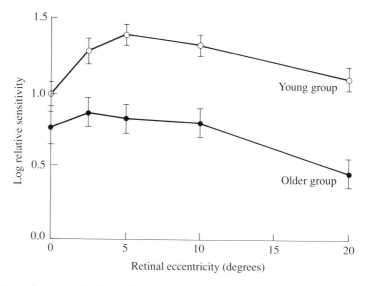

Fig. 4.4 Log sensitivity (relative units) as a function of retinal position in degrees. The open circles refer to the younger of two age groups. After Haegerstrom-Portnoy (1988).

radiation reduces the sensitivity of those spectral mechanisms which are not the instantaneous object of interest: this ensures that the sensitivity of preferably a single mechanism may be left unimpaired and available for testing.

Comparative measurements were made of scotopic thresholds with stimuli of wavelengths of 450 and 656 nm respectively; absorption being assumed negligible for the latter, the difference between the two thresholds was compared with the corresponding absorbance difference of rhodopsin (see p. 90), and thus yielded a measure of pre-retinal absorption at 450 nm (Fig. 4.5). Once again, pupillary diameter was not measured, and the above-mentioned uncertainty regarding the adequacy of the control of pre-retinal absorption is unresolved also in this study. Note that pre-retinal absorption was measured presumably with dilated pupils; Fig. 2.19 suggests that for wavelengths shorter than 460 nm a small but systematic error is introduced when corrections appropriate to large pupils are used in small-pupil conditions. This reservation is unlikely to apply to results obtained in an analogous study with a test radiation of 480 nm (Haegerstrom-Portnoy *et al.* 1989), which show a similar age-related loss in short-wavelength sensitivity corrected for pre-retinal absorption.

On the above evidence there is some doubt as regards the significance of Johnson *et al.*'s conclusion that a rise in short-wavelength threshold, particularly of older observers, is evidence of cumulative retinal damage. However, they also noted that the corrected sensitivities showed a greater scatter than the

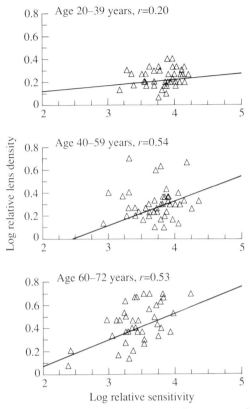

Fig. 4.5 The logarithm of the lenticular absorbance in relative units as a function of the photopic short-wavelength sensitive mechanism as determined for three age groups. After Johnson *et al.* (1988).

uncorrected ones. This is not altogether surprising because the corrected values depend on additional threshold values the errors of which are unlikely to run in tandem with those of the uncorrected data. The correlations between the results for lens absorption and the (corrected) sensitivity measurements were positive, being lowest in the youngest of three age groups. The authors conclude that this raises the possibility that a more absorbent lens protects the retina (Fig. 4.5), much as the macular pigment is thought to do (Haegerstrom-Portnoy *et al.* 1989).

Confining their attention to an age range between 60 and 87 years and stipulating that vision should be at least 1.0 in the better eye, Eisner *et al.* (1987) studied foveal thresholds with two stimuli, namely 440 and 490 nm, superposed on a background 580 nm; test-fields of 3 ° and 1 ° were used in that order. S-cone responses were shown to be isolated. Measurements were made also of photopic dark adaptation and the absolute foveal threshold, and the time constant of the recovery of sensitivity following exposure to an adapting stimulus was also determined. Anomaloscope settings were studied with two field sizes, namely 5.8 ° and 1.1 ° respectively.

As expected, S-cone thresholds rose with age, but did so almost three times as fast in women as in men. This difference appeared, however, only in the higher age groups. It is probable that the authors' correction for lenticular absorbance is too low since they used an exit pupil of 1.23 mm (in diameter?). Figure 2.19 shows that published data would represent an underestimate at least for 440 nm. At 660 nm, the absolute threshold rose with 0.09 log unit in 10 years in both men and women. The photopic time constant of threshold recovery did not vary with age (see Sucs' above result for rods).

Younger observers in this population aged 60 and over were more sensitive to the size of the test-field in the anomaloscope measurements than were older ones. There is a weak but significant negative correlation between this difference and age, which the authors attribute tentatively to a 'reduced quantum catching ability of the foveal cones' or a lower cone pigment density (Kilbride *et al.* 1986; Keunen *et al.* 1987). Since the authors believe that some of their results were affected by rod intrusion, it may be that the luminance level of the anomaloscope may have been too low for some of the observers: there is no evidence to suggest that it was related to the observers' thresholds (see p. 174).

These detailed results return us to the question raised on p. 5, namely whether representative data for a variable should be sought or the best value that the species can achieve should be determined. Although the observers were examined ophthalmoscopically, and drusen and pigmentary changes were mentioned, no quantification or correlation with age was attempted. This may be significant because Massof *et al.* (1989) reported more than five times higher foveal thresholds for patients with drusen than young normal adults. On balance it would seem that both rod and cone thresholds are holding their own through-out life, and the lack of correlation between threshold and visual acuity reported also by Massof *et al.* may be of considerable interest for the understanding of visual senescence (see p. 239).

4.4 Spectral sensitivity

Verriest (1972) measured the spectral foveal sensitivity curve by means of a flicker photometer in both phakic and aphakic observers, the latter covering an age range from 10 to 78 years. Even though the luminance level for a large spectral range amounted to no more than 55 troland, the method involved photopic conditions, in that the threshold criterion was the absence of the sensation of flicker in a situation in which a spectral test-field alternated with a constant white control field.

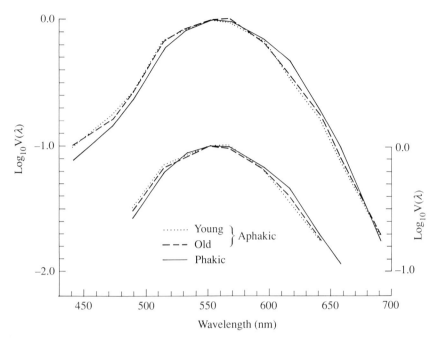

Fig. 4.6 The logarithm of the spectral sensitivity [Vλ] as a function of the stimulus wavelength. The upper group of data were measured at a retinal illumination level of 55 troland, the lower one at 415 troland. The mean ages of the aphakic groups were 32.7 and 66.5 years respectively. After Verriest (1972).

It is noteworthy that there was no difference in sensitivity at short wavelengths (Fig. 4.6) when young (28–56 years) and old (57–78 years) observers were compared. As expected, the phakic values (bulked for all ages) are lower than the aphakic ones at short wavelengths, but exceed them systematically between 595 and 658 nm. A significant relative drop occurs again at 700 nm. These zig-zag variations, the importance of which Verriest seems to be overestimating, almost certainly result from the standardization of all the curves at 555 nm. If regard had been paid to their absolute, as distinct from only their relative, values, information useful for the resolution of some of the attendant problems could have been preserved.

This stipulation can be seen fulfilled in the extensive study due to Werner and Steele (1988). The authors used the above-mentioned method due to Stiles, and isolated the $\pi(1)$, $\pi(4)$, and $\pi(5)$ mechanisms, which peak at approximately 440 nm, 540 nm, and 575 nm respectively. The tests were extended to 76 observers aged between 10 and 84 years. At the shorter wavelengths, not all the measurements could be performed by some of the more elderly participants,

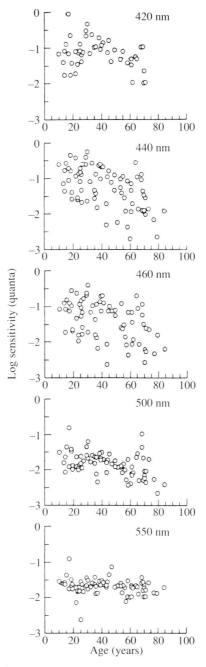

Fig. 4.7 The logarithm of the sensitivity of a foveal short-wavelength mechanism isolated by the Stiles method, and plotted as a function of age. Note that there is a tendency for the dependence on age to vary inversely with the wavelength. Arguably, the function is linear for wavelengths greater than 440 nm. The decline is attributable in large measure to lenticular yellowing. After Werner and Steele (1988).

perhaps because of heavily absorbing crystalline lenses. However, the preservation of absolute values enabled the authors to present individual threshold measurements as a function of age with wavelength as a parameter (Fig. 4.7). The regression which they calculated show a systematic negative slope which varies between 440 nm and 550 nm inversely with the wavelength.

The situation is less than clear at 420 nm. The authors say that no significant improvement was obtained when they calculated a non-linear regression, but this is almost certainly due to the outlier at 15 years. Apart from this, the distribution looks parabolic particularly at this wavelength, with a peak lying in or near the fourth decade.

In Fig. 4.8 the authors show a plot of the peaks $\pi(4)$ and $\pi(5)$ at the top and bottom respectively, plotted against that of $\pi(1)$. This is interesting because the slopes of the two regressions are approximately 0.7, i.e. sharply lower than unity. But this implies that the age-related drop in the short-wavelength threshold is 50 per cent faster than the other two. This would provide more evidence in favour of a belief in the special vulnerability of the mechanism operating at that threshold (see p. 180). The data were corrected for pre-retinal absorption by a method related to type (4) (p. 90), but may be insufficiently compensated for lenticular yellowing because younger observers tend to have larger pupils than older ones (p. 93). At a wavelength of 440 nm such a correction is unlikely to exceed 25 per cent (Fig. 2.19), but this is sufficient to make one defer one's definitive judgment on this important matter.

In a different type of study, Werner *et al.* (1990) used the same method in an examination of the visual thresholds of eight aphakic observers with implants after bilateral operations for cataract. The implants were made of polymethyl methacrylate (PMMA) which is fairly transparent to the near ultraviolet part of the spectrum. This ranges from about 320–400 nm, and is transmitted fairly readily by the cornea, but absorbed increasingly by the ageing crystalline lens (p. 92). Evidently the absence of even a normal, non-cataractous lens means that that the barrier between the photic environment of the eye and the retina is lower for potential hazards than would be true under normal conditions. During the last few years more and more attention has been drawn to the implied hazard (Kirkness and Weale 1985), and manufacturers are now producing PMMA with UV-absorbing chromophores (the permanence or otherwise of which is still uncertain).

Werner *et al.*'s observers were provided with both types of implant, one in each eye, so that one retina was exposed to the putative hazard attributed to short-wavelength radiation while the other was protected from it. The protection afforded by the additive was significant: the authors calculated that the implant containing it transmitted only 1 per cent of the incident ultraviolet radiation, whereas the earlier untinted type transmitted 86 per cent. The latter had been implanted on average 5 years before the tests, and the insertion of the newer types preceded the study by 2.3 years. It was assumed that the spectral

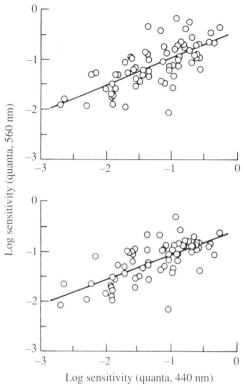

Fig. 4.8 The logarithms of the sensitivities of the retinal mechanisms sensit-ive to medium (top) and long (bottom) wavelengths as a function of the logarithm of the sensitivity of the mechanism sensitive to short wavelengths. After Werner and Steele (1988).

distribution reaching the retinae of the unoperated eyes between the two operations was similar to that reaching them through the tinted implant. The reason is that the absorption characteristics of the latter have to try to match those of the normal crystalline lens if the latter exerts a protective filtering function. It follows that one retina received almost two orders of magnitude more UVA radiation than did the other protected one.

The ratios of the thresholds measured in the exposed and protected eyes are shown in Fig. 4.9; the basic measurements refer to the wavelengths of maximum sensitivity of the three π mechanisms mentioned on p. 181. Those for $\pi(5)$ and $\pi(4)$ do not differ significantly from unity, but, at short wavelengths, the unprotected eyes show an increase of 75 per cent. The authors mention a great inter-observer variability, and say that in six of the eight observers the rise in threshold was statistically significant: anecdotal evidence suggests that the

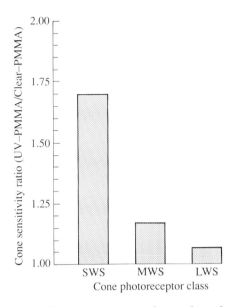

Fig. 4.9 A comparison of the sensitivities of retinal mechanisms responding to short, medium and long wavelengths respectively, as measured in patients who had a different lens implant in each eye. One type absorbed ultraviolet light (UV-PMMA), the other (Clear-PMMA) did not. The apparent effect due to UV irradiation was most marked for the short-wavelength mechanism. After Werner *et al.* (1990).

degree of the rise may correlate negatively with the wearing of sunglasses. In this instance senescence is likely to have affected both retinae equally, and the results are consistent with the view that what appears to pass for senescence as regards the rise in threshold of one of the blue-sensitive visual mechanisms may in fact be due to environmental photic pollution. The authors estimate that five years of exposure to unfiltered UVA radiation cause a rise in threshold equivalent to 30 years of ageing.

In conjunction with the results of tests mentioned earlier these conclusions suggest that ultraviolet radiation may, indeed, constitute a hazard at least in some cases. But it would be too far to go at this juncture to imply that it actually damages the retina or even that it may in some way lead to conditions favouring the onset of age-related maculopathies (see p. 164). Werner *et al.* are never-theless right to draw attention to the need for eye-protection in some geographical locations. What they do not say explicitly, and what is difficult to submit to experimental tests, is that steps taken to protect the eyes from photic hazards only in middle life or later are probably pointless. Attention was drawn earlier to the large numerical aperture of childrens' eyes (Fig. 3.23). Even if parents may be understandably unwilling to guard young eyes with effective sunglasses, maturing adults should at least be informed that the avoidance of cumulative effects in old age may require long-term protection beginning when we are young.

4.5 The visual field

The concept of the visual field seems relatively simple: it is looked on as the circumference of the two-dimensional projection of the external world onto our retinae. This is why instruments used to determine the size of the field are called perimeters, i.e. they measure the circumference.

The basic measurements assume just this, for they are expressed in terms of angular radii recorded along various (usually four) meridians: traced from the fixation area of a stationary eye they are defined severally as the furthest distance up to which a suitable small test target is visible. In this simple, essentially clinical concept, the stimulus intensity is fixed, and in general supra-threshold within the field, except on the blind spot; it defines the threshold at the limits of the field. In normal eyes there is a variation of sensitivity along the various radii; but a drop to zero before the normal limit of the field is reached betokens a pathological condition which may be retinal, as in glaucoma, or more central, as in the presence of a neoplasm somewhere along or in the visual path.

During the last few decades considerable refinements of the above basic concept have taken place. In particular, methods have been developed for the exploration of retinal performance within the limits of the field by a variety of techniques and subjective criteria. The subject does not fall within the ambit of this book, except insofar as all diagnoses of the abnormal have to rely on age-related information on what is normal. Some attention has therefore to be given inevitably to the provision of this important baseline. At the same time, it should be noted (see Chapter 1, p. 5) that a clinical judgment of what appears to be normal may actually be found to be abnormal when stringent standards are employed. The dilemma of whether age-norms should be based on some notional average or an equally notional optimum is as little resolved in ophthalmological as in general gerontology. There is little doubt that if those concerned with the provision of standards for visual fields were more aware of this problem the vexed question of false positive responses would be greatly simplified.

4.5.1 *Some physical determinants of field size*

The geometrical extent of the visual field is governed by at least four factors.

First, there is the anatomy of the eye, of the orbit, and of the nose, and also the size of the pupillary aperture. To the extent to which they change in an age-related manner they may affect the apparent size of the field simply on a physical basis. For example, it can be shown that the limit of the field on the temporal side increases with the size of the pupil; consequently senile miosis (p. 48) is likely to reduce it even in the absence of other modifying factors (Fisher 1968). The position of the eye within the orbit also plays a role, and has been a contentious matter because of the difficulty of determining a baseline for the corneal vertex which is used to determine exophthalmos and endophthalmos. Fisher (1968) used the lateral orbital margin for this purpose and found that for subjects below the age of 30 years the distance of the corneal vertex was on average 14.4 mm compared with 15.8 mm for those over 65 years of age. Moreover, in the elderly the globe moves downward and laterally by about 1.5 mm.

Secondly, the size of the field is determined by the state and the sensitivity of the retina and visual pathways, whence the usefulness of the concept in clinical ophthalmology and in neurology. In this connection one distinguishes between scotomata, or dark (i.e. blind) areas, on the one hand and field constriction on the other. For example a solar or laser burn may cause relative or absolute loss of vision in a circumscribed retinal region: an object imaged on this spot may therefore be invisible. The notion of field constriction is easy to picture in the drastic case of tunnel vision. Such an extreme is age-related only in pre-existing conditions, as in retinitis pigmentosa, but does not appear in the normal course of senescence.

Thirdly, and this is a point frequently overlooked in the clinic, the field may also depend on the energy available for stimulating the retina. For example, in one type of cataract when the lens is dark brown or brunescent, the patient's vision may be impaired not because of any structural alterations in the crystalline lens but simply because not enough light can reach the retina on account of lenticular absorption. If such a patient's field were to be measured it would be found to be grossly constricted because available instruments do not possess a hundred- or a thousand-fold reserve of stimulus energy to draw on in such a case. This is an extreme example, but it serves to illustrate an occasional limitation of the usefulness of field measurements.

Finally, the extent of the visual field also depends on the spatial and temporal configuration of the stimulus used to explore it. This is nothing new. The old perimetric masters were well aware that a large stimulus was conducive to the measurement of a larger field than could be achieved with a small one, but this was largely due to the use of fixed intensity stimuli. More recently, this old problem reappeared in a new guise when Collins *et al.* (1989) determined the extent of the horizontal field in two age groups of mean ages 22.1 years and 54.2 years with two König bars separated by gaps of 2.4 and 4.8 minutes of arc respectively. The older group had a more constricted field for the smaller target than did the young one: there was no statistically significant difference between them for the larger target. It is probable that the different results are more likely to be attributed to the stimuli not having been related to the observers' thresholds than to some aspect of neural ageing, which this study neither proved nor disproved (see p. 174).

All the above circumstances conspire to the recording of field constrictions with advancing years in normal and pathological eyes, but an increased understanding of some of the underlying problems has led to the development of more detailed measuring techniques so much so that the tracing of the mere outline of the visual field is now obsolete.

4.5.2 *Aspects of recent field measurements*

The introduction of computerized perimetry has been fundamental in the progress made. As noted above, full attention is now paid to the characteristics of internal regions of the field by means of threshold measurements or the statistical assessment of retinal performance in any one particular locus. There are, for example, several sampling instruments in which a number of discrete and distributed tests are applied simultaneously, and the patient is asked to state the number he or she has seen. Again, when fixation is maintained, random scanning of the visual field can be performed automatically and the response recorded and analysed by a computer.

This implies that visual field performance and the integrity of the retina can be quantified with indices which represent the patient's bulked responses. In this manner a value may be obtained for the surface of the field, which can be expressed for example in mm^2. Adherence to a rather old fashioned unit, namely the decibel (dB), has led to the adoption of the square dB. It will be recalled that the decibel is equal to 0.1 of one logarithmic unit, which, in turn, corresponds to a factor of 10. However, retinal sensitivity can also be taken into account in which case the measure used is the volume of the field, and this is expressed in mm^3 (or alternatively cubic dB). The concept of the volume is based on the notion that a good performance is normally linked to a high sensitivity; for a fixed retinal surface the volume will be greater if the sensitivity is higher rather than low (Jaffé *et al.* 1986). Note that the dB is not specifically linked to threshold measurements; it represents the logarithm of a fraction and can therefore inform on a relative distance or angular separation, etc.

This is illustrated in the computer-generated three-dimensional representation of a normal field (Fig. 4.10). The height is expressed in dB of sensitivity so that 36.5 is proportional, or corresponds, to 4467 reciprocal photometric units (lux). The central bulge corresponds to the sensitivity of the macular region which is dominant in the light-adapted eye (in the dark-adapted state the sensitivity is doughnut shaped: a relatively insensitive macula is surrounded by a ring of high sensitivity because this follows the concentration of rods). The bucket on the left of the plot indicates zero sensitivity at the blind spot; as the scale is logarithmic

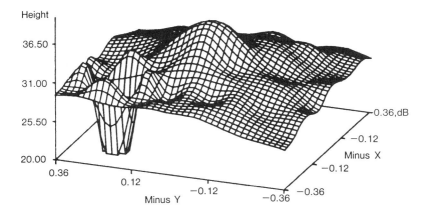

Fig. 4.10 A three-dimensional representation of the normal visual field as generated by a computer. The field is co-extensive with the co-ordinates of x and y, while the sensitivity, measured in relative units, is plotted along the z-axis. After Jaffé *et al.* (1986).

there is a drop to minus infinity. The horizontal scales are logarithmic instrument constants, easily converted to retinal or field co-ordinates.

Jaffé *et al.* measured the above and determined the variation with age of the mean sensitivity, of the surface, and of the volume of the plot (Fig. 4.11*a*, *b*, *c*). The slope of the sensitivity function is approximately 0.0074 log units per annum and agrees well with the value for a long wavelength in Table 4.1 because Jaffé *et al.* used white light which is not very sensitive to lenticular yellowing (Weale 1982*a*). The number of points is insufficient to determine whether the three regressions are linear or whether a plateau or even a peak may occur among the points obtained for the younger observers (see Iwase *et al.* 1988, mentioned below).

The above slopes are not easily explained. There was no physical control of the pupillary area; indeed, the authors affirm that they could not see any age-related change amongst their patients (whose ages ranged from 24 to 72 years). None of the pupillary diameters was smaller than 3 mm, the mean being 5.5 mm. As the drop in sensitivity could be explained by a reduction in pupillary radius from 2.5 to 2.1 mm it may be that the 25 observers studied represented too small a number for the well-established phenomenon of senile miosis (Fig. 2.1) to be revealed. Although the authors think that the cornea might be implicated, no quantitative evidence is quoted to support this speculation, and they incline to the view that cell death in the retina (see Gartner and Henkind 1981) and in higher centres may be able to explain their observations.

Iwase *et al.* (1988) studied a much larger number of observers, aged between 10 and 82 years, with a Humphrey Field Analyzer, and, while not trying to

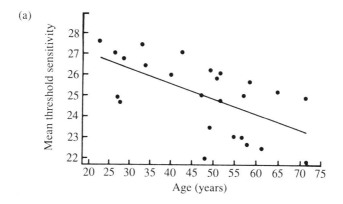

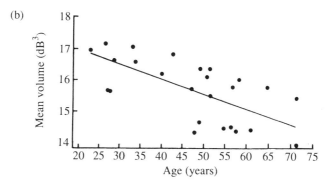

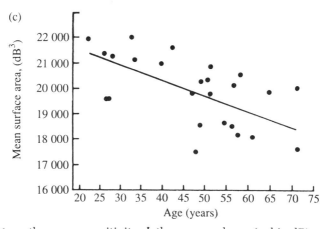

Fig. 4.11   *a* the mean sensitivity, *b* the mean volume (cubic dB), *c* the mean surface area (dB²), all of the visual field as a function of age. The meaning of these quantities is explained by Fig. 4.10. After Jaffé *et al.* (1986).

explain the cause of such decreases in sensitivity and volume as they observed, made two valuable points. There are considerable regional differences in the age-related variations of some parameters; bulking data obviously involves the loss of this information. The authors noted that the variance of their results was greater than expected in older observers at an eccentricity of 21 ° and beyond. Secondly, the fact that they used almost six times as many observers as did Jaffé *et al.* enabled them to reject linear regressions in the description of their data. Both sensitivity and volume remain approximately constant up to the fifth decade with a decline setting in only then.

Although the authors state that they do not believe that their test population was different from the ones studied by previous investigators, because the criteria for enrolment into and exclusion from the study were more or less the same and the number of enrolled subjects similar or larger, the fact remains that they do not refer to any other comparable Japanese study: it may be that there are ethnic differences to be uncovered, but we are not going to resolve this with our eyes closed to even the possibility of such being the case.

A Humphrey Field Analyzer was also used in a study longitudinal over 18 months (Katz and Sommer 1987). The mean age of their observers ranged from 26 to 76 years, and averaged 50 years, i.e. about 10 years higher than the mean of Iwase *et al.* Katz and Sommer found that the variability of thresholds over time increases with age and, like Iwase *et al.*, that it varies with the location of the test. In younger eyes the standard error ranged from 0.12 to 0.28 log units, whereas in older ones it could be as high as 0.83 log units, which corresponds to a factor of almost sevenfold. As regards actual threshold measurements for younger eyes, at a particular location the change in threshold could be 0.56 log units or 3.6-fold and still lie within the 95 per cent confidence limit of the preceding measurement. In contrast, older observers can report a variation of as much as 1.66 log units, or 46-fold and still be within the normal variation. As observed by Donovan *et al.* (1978), there is a thin line between a large variability and guesswork.

Special attention was paid to the central area by Williams (1983) who used a Goldmann perimeter linked to an areal integrator. The area of the field appears to decrease linearly with age although the data do not rule out the presence of a peak in the third decade. But what is more noteworthy is that the variance of the field areas is approximately independent of age. However, this once again conceals great local variations. Williams shows isopters, i.e. closed loci of constant thresholds, for normal 24 and 75 year-old observers (Fig. 4.12). The younger field was more than three times as large as that of the older observer. Yet the principal loss, equal approximately to half the total difference, was confined within a lateral angle of about 60 °. The data do not permit one to say whether it occurred on the nasal or temporal side of the field. Outside the angle, i.e. over some 300 °, the isopter constricted in a regular manner by 8−10 ° as between the old and the young field.

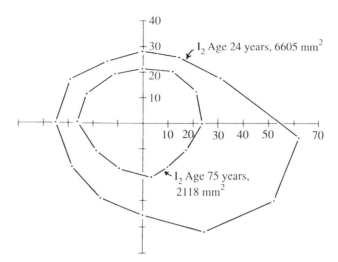

Fig. 4.12 Two normal visual fields recorded with a Goldmann perimeter for 24 and 75 year-old eyes respectively. The figures refer to areas occupied by the plots on Goldmann recording charts. After Williams (1983).

The nature of field losses has been much debated and, although Williams' result has been ignored, it is crucially important to repeat his simple study. The reason is that it appears to reveal both general and special field modifications. The more regular nature of the isoptric constriction could be due to a change in sensitivity or to an effectively reduced stimulus in the older eye as a Goldmann instrument was used in which the target intensities are preset. But it is hard to see how the laterally angular loss can be due to a physical cause. It is as though a large bundle of optic nerve fibres had vanished in later life. It is, however, possible that, though normal, the younger observer would always have produced the elongated isopter shown in Fig. 4.11.

The possibility that age-related field losses in eyes free from all pathological signs may be due to neural modifications (cell death) was considered in great detail by Johnson *et al.* (1989). They modified a Humphrey Field Analyzer so as to ensure a high level of light adaptation; the use of a large test-field was thought to reduce the effect of pupillary miosis. An artificial pupil might be thought to have provided absolute control over this variable. They also studied incremental thresholds with stimuli free of wavelengths shorter than 530 nm, so as to minimize variations in pre-retinal absorption. The average loss in sensitivity they recorded was 0.8 dB per decade for three conditions, namely a white test on a white background, and an intense yellow and a feeble yellow test on a yellow background. This is equivalent to a loss of 17 per cent in ten years.

It may be mentioned incidentally that a comparable study of a group of observers with at least one implant might provide an additional and independent control of the role, if any, played by lenticular irregularities in the putative modification of the visual field.

Now the results obtained by Johnson *et al.* are not best described by a linear regression. The main losses appear to occur after the age of 60 years. This makes it unlikely that senile miosis is involved because this continues fairly uniformly throughout most of life; it might account for the slow decline earlier on, but is unlikely to do so for both the changes before and after 60 years. Similarly, whatever scatter may develop in the lens does so gradually, and is unlikely to play an important role in connection with stimuli devoid of radiations containing short wavelengths. Johnson *et al.*'s conclusion that the changes in the visual field they have observed have a neural basis thus appears to be valid. When one considers the smallness of the changes that are left when care is taken to control physical factors, the importance of doing so when field testing is done in a clinical context becomes obvious.

Therefore the indiscriminate comparison of an age-related norm with natural pupils and a group of glaucoma patients several of whom 'were receiving miotics' is likely to produce a scatter which may disguise valuable information. This potential loss is aggravated when no attempt is made to express results in units which readily relate to those used in other studies (Holmin and Krakau 1980). In any case it would seem that, looked at from the point of view of eyes being used rather than just tested, clinical perimetry underestimates some of the field handicaps apparently associated with old age.

This transpires from a study by Ball *et al.* (1990) who tested two groups of mean ages 21 and 70 years respectively. The central 30 ° of the visual field was measured with both a Goldmann and an Octopus perimeter. The former is a static instrument and determines isopters whereas the latter serves to measure threshold within a given field. The useful field of view was also determined. The observers were instructed to fixate a target (which may have had a task to solve associated with it) and another target appeared unpredictably outside the fovea: this had to be located both in the presence and the absence of a distracting stimulus.

As might be expected, the younger group did better than the test group on all counts. However, the presence of distractors had an adverse effect on the older observers, particularly at greater eccentricities, at which performance tended to approach chance. The study establishes the value of the concept of the useful field of view, but there is room for argument as regards the applicability of some of the statistical methods used. It is often overlooked that correlation coefficients can be determined meaningfully only for data distributed approximately uniformly along the range of the study. Dumb-bell distributions in which there is a cluster of results each at widely separated ends are likely to yield high but misleading values for the coefficient of correlation, and comparisons of mean

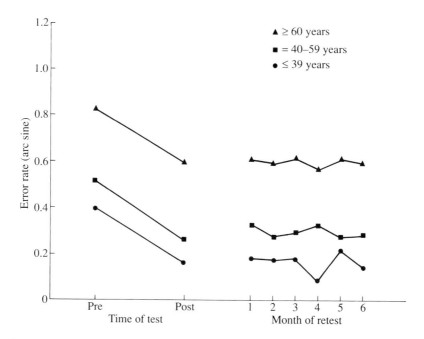

Fig. 4.13 Error rates obtained for each of three age groups as a function of the time of testing. The metric of the ordinate is the arc sine of the square root of the percentage errors made in the location of a target in the presence vs absence of a distracting stimulus. After Ball *et al.* (1990).

values are free from this defect. There is little doubt, however, that Ball *et al.*'s conclusions would safely rest also on such a foundation.

It is interesting that the degree of usefulness of the field of view of neither older nor relatively young observers is definitive. It can be improved by training. Ball *et al.* (1988) tested three age groups of mean ages 25, 45, and 69 years respectively, using a method similar to the one underlying the above study. After baseline results had been obtained, the observers took part in five training sessions, when they were presumably informed of their responses, and then invited to return for once a month for 6 months, when they were tested without training. The results speak for themselves (Fig. 4.13): training led to an improvement in the error rate which was independent of age, and the benefits of the training persisted for at least half a year in all three groups.

This important observation is relevant to studies of applied perimetry such as have been pursued in connection with the relation between field loss and driving performance (Johnson and Keltner 1983). Automated perimetry was done on over 17000 volunteers divided into 5 year groups from 16 to > 65 years.

Subjects with abnormal fields were investigated for recorded driving convictions and accidents, particular attention being paid to the possibility that a major portion of the field(s) was impaired. Only when the defects were bilateral was there a significant correlation between vision and driving performance: both the accident and conviction rates were more than twice as high in this group as in age- and sex-matched control groups. The authors believe that the reason why this result differs from those of other studies is not only that in this case trained personnel were conducting the tests but that also attention was paid to the retinal periphery rather than predominantly to the central field.

It is noteworthy from the purely gerontological point of view that abnormal fields were found in 3.3 per cent of the total sample, with 13 per cent in those over 65 years old. Severe defects were found in 0.5 per cent of the total. In 1.1 per cent of all the population losses were binocular and, in 0.3 per cent of all, such losses were severe. It should be noted that this population was not selected as regards the presence or absence of pathological signs or symptoms except that visual requirements for holding a driving licence were complied with by implication, and verified by means of answers to a questionnaire. Provided acuity criteria were satisfied, the presence of glaucoma, cataract, hemianopia, etc. were not considered to be a disqualification for full participation in this study.

4.6 Glare, light adaptation, and related effects

Up to this point we have considered aspects of vision which are determined by the visual threshold. It can be argued that most, if not all, quantitative subjective tests are based on measurements of absolute or differential thresholds, matches being a subset of the latter. However, when it comes to subjects like glare, criteria become harder to define and to convey. For example, there are those who attempt to define disability glare, but overlook that disability may depend on motivation. The disability may be task-orientated, but even then it is improbable that an absolute criterion can be determined. However, if the criterion is ephemeral measurement loses much of its objectivity. This is plainly less of a problem when the criterion is simply 'to see or not to see' (see also Sturr *et al.* 1987).

Experiments involving timing fall into the category where hope is expected to triumph over experience. The judgment of whether one of two stimuli precedes the other, or whether they are coincident, depends for example a great deal on the precision of fixation. There are very few experimenters who satisfy themselves not only as regards their observers' ability to fixate steadily for as long as may be necessary − a difficult task at the best of times − but also of the precise retinal location of a test stimulus. The matter is usually taken on trust, and, in the absence of amblyopia or some muscular imbalance, the trust is usually justified; but trust it remains. One should not allow oneself to be misled by the existence of such crude controls as the indication of the blind spot on perimetric charts: the blind spot is of the order of 2 ° in angular diameter: successful fixation may have to depend on 1 or 2 per cent of this.

4.6.1 *Transient light adaptation*

These reservations serve to underline that transverse studies, which form the major portion of the relevant gerontological research, have to contend with apparently unsystematic variations in the type of criterion that is used to arrive at quantitative assessments of subjective phenomena (Morrison and Reilly 1986). The problems are well illustrated in a study of early light adaptation done on three groups of observer with mean ages of 27, 48 and 65 years (Sturr *et al.* 1985). It was based on the visibility of a test-target presented at various times before or after the appearance of a large adapting field, whence the reference to early light adaptation. In Crawford's (1947) pioneering experiment there appeared a paradox, sometimes referred to as backward masking: under certain conditions the threshold of the test-field appeared to rise as it were in anticipation of the onset of the adapting stimulus which gave rise to negative values for times of onset. The explanation of this is based not on some type of neural foresight but rather on the fact that receptors tend to have a longer latent period for weak than for strong stimuli. Thus the test-stimulus must have followed the appearance of the adapting field, but, by virtue of being more intense, its signal was conducted with higher frequency potentials and therefore was perceived more quickly than was true of the adapting stimulus.

An involved test situation such as the above offers plenty of potential for complications. For example the on-response, i.e. the initial rise in the threshold of the test-stimulus, varies inversely with the speed with which the adapting field is presented. In Sturr *et al.*'s study a zero difference between the onset of the two stimuli produced a characteristic response function in observers in their twenties, but this was both attenuated and slowed down at twice that age. Thus the youngest group showed a high threshold for coincidence between adapting and test stimuli with an exponential decrease as the interval between the two is increased (Fig. 4.14). By contrast the central group showed a lower threshold for coincidence than did the younger one but a rise to a peak was reached after 0.04 seconds. This was accentuated in the oldest group. These results appear to lay a possible foundation for changes in criteria amongst different age groups.

Sturr *et al.* suggest that the results can be explained in terms of the onset of the adapting field being able to trigger two different responses, namely transient or sustained trains, and that neural communication channels may become more rarified with advancing years. It would appear that, in the first instance, their result may be explicable on a technical basis (see p. 174). The experimental conditions were determined by results of an earlier study done on young observers. This determined the parameters of the adapting light, which was

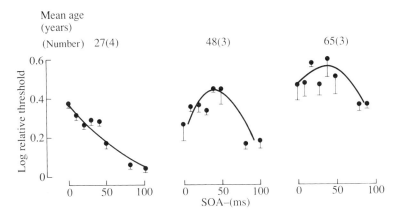

Fig. 4.14 Log relative test thresholds as a function of the delay between the presentation of the test and adapting stimuli necessary for a sensation of apparently simultaneous presentation to be achieved. SOA: stimulus onset asynchrony. The figures indicate the average age of, and number in, each group. After Sturr *et al.* (1985).

white and of fixed luminance. The adapting luminance was consequently un-related to the observers' thresholds although an artificial pupil was used. Lenticular absorption plays a small, but not negligible, role insofar as retinal stimulation with white light is concerned. Previous calculations of this effect were made in ignorance of the data underlying Fig. 2.19. It might well be the case that, had Sturr *et al.* increased the adapting stimulus so as to relate it to the visual thresholds of the higher age groups, an exponential decline might have been observed for them as well as for the young group. Moreover, the absence of any data for negative onset times (see above) hampers a more detailed analysis of these important results.

Some of these reservations received an answer in a more recent study done in the same laboratory (Sturr *et al.* 1986) in which three groups with slightly higher average ages than the above were studied with adapting fields the luminance of which was variable, as had been done earlier by Till (1978) with binocular stimulation for a smaller group of observers. In one test, detection thresholds were obtained (a) for a transient situation when adapting and test field were presented simultaneously, and (b) for a steady state when the observer's fovea had been adapted to the adapting field for three minutes. Over all, the authors studied four adapting luminance levels ranging over a factor of 30. Whereas (b) revealed no age-related change, (a) showed a steeper rise for the youngest as compared with the oldest group (see eqn 4.1): the central age-group fell between the two but did not differ significantly from either.

In order to compensate for any likely understimulation of the retina in the old groups, the authors extended the tests to two new groups of average ages of 24 and 66 years respectively, increasing the adapting luminances for the older group by a factor of three in relation to those for the younger one. The above results were confirmed: the steady state showed similar threshold rises for both groups, but the transient one produced a greater one in the younger observers.

The results suggest that the visual system has a greater response gain in youth than later in life. They are complemented by a study which involved a determination of the time interval during which tachistoscopically presented green and red stimuli were fused to produce a sensation of yellow. The only luminance levels selected were 3 and 7 ml, but the two age groups tested were well separated, with mean ages of 19.08 and 68.42 years respectively (Kline *et al.* 1982). At interstimulus intervals **t**, ranging from 0 to 50 ms, the young group consistently yielded lower numbers of fused responses of yellow, the difference between the two age-groups being significant for $\mathbf{t} > 30$ ms ($p = 0.001$). Not surprisingly, the luminance level was unimportant. Like Sturr *et al.*, the authors suggest that the difference between the two age-groups points to an age-related decline of the operation of transient visual channels.

In a brief review of the evidence Kline and Schieber (1981) list the following results in support of the idea that transient visual mechanisms age relatively faster than sustained ones: an age-related loss in the ability to detect stimulus intermittency (flicker), a reduction of dynamic visual acuity, experiments of the type just discussed, and the fact that older groups with good contrast sensitivity at high frequencies have a comparatively low sensitivity at low frequencies. More recent studies (Owsley and Burton 1992) cast some doubt on the magnitude of this difference, but an extension of this latter study to higher spatial frequencies might perhaps help to validate the last piece of evidence quoted by Kline and Schieber.

The matter is of considerable physiological interest, as different types of retinal ganglion cell appear to dominate steady and transient responses respectively. There are also temporal and spatial frequency connotations to this correlation (see p. 205). The results of a study involving brightness judgments at supra-threshold levels (Sturr *et al.* 1987) are consistent with the notion that there is an age-related rarification of neural units mediating transient responses. At relatively low luminances, an increase in luminance for presentations ranging from 10–1000 ms, evoked a steeper increase in log brightness judgment in the younger of two age-groups (mean ages 24.8 and 67.6 years, respectively). However, the slopes of the two groups were similar at the higher luminance levels. Rather surprisingly, the duration of the stimulus was without effect on the results (see Crawford 1947).

Coyne (1981) studied a variant of the above method, having included onset-times for his threshold stimuli which preceded the presentation of the adapting stimulus. Like other authors before him, he refers to negative values for the time of onset as backward masking, a designation which we noted on p. 196 could be misunderstood. Three age-groups of mean ages of 25, 65, and 74 years were presented with black letters on white backgrounds, viewed through an artificial pupil as large as 3.5 mm in diameter. The criterion of detection was the correct identification of four consecutive letters. Both the adapting, i.e. masking, and the threshold luminances were fixed. As pupil diameters in the upper age echelons may well have been smaller than the artificial pupil used it is difficult to interpret the result, namely that the time needed to avoid masking rose from 24.5, through 52.2 to 69.5 ms. Although this is likely to contain a real component, part may be artefactual and due to inadequate stimulus control. However, changes in threshold criteria cannot be altogether ruled out.

Indeed, Till and Franklin (1981) used an experiment on backward masking with the specific objective of distinguishing between criteria based on central and peripheral processes respectively. More specifically, optical masks were used to separate the two. After a suitable standardizing procedure, either a target presenting random noise or one made up of randomly placed 'letter fragments' followed a sequence of a 2 second presentation of a fixation field, a structured target consisting of two letters, and a dark interstimulus interval. Target durations were varied so as to establish a critical one at which masking was avoided when the physical interval between the adapting and the test stimuli was zero. Masking was held to be abolished when the observer correctly identified four consecutive letter pairs for a given interstimulus interval.

The random noise masks affected thresholds of young (18–21 years) and old (58–70 years) observers similarly: the critical interval decreased rapidly as the target duration rose from 4 to 24 ms, after which it remained constant. However, the structured mask achieved a marked separation between the two age groups: for equal target durations, the critical intervals were much higher for the older group, who showed a linear decrease with increasing target duration, whereas the results of the young group were more nearly exponential. The authors deduce from this that age differences in central processing are larger than is true of peripheral ones.

4.6.2 *Glare*

The connotation of glare is with a reduced capacity to perform some task rather than with an extreme of light adaptation: it is as though it reflected an applied aspect of an academic subject. The reason is probably semantic. One speaks of the glare of headlamps of oncoming vehicles, the glare of the sun streaming into a bedroom when one has just woken up, etc. As glare is not amenable to a specific quantifiable definition, one accepts that the stimuli giving rise to this sensation as continuous with the gamut used in the study of light adaptation. Thus Collins (1989) used a floodlight with a 500 watt tungsten halogen bulb as a glare source in a study of glare sensitivity of observers ranging from 16–79 years in age. The criterion task involved the detection of five different contrast targets in turn following a 10 second exposure to the glare source. The time required for the contrasting targets to be perceived was recorded: it varied inversely with their physical contrast.

In order to eliminate the effects of differently sized pupils and unequal media absorbance, Collins determined a baseline in the form of an individual *ad hoc* measurement of each observer's contrast threshold before the glare exposures. This value was subtracted from the values recorded for the glare experiment. The corresponding glare recovery time was found to be about 30 seconds and independent of age up to the mid-fifties, and to rise thereafter to about 70 seconds for the highest age-group. We shall see in a moment that such an age-variation appears to differ from both earlier and contemporary studies which show rises in recovery times starting earlier in life. One reason for this may be the way the baseline measurement has been used.

Optical theory (see Driscoll and Vaughan 1978) shows that contrasts are multiplicative, not additive. This is evident from the definition of the modulation transfer function which is the ratio of the contrast (at a given spatial frequency) of an image to that of the object giving rise to it. The modulation transfer function varies with the wavelength of the radiation used in image formation and also the numerical aperture of an optical system. Therefore the human pupillary diameter or the transverse sectional area of the light beam in its plane, whichever is the smaller, has to be taken into account. But the appropriate standardization is done by division, which is why the validity of Collins' conclusions based on 'corrected contrasts' is circumscribed.

4.6.3 *Another digression on the role of the pupil*

The pupil of the eye fulfils two functions, as is true of the limiting aperture of any image-forming device. It controls the radiational flux or the number of quanta involved in the formation of the retinal image, and it also acts as a spatial filter. The former function is easily mimicked with a camera. The latter rests on the approach to image formation based on diffraction theory (Driscoll and Vaughan 1978), and was alluded to above (p. 62). An image can be represented by a spatial power spectrum which informs on the relative amounts of spatial frequencies of different magnitudes it contains. For example a thin line is represented by a narrow band of high spatial frequencies, much as is true in subsequent references to vernier acuity (p. 207). The spectrum of an image of a broad silhouetted tree trunk will on the contrary contain a considerable low-frequency content though the edges contribute also high frequencies.

By acting as a spatial filter, an aperture transmits some frequencies better than others. When a system is diffraction-limited it offers the most effective transfer of contrast, i.e. its imaging properties are optimal for a given set of physical parameters. As mentioned above, these include the wavelength of the radiation and the numerical aperture of the system: this in turn is a function of the area of the aperture and the effective focal length of the system. The smaller the aperture the wider the spatial spectrum it transmits, which is why a pinhole device can dispense with the need for a lens. In general, spatial frequencies greater than a limiting or cut-off frequency are not transmitted. Campbell and Green (1965) have shown that the emmetropic human eye is diffraction limited.

If a pencil of light traversing the pupil, for example in Maxwellian view, is smaller than the natural pupil then the size of the latter becomes optically irrelevant: the transverse dimensions of the beam are the governing parameters as far as the quality of the retinal image is concerned. This notion has caused problems in some laboratories (see Alpern *et al.* 1983, 1987; Nordby and Sharpe 1988), and appears to have been overlooked also in studies of visual senescence. In the latter case the problem arises from senile miosis (Chapter 2). Older pupils are smaller than young ones. They therefore admit less light into the eye. The progressive age-related change is, however, important principally in measurements involving, or directly depending on, an absolute visual threshold.

The reason that it is relatively less important in contrast measurements is that, by being a better spatial filter, an older pupil should in theory lead to the production of better retinal images than is true of a younger large one. As human contrast sensitivity drops with luminance even under photopic conditions (Van Meeteren and Vos 1972), senile miosis leads to opposing effects which may cancel each other in certain circumstances. It will help if this is borne in mind in the subsequent considerations of the senescence of contrast vision.

4.6.4 *Glare and intensity*

While the study by Gomez-Ulla *et al.* (1986) on the recovery from glare is free from this problem it presents a new one. The glare source was an electronic flash and the criterion task consisted in resolving that line on a Snellen chart which the observer had been able to resolve prior to being dazzled; as in the studies considered above a well-defined baseline was being used. The recovery times for the younger observers were about half as long as those measured by Collins, indubitably because the latter used a stronger glare source. The age-related rise starts some fifteen years earlier (Fig. 4.15), as observed in other studies (see Reading 1968).

The authors were interested to discover whether the recovery times for near and distant objects were similar: Fig. 4.15 shows that they appear to be shorter for a short viewing distance. The two conditions yield significant differences only for the younger age groups: for the first decade $p < 0.001$ whereas for the last one it is approximately 0.3. If the presbyopic observers did not wear corrections for near vision for the shorter distance (no information is given on this point) the lack of change in recovery to macular dazzling canot be surprising. The authors seem to have underestimated the role played by miosis

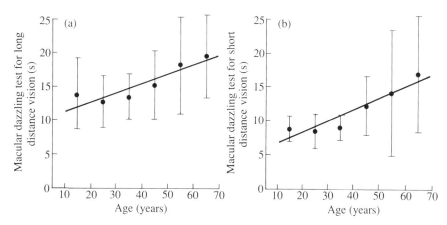

Fig. 4.15 Recovery times (mean ± SD) from macular dazzling as a function of age for **a** far and **b** near vision. After Gomez-Ulla *et al.* (1986).

during accommodation. They stress that the physical conditions in the two experiments were not matched (nor were similar methods employed), so that the significance, if any, of the different results remains uncertain.

An even weaker glare source, namely a penlight, was used in an imaginative study in which subjective glare (or photostress) recovery times were compared with the recovery rate of visually evoked response amplitudes, with pre-glare readings providing baselines for each test as above. The feebleness of the glare source may well explain why observers in the first three decades of life yielded recovery times of 10 seconds or less. Lovasik (1983) rightly forebore to fit a linear regression to his data (Fig. 4.16), but it is clear that the use of his exponential tends to obscure that, amongst the very young, so many points lie above the curve as to suggest the use of a parabolic function: it may well be that there is a minimum during the third decade, more than a hint of which appears also in Fig. 4.15.

The part of the experiment involving visually evoked potentials revealed rapid recovery rates for the young, but slow ones for the old. However, the author departed fundamentally from the pattern set in the subjective part of the study in that subjects were instructed to fixate a reversing checkerboard with elements subtending at the eye angles of 14 minutes of arc. This was a large, arbitrary and fixed multiple of some average Snellen reading of the subjects, all of whom had a visual acuity of 1.0 or better in the test eye. For the two parts of the study to be more nearly comparable a variable checkerboard would be required, and each participant would have to determine that configuration which yielded a standard visually evoked potential (cf. Trick *et al.* 1986).

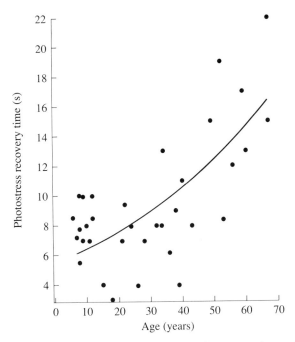

Fig. 4.16 Recovery time from photostress as a function of age. After Lovasik (1983).

It is unlikely that the glare source could photolyse enough visual pigment for these results to be accounted for in this manner. They are explicable on the basis of a conventional relation between visual acuity and stimulus intensity expressed in terms of individual thresholds; this would give rise to the greatest drop in visual acuity in cases where the latter is high. It might also explain why the recovery rate was fast in the young and vice versa. It may further provide a tentative link with visual acuity peaking at ages apparently showing the shortest subjective recovery times (Fig. 4.16).

The caveat made above (p. 196) in relation to the reliance one has to place on an observer's or patient's ability to fixate is emphasized by an application of some of the above methods to those suffering from age-related (and pre-age-related) maculopathies. In this condition there is a rise in threshold of both rods and cones. At first sight, it may not be clear whether this is due to a loss of gain, a reduced capture of quanta, receptor loss or perhaps some combination of these and other factors. However, the fact that contrast sensitivity and visual acuity are reduced in those cases of age-related maculopathy which show pigmentary changes (Sarks 1976, Collins and Brown 1989) and the histological picture (Chapter 3) implicate receptor loss as a primary cause. This would affect visual acuity adversely more in the retinal centre than in extra-foveal regions, and therefore impede fixation.

It would seem to follow that, unless independent evidence is obtained as regards the part of the retina that is stimulated, an abnormal recovery time following glare can be due to (i) the glare source being subnormal in comparison with its value in non-pathological controls, (ii) a non-central area being sampled, (iii) a genuine difference between pathological cases and normal controls. Collins and Brown used the method reviewed above (Collins 1989) and found that, particularly at low 'corrected' contrasts, maculopathy is associated with greatly extended recovery times. Thus whereas normal patients showed average maximum recovery times of 32 seconds, the corresponding value for pre-age-related cases was 190 seconds, and for age-related cases 525 seconds, considerable variances being associated with all these results. Glare recovery times thus seem to be sensitive statistical indicators of the state of the retina, but considerable overlap may be found for high contrast targets.

4.7 Contrast sensitivity: spatial and temporal parameters

4.7.1 A relation to incremental thresholds

A close link between incremental thresholds and contrast sensitivity was mentioned on p. 170. It becomes apparent as soon as a scale is adopted for the measurement of contrast.

A variety of definitions have been used in the past, but all of them are functions of the ratio of the contrasted luminances (or radiations). The equation used by most workers in vision expresses the physical contrast C between two luminances $I(1)$ and $I(2)$ in the form of

$$C = [I(1) - I(2)]/[I(1) + I(2)] \qquad (4.6)$$

This can also be expressed as

$$C = \{[I(1)/I(2)] - 1\}/\{[I(1)/I(2)] + 1\}$$

which shows the involvement of the ratio of the stimuli, and, incidentally, emphasises that, if the geometry and spectral distributions of the two stimuli are similar, no correction for optical factors is required.

In order to relate C to observations on incremental thresholds we put $I(1) - I(2) = \Delta I$, and can also set $I(1) + I(2) = 2I(1) + \Delta I$. It follows that

$$C = \Delta I/[2I(1) + \Delta I] \qquad (4.7a)$$

and, if ΔI can be neglected in comparison with $2I(1)$,

$$C = \Delta I/2I(1) \qquad (4.7b)$$

This formulation indicates that with a stimulus varying periodically either in the spatial or the temporal domain **I** represents a constant background and ΔI/2 the amplitude of modulation.

In any one context it is important to be sure how contrast has been defined. Contrast sensitivity **S** is simply the reciprocal of threshold contrast. Reference to eqns 4.4 and 4.5 shows that the variation between contrast and luminance can be predicted.

It is easily seen that when **I** is very small

$$0.5\log S = \log[\mathbf{pR(max)}/\Delta\mathbf{R}] + \text{plog}(\mathbf{I/K}) \qquad (4.8a)$$

and when **I** is very large

$$0.5\log S = \log[\mathbf{pR(max)}/\Delta\mathbf{R}] + \text{plog}(\mathbf{K/I})$$
$$\sim \log[\mathbf{pR(max)}/\Delta\mathbf{R}] \qquad (4.8b)$$

At low levels, when an increasing luminance is divided by a constant threshold, the function for the sensitivity rises (see Fig. 4.21); in the region of the validity of the Weber-Fechner law, the function reaches its peak. The reason for this is to be found again in Fig. 4.1: beyond this point, Δ**I** increases toward the saturation of the response. In other words, contrast sensitivity becomes constant as shown in eqn 4.8*b*. Age-related changes in incremental thresholds would therefore be expected to be reflected in appropriate studies of contrast sensitivity.

4.7.2 *Basic data*

Ever since Robson's pioneering study (1966), in which he demonstrated the role of the interrelation between spatial and temporal modulation in the measurement of contrast thresholds, the separation of the two might be thought to have been avoidable. However, clinical practice, in which a patient's visual acuity is assessed without being timed, may well have founded an early tradition hard to eradicate.

This is not an academic point. It was emphasized in connection with adaptation (p. 174) that it is important to relate adapting stimuli to an observer's threshold (Weale 1985*c*, 1991*b*), as is implicit also above in eqn 4.4*a*. This requires the exercise of care in the interpretation of data obtained on different age groups with constant physical parameters unrelated to group thresholds. However, a visual stimulus is defined not only by its intensity but also by its duration, and, unless this is similarly standardized (apart from being defined), doubtful conclusions may be drawn from any one set of gerontological experiments. Higgins *et al.* (1988) fixed the exposure of their grating target to 700 ms when measuring contrast thresholds by forced-choice, and demonstrated that the results so obtained differ from those derived from continuous adjustment, perhaps, they concluded, because 'eye movements mights introduce temporal components of differing consequences to young and older subjects'.

Acuity measurements, involving targets of fixed physical contrast but variable angular subtense, are still widely used, and used as criteria for other studies. Thus Johnson and Choy (1987) attempted to specify age-related norms for the testing of visual function on the basis of data they selected from the literature, and observed that the age of onset of visual acuity loss occurs at the age of 60 years, i.e. '10 years later than the time at which other visual functional measures start to degrade'. They attribute the observation, which they dub as being an apparent inconsistency, to visual acuity of 1.0 being defined as normal. At the same time, they show stereo-thresholds showing a parabolic age-related function with a minimum at the age of approximately 25 years (see p. 228). This is based on observers having normal (0.5 or better) visual acuity, a criterion that often ignores gender differences (Lavery *et al.* 1988*b*). Often patients who are allowed an unlimited time, and turn their heads about more than one axis, will ultimately give a correct answer. This can hardly be, yet is, classed with an immediate response. It is evident that, once again, the problem is the dilemma between gerontological data describing an average of sorts (p. 4) or the optimum that can be detected in any one set of circumstances.

This problem received some attention in a study which dealt quantitatively with the question of how visual acuity should be defined. The letter test presents targets, the number of which varies inversely with their size, and some workers accept partial success, some insist on 100 per cent for a line and ignore anything less than that, etc. Frisén and Frisén (1981) demonstrated that a criterion involving, say, 50 per cent correct responses was more satisfactory for example from the point of view of re-testing than is true of higher percentages. In particular 100 per cent is to be deprecated in detailed studies. They also showed that early foveal changes, which are of obvious gerontological interest, are unlikely to be detected in the absence of targets corresponding to a nominal acuity of 1.0; finer detail is needed.

The recognition that high contrast targets can lead to misleading conclusions is brought out in a study by Adams *et al.* (1988) who measured acuity as a function of contrast (which is the reverse of the conventional method of studying contrast thresholds), of background luminance, and of age. Acuity decreased with contrast, particularly at low luminances, and more so for older observers. The authors plotted their data with log contrast as the independent variable and showed that both the luminance parameter and age could be described by simple scaling, i.e. by factoring contrast. Equation 4.3 shows that factoring contrast is equivalent to doing so with incremental thresholds.

The importance of statistical assessment transpires also from a study on vernier thresholds (more often as not carried out in disregard of any role that contrast might play). Measurements of vernier acuity used to involve, traditionally, the determination of the least lack of alignment of two originally collinear targets. However, the criterion task may conversely involve the alignment of two lines: the mean setting following a number of settings represents vernier acuity (Odom *et al.* 1989), and its standard error offers a separate assessment. Acuity as such does not vary greatly over a mean age span from 25 to 68 years. However, the mean error trebles during the fourth decade of life (see p. 7), being apparently constant before and thereafter. The significance of this type of measurement is that very high spatial frequencies play a crucial role in the task (but see Tyler 1973), and the observation that there is no significant change over more than four decades is particularly interesting in view of the fact that other indices of spatial resolution do vary with age (see Fig. 4.17).

Using natural pupils, McGrath and Morrison (1981) carried out one of the most extensive studies on age-related changes in contrast sensitivity. Some representive results are shown in Fig. 4.17: the logarithm of contrast sensitivity is plotted as a function of the spatial frequency in cycles per degree. It will be recalled that in these studies the observer is faced with a grating, the luminance variation of which is usually sinusoidal. The spacing of light and dark bars is periodic; the distance between two luminance maxima is called the spatial wavelength. If it is λ and the viewing distance is $\mathbf{D}$ then the angular subtense of one period is $\lambda/\mathbf{D}$ radians. The spatial frequency is the reciprocal of this, namely $\mathbf{D}/\lambda$ cycles per radian. This value is readily converted into cycles per degree.

McGrath and Morrison's results are collected in Fig. 4.18 in which the open symbols represent data obtained from men and solid ones from women except in the plot of contrast sensitivity (b) where they are merged; the filled triangles represent here data due to observers taking the sedative valium. The authors note that high peak contrast sensitivities were not observed amongst their youngest observers. The logarithms of the points shown in the plot of upper frequency limit (f) were analysed in detail, and shown to be described by two sets of regressions, namely one with zero slope up to the age of 40 years and over, and two in agreement with those derived by Weale (1975) for visual acuity, which is related to the upper frequency limit measured by McGrath and Morrison. Arguably, a parabola would provide a statistically significant fit for all these data.

It may be mentioned incidentally, that the above authors did not find any difference due to gender, but Korth *et al.* (1989) report that there are particular losses above the age of 50 years in females, for example with a frequency of 1 cycle/degree counterphased at 10 Hz and 11.3 degrees off centre. The Framingham Study (Kahn *et al.* 1977) found that women above the age of 60 years tend to have slightly lower visual acuities than do men.

Separate measurements of their observers' pupil diameters enabled McGrath and Morrison to address the question of how far optics could explain their results. A random element was introduced by the background illumination being

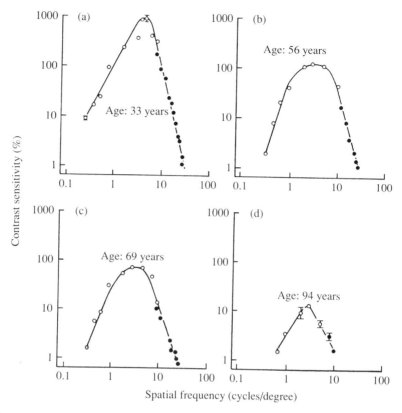

Fig. 4.17 Contrast sensitivity as a function of spatial frequency for four observers of different ages. Open circles, near viewing distance; solid circles, far viewing distance. After McGrath and Morrison (1981).

adjustable according to each observer's wish, but this did not seem to affect the diameter of the pupil. The authors point out that contrast sensitivity declines with age, notwithstanding the existence of senile miosis, which is linked to a decrease in the upper frequency limit, contrary to what is to be expected on the basis of diffraction theory (p. 210). It is important to be clear about this. Campbell and Green (1965) having shown that human contrast sensitivity is diffraction-limited, then, if luminance is controlled, the upper frequency limit should rise with age. However, it is found to fall (Fig. 4.18*d*). This does not disprove Campbell and Green's conclusion, but suggests that other variables may be involved.

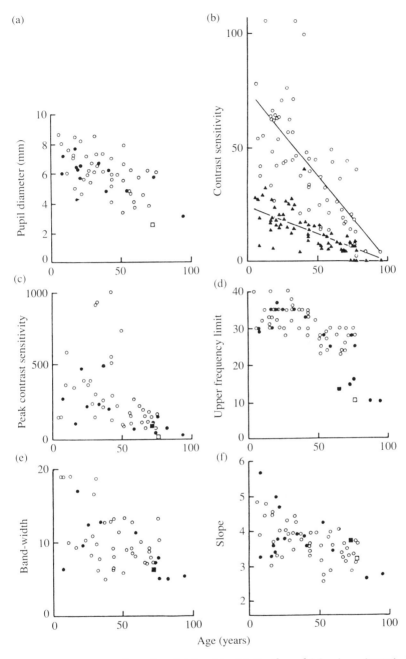

Fig. 4.18 Summary of results obtained by McGrath and Morrison (1981). (a) pupillary diameter, (b) contrast sensitivity at 10 cyles per degree, (c) peak contrast sensitivity, (d) maximum spatial frequency to be resolved (cycles per degree), (e) band-width (cylces per degree), and (f) slope of regression of log(contrast sensitivity)/log(spatial frequency) (see Fig. 4.17). After McGrath and Morrison (1981).

4.7.3 *The role of physical factors*

As there are demonstrable age-related changes in factors which control − or are believed to control − contrast sensitivity, a great deal of effort has gone into attempts at pinpointing them. The problem here is analogous to, though not identical with, that considered earlier in connection with thresholds (p. 175). For example, the ability of the crystalline lens to absorb light is less of a concern than is its propensity to scatter it, and thereby to cause a deterioration of the retinal image, or, to substitute a quantitative term for a qualitative one, a reduction in the modulation transfer function of the eye (see p. 200).

Indeed, a paper by Kay and Morrison (1987) specifically addresses the effect of optical variables of contrast sensitivity. As expected, defocusing of the image greatly reduces contrast sensitivity. The effect of the pupil was examined in mesopic conditions (3.8 log units above the foveal threshold as determined for each of 12 observers in the age range of 18−40 years). Contrast thresholds were determined for a variety of out-of-focus conditions, both with natural and dilated pupils. No significant role of pupil diameter could be detected, and the authors surmise that the balancing act mentioned on p. 208 was probably in operation.

Sloane *et al.* (1988*a*) similarly conclude that senile miosis cannot explain the lower sensitivity which they observed for older observers (mean age 73 years). Dilation of the older pupil to the size measured in a younger group (mean age 24 years) failed to improve the contrast sensitivity of the seniors. The authors suggest that 'increased intraocular light scatter and increased light absorption in the aged eye contributed to older adults' contrast sensitivity deficit', even though they have shown that Hemenger's hypothesis (1984) in support of this view is not borne out by a number of reliable experiments. An analogous study, in which contrast sensitivity was measured at various intermittencies (Mayer *et al.* 1988) and in which the senile deficit in retinal illumination was compensated, showed that there is an age-related decrease in sensitivity to intermittent stimuli, particularly at intermediate temporal frequencies.

On the other hand, Wright *et al.* (1985) emphasized that senile miosis reduces retinal illumination so as to account for 0.19 out of 0.31 log units of reduced contrast sensitivity over six decades which they observed at a spatial frequency of 12 cycles/degree. The relevant variation of contrast sensitivity with luminance, calculated from data due to Van Meeteren and Vos (1972) and others (Weale 1987), is shown in Fig. 4.19: note that $\Delta\log S/\Delta\log I$ reaches unity only just before the cut-off frequency is reached, and remains otherwise below this value. Wright *et al.* did not consider the above-mentioned balancing improvement to be expected on the basis of diffraction theory.

The role of the lens was studied directly by Owsley *et al.* (1985) who ingeniously compared contrast sensitivity in older aphakes (mean age 70 years) wearing implants with values obtained in similarly old phakic adults (mean age

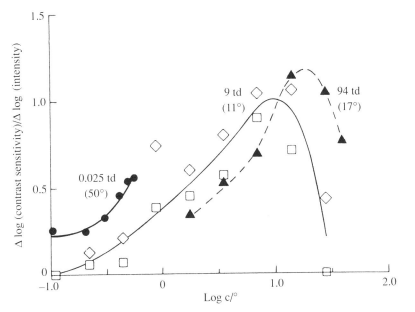

Fig. 4.19 The change in log(contrast sensitivity) with log(intensity) as a function of spatial frequency for three luminance levels. The figures in brackets indicate the field size subtended by the grating screen at the observer's eye. Data: Fiorentini and Maffei (1973): ○; Van Meeteren and Vos (1972): ▲; Weale (1987): ◇, □; (td: troland). The extent to which luminance level and diffraction balance each other is therefore likely to vary from case to case. After Weale (1987).

71 years) with no known ocular pathology, and also with results on young observers (mean age 21 years). Figure 4.20 shows unambiguously that the older group exhibits a deficit in comparison with the young controls, and that this does not depend on whether the observer is phakic or not.

A similar study with a comparable result was reported by Jay *et al.* (1986) and by McGrath and Morrison (1981). The former was based on measurements of Snellen acuities, which correspond to values measured near the high-frequency minimum of the sensitivity function. Two groups of patients were examined, both after cataract extractions. Group A (mean age 68 years) had implants. Group B wore correcting spectacles; their mean age at the time of the operation had been 62 years, and the final follow-up was done 14 years later. The best Snellen acuity was recorded as a function of age 3 months post-operatively in both groups, and in group B at the final follow-up. The authors found no significant difference between the changes in visual acuity as a function of age in group B, based on the transverse and longitudinal (follow-up) approach respectively. The regressions were also comparable with those obtained by

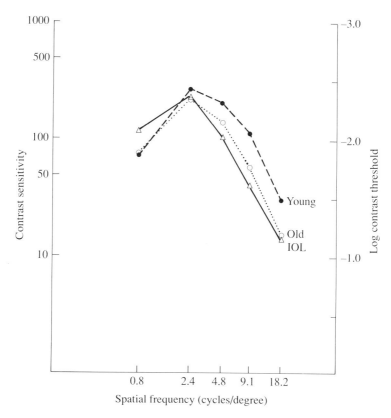

Fig. 4.20 Contrast sensitivity as a function of spatial frequency (cycles per degree) as measured in three groups of observer: young (mean age 21 years), old phakic (mean age 71 years), and old aphakic with intraocular implants (IOL) (mean age 70 years). The difference between the two groups of phakic observers is therefore unlikely to be due to age-related lenticular scattering of light. After Owsley *et al.* (1985).

Morrison and McGrath (1985) who used an interferometric method minimizing the effect of refractive anomalies (but not wide-angle light scatter).

To be precise, the authors compared results obtained from gratings produced with coherent and incoherent radiations respectively. A helium−neon laser ($\lambda = 632$ nm) was used for the former, and a cathode-ray oscillograph for the latter. The advantage of interferometric measurements with coherent light over those based on conventional imaging methods is that the former are only minimally affected by refractive anomalies. Contrast sensitivity measured with the laser interferometer was found to decrease with age systematically much as was found with the cathode-ray oscillograph. The ratio of the two values which is a measure of the optical quality of the eye did not change with age (but see Elliott (1987) who found in a smaller number of observers that there was a slight dependence of this ratio on spatial frequency). In healthy eyes the quality of the optical media does not therefore seem to change with age significantly, a result consistent with measurements of the cut-off frequency (p. 201) on excised human lenses of various ages (Weale 1983).

It would seem to follow from these studies that, given healthy eyes, there appears to be a decline in the optical resolving power of the eye from a value of approximately 1.2 at the age of 40 years to approximately 0.4 at the age of 90 years, which is not attributable to lenticular changes. It is also evident that senile miosis cannot be invoked to account for this. We are still faced with the question whether the observed decline is due to methodological factors (Owsley and Burford, 1992), to effects due to observer selection (see Morrison and McGrath 1985) or, indeed, to age-related changes in the visual nervous pathways.

4.7.4 Nervous aspects

One of the basic differences between conventional measurements of visual acuity and tests of contrast sensitivity is frequently ignored. Visual acuity is almost invariably measured in the fovea, whereas grating targets equally frequently extend far outside the foveal contour. When the screen displays a high-frequency pattern the foveal region is easily visualized. Indeed. a commercial auto-tester based on interference fringes operates on this basis. At low spatial frequencies there is unlikely to be a problem, but the extent to which the fovea dominates the extra-foveal contribution to an overall response may well be age-related (Ball *et al.* 1988).

For this reason, studies devoted to the retinal periphery can be particularly informative. Nervous summation prevails in this region to a far greater extent than is true of the fovea. This applies to both the spatial and the temporal domains: visual resolution and sensitivity to intermittent stimuli are lower in the periphery than in the retinal centre. For example Crassini *et al.* (1988) report that, except for a spatial frequency of 0.2 cycles per degree, contrast sensitivity is higher in the foveae of both young (mean age 20.4 years) and older (mean age 64.4 years) observers than is true of locations 10 degrees off centre; also that as regards both locations younger observers performed better than the older ones.

An interesting variant involved the same observers in a test based on a screen divided vertically into two equal halves with slightly different luminances separated by a sharp, i.e. high-frequency, edge. The task consisted in deciding which half was the lighter of the two. If the younger group were more sensitive to contrast at high spatial frequencies, then they might be expected to perform this task better than their elders: this proved to be the case particularly in the extrafoveal tests. The result was shown to be contingent on the presence of high spatial frequencies, since a repetition of the test with a semi-sinusoidal luminance distribution across the boundary between the two fields failed to reveal any difference between the two age groups. However, the authors stress that the use of limited fixed contrast ratios reduced the extent to which these results can be generalized.

It is important to emphasize that Sloane *et al.* (1988*b*) studied the age-related deficit of contrast sensitivity within a luminance range of 3.5 log units between 0.034 and 107 cd/m^2 and a number of intermittencies, so making it possible to relate their results (Fig. 4.21*a*) to eqn 4.1 above. What they observe is that, at a spatial frequency of 0.5 cycles/degree, contrast sensitivity rises to a maximum for both of two age groups (mean ages 23 and 74 years). Both at this frequency, and at 2 cycles/degree the older group exhibited a greater rise in contrast threshold with luminance than the younger group. At higher spatial frequencies, this distinction between the age groups disappeared, the two functions showing merely a relative horizontal (less probably, vertical) displacement; if there were only one cause for this, the authors believe that the result could be due to differences in ocular absorbance or retinal quantum absorption, a point that can be tested with an aphakic population.

When the measurements were repeated with an intermittency of counterphasing increased from 0.5 to 7.5 Hz, the difference in slope had vanished, the functions for both age groups being superposable at all of the four spatial frequencies by a vertical displacement (Fig. 4.21*b*). According to the authors, a single cause, namely ocular scatter, would explain this. They make the telling point that one cannot invoke physical factors which act under all conditions to explain some but not other results. Their data impel one to the inescapable conclusion, that the use of the luminance parameter is a powerful tool for the study of age-related variations in contrast thresholds.

It is possible, however, that a different temporal modulation might have clarified the picture even further. Thus Owsley *et al.* (1983) have shown that gratings moving with an angular velocity of 4.3 degrees/s considerably lower the contrast threshold, particularly for young observers. Moreover, Nameda *et al.* (1989) found that a low frequency intermittency reduces the contrast threshold in the spatial frequency region of 1–2 cycles/degree more for 60 year-old observers than for 20 year-old ones. While drift and intermittency have to be distinguished from each other they both interact in an age-related manner with contrast perception.

The similarity of the spatial and temporal domains was demonstrated by Elliott *et al.* (1990), who measured both types of sensitivity for the mean ages of 23.2 and 69 years. They found that a sensitivity deficit is associated with age only with medium and higher frequencies. Retinal illumination was without effect at the luminance level (300 cd/m^2) used: when the younger group mimicked the reduction in retinal illumination supposedly experienced by the older group they suffered no change in sensitivity compared with their normal results. As the healthy state of the eyes of Elliott *et al.*'s observers made it unlikely that intra-ocular scatter could play a significant role, the authors attribute the parallel changes observed in the two domains to neural attrition.

This is also the broad conclusion reached by Nameda *et al.* (1989), who analysed both domains of contrast sensitivity with a laser interferometer thereby minimizing effects due to refractive irregularities (see Morrison and McGrath 1985). At 160 td the retinal illumination was relatively low, but the use of exclusively red light will have probably insured that only the long-wavelength sensitive mechanism was being examined. The gratings drifted with angular speeds between 1.25 and 3.15 degrees/s. A total of 19 observers in the age range from 24 to 63 years took part, and results for the extreme age groups are shown in Fig. 4.22. The lines marked 'flicker' appear as rectilinear projections, B, in the frequency plane, and those shown as having been obtained with a constant velocity 'v: const.' are called A, appearing in the same plane. Note that, while the former are fairly similar in the two age groups, there are marked differences in the latter. These arise almost exclusively from the drop in sensitivity of the older group when it comes to low spatial frequencies that are drifting and presented at temporal frequencies higher than the lowest ones; note that the data for the older group are presented on the left of Fig. 4.22. The authors' attribution of the deficit to lenticular yellowing is remarkable in that the conventional wisdom would have it that their long-wavelength stimulus would be unaffected by lenticular absorbance even though their stimulus intensity was 'corrected' for this factor with data obtained on extracted cataractous lenses of mostly 70-year-old Japanese subjects. While it is probable that the absolute values in Fig. 4.22 have to be received cautiously, the differences in the shapes of the functions as between young and old are likely to be valid.

A comparison between contrast threshold and supra-threshold data in the age range between 13 and 67 years (Tulunay-Keesey *et al.* 1988) showed that matches made between the contrasts of a test stimulus and a standard were not subject to any age-related variation in either frequency domain. Intermittency did not affect the issue although it will be recalled that drift (Owsley *et al.* 1983) played an appreciable role (p. 214). These results may be juxtaposed to those due to Buckingham *et al.* (1987) who tested age-groups between 20 and 80 years and measured the smallest amplitude in the oscillation of a grating target that can be perceived. It was found that there is an age-related increase in this quantity which is independent of the oscillation frequency. Elliott *et al.* (1989) critized this study on the following ground. In hyperacuity tasks − for this is what is involved because displacement thresholds of 10 or 15 s of arc are being recorded − low frequency oscillations (approximately 2 Hz) require a stationary fiducial mark to be available. At higher frequencies this can be dispensed with, presumably because position memory is involved. Buckingham *et al.* used no

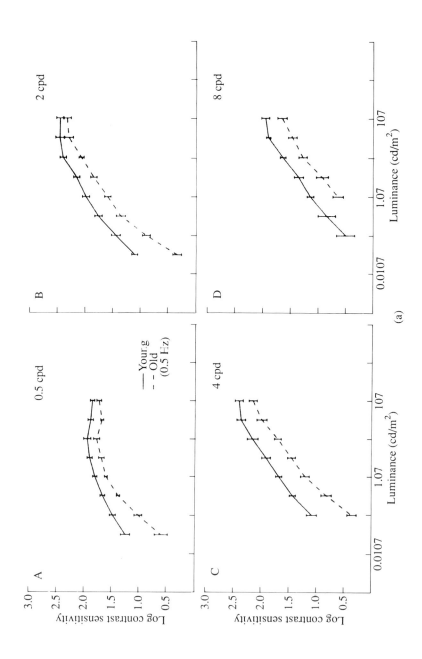

(a)

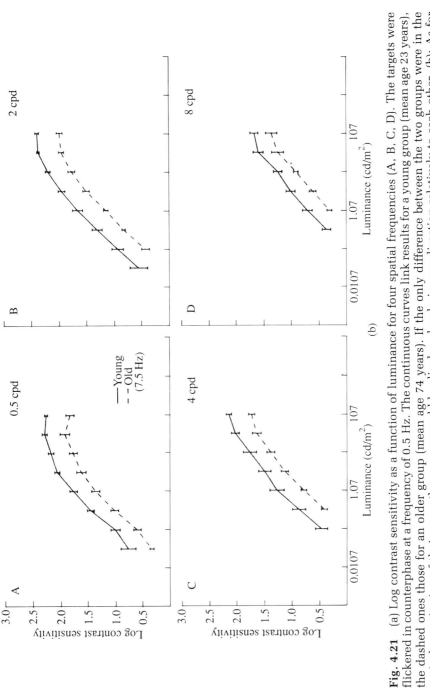

Fig. 4.21 (a) Log contrast sensitivity as a function of luminance for four spatial frequencies (A, B, C, D). The targets were flickered in counterphase at a frequency of 0.5 Hz. The continuous curves link results for a young group (mean age 23 years), the dashed ones those for an older group (mean age 74 years). If the only difference between the two groups were in the optical constitution of their eyes, the curves would be displaced only in one direction relatively to each other. (b): As for (a), except that the target was flickered at the higher frequency of 7.5 Hz. All the relative displacements appear to be vertical.

After Sloane et al. (1988b).

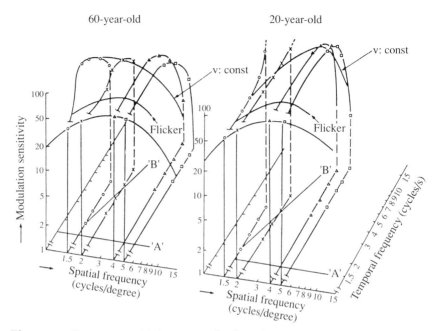

Fig. 4.22 Contrast sensitivity (vertical) plotted as a function of spatial (frontal plane) and temporal (sagittal plane) frequencies. Left: data for a group of average age 60 years. Right: date for a group of average age 20 years. For details see text. After Nameda *et al.* (1989).

such mark, thereby losing one of the advantages of hyperacuity measurement in that it is relatively unaffected by optical irregularities, and hence by any of their age-related changes. Elliott *et al.* found that oscillation thresholds increased with age twice as fast as the minimum angle of resolution measured on the same population, and concluded that this could not be due to a progressive reduction in the optical quality of the eye. This left only the neural paths for impugnment.

The above studies seem to confirm a point made earlier, namely that drift and intermittency play different roles. As there is a well-established relation between the latent period of vision and sensitivity to intermittent stimuli (Enroth 1952), the existence of a link between spatial frequency (at constant contrast) and reaction time cannot come as a surprise. A young age-group (mean age 18.3 years) yielded statistically significant correlations between spatial frequency (5–12 cycles/degree) and reaction time, but an older one (mean age 64.4 years) did so only for 6 cycles/degree (Kline *et al.* 1983).

Threshold contrasts measured for various ages at 0 Hz and 4 cycles/degree — where they tend to be minimal — are shown in Fig. 4.23. The parabolic trend of the data is unmistakeable. Wilkins *et al.* (1988) observed something similar

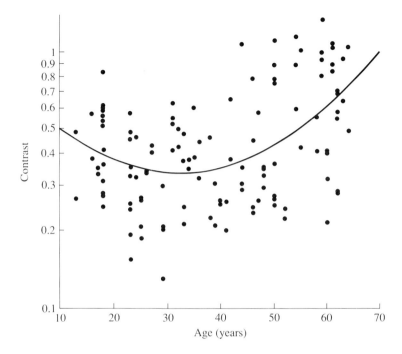

Fig. 4.23 Contrast thresholds measured at a spatial frequency of 4 cycles/degree and 0 Hz (where they are minimal) plotted as a function of age. After Tulunay-Keesey *et al.* (1988).

in a study which involved low contrast targets of an angular subtense to which the human mechanism is maximally sensitive. The method, designed for clinical use, successfully distinguishes normal from diabetic, glaucomatous, and demyelinated visual pathways, and yielded a variation with age which peaked during the third decade of life. The authors disclaim that this is statistically significant, but their disclaimer is arguable.

There are authors who find it difficult to accept this type of result which has, in fact, surfaced repeatedly. For example, Morrison and McGrath (1985) write about their own observations that 'such anomalies are likely to arise from a deficiency in attention or inexperience in applying themselves to the task of visual discrimination rather than from the immaturity of the visual system itself'. If this were, indeed, the case then an age-related analysis of the associated variation rather than loose speculation would be more likely to resolve the matter. It would be remarkable that attention should be improving up to the 30s and 40s if not beyond (see McGrath and Morrison 1981), yet we do not hesitate to trust members of these age groups making judgments based on contrast that may determine life or death for hundreds of air passengers, not to mention make make or break for expensive instruments of space and war. Moreover, if the polynomial in Fig. 3.1 has a realistic basis, then we are presented with an objective substrate for the above optima in sensory performance: they appear to coincide roughly with the peak of myelination in Gennari's line, a structure which represents an integral part of the human visual system.

It may be added that the matters of attention and of maturing sensory discrimination pose some questions also in the field of colour vision which have yet to be answered.

4.8 Colour vision

4.8.1 *Normal changes*

Some consideration of the senescence of retinal mechanisms subserving colour vision has already been given in sections 4.3 and 4.4. It was noted that there was virtual unanimity on the existence of an age-related rise in threshold of the short-wavelength mechanism, whereas there is a lack of consensus on the situation at longer wavelengths. There is little doubt that future attention to absolute, rather than just relative, values might supply some of the missing information. Moreover, a number of assumptions have to be made in order to draw conclusions about colour vision on the basis of the spectral functions of mechanism sensitivities. So far it does not appear to have been demonstrated that those holding for a typically young eye are necessarily valid throughout life. To be specific, Stiles' development of the Helmholtz line-element (1946) is based on the Fechner functions of the principal three mechanisms identified by measurements of incremental thresholds (p. 170), and convertible to colour mixture functions by means of linear transformations. The question of age-related variations, if any, of incremental thresholds are outlined on pp. 177 seq., and this is where the matter rests.

It will be recalled that one of the ways of studying colour vision is by means of colour matches. A chromatic test stimulus is presented in one part of the visual field, and the observer's task is to match it with a suitable mixture of three variable, but chromatically or spectrally constant, superposed matching stimuli juxtaposed to it. It is at once apparent that the test stimulus can be conveniently partitioned into three sections, each of which forms a contrast to each of the three matching stimuli. It is therefore possible to view a match in terms of the superposition of three contrasting heterochromatic fields, each of which is expressible as a multiple of its own contrast threshold (Weale 1986*b*). For a perfect match the sum of the three contrasts must equal zero. Since these contrasts are heterochromatic such a method requires appropriate corrections to be made for pre-retinal spectral absorption even though they cancel in the special case when the test stimulus is spectrally pure.

This approach also shows that colour matches can be affected by age-related effects in at least two ways. First, there is the yellowing of the lens compounded by complications arising from various pupillary diameters (p. 93). These have been shown to affect both anomaloscope settings and results obtained with the Farnsworth 100-hue test (Lakowski and Oliver 1973) by amounts which the authors find surprising. It will be recalled that this test consists in an observer having to sort coloured chips in the correct chromatic order: errors are scored, the sum-total informing on the quality of the observer's colour vision. More specifically, if errors tend to be confined to certain chromatic locations, or axes, information can be obtained on the defect affecting performance.

Now Lakowski and Oliver based their expectations on the pupil acting simply as a luminance control, whereas it would seem to follow from considerations of the Stiles–Crawford effect that the ratio of the matching stimuli in the anomalo-scope is liable to change (Reeb 1957). Secondly, contrast thresholds are involved and there is abundant evidence that achromatic ones vary with age, the extent of any change depending on the spatial frequency. Consequently, it is likely that chromatic ones are probably going to be affected, and to depend on the size of the target used. It is seen, therefore, that if there are neural effects in the perception of contrast, they may extend to the perception of colour quite apart from any changes that may occur for example in the cones and the pigments contained therein (Chapter 3).

One of the more comprehensive studies giving, as it were, a global view of the changes accompanying senescence is due to Knoblauch *et al.* (1987). Using the Farnsworth 100-hue test, they used both age and luminance as parameters (Fig. 4.24), and showed that reducing the illumination affected the performance of a young eye much as did senescence when the illumination was kept physically constant (see p. 210). It will be recalled that one of the attributes of this test is that the accentuation of the error score along an axis may diag-nose a colour defect. Since errors are added radially in what amounts to Newton's colour circle (Fig. 4.24), the elongation of the error locus along the near vertical indicates that both parameters point to a reduction in the short-wavelength response, i.e. tritanopia, as first demonstrated by Verriest *et al.* (1962).

Harper *et al.* (1988) have used both the 100 hue test and a reduced (15 hue) test, due to Lanthony, in order to compare phakic and aphakic groups of average ages 65.8 and 67.7 years respectively. They failed to demonstrate with either test any significant difference between the two groups. The 100 hue test was used also on Japanese observers aged between 11 and 68 years. Like Verriest *et al.* (1962), Noyori *et al.* (1987) observed a minimum of errors in the early 20s (Fig. 4.25), and it is pertinent to ask whether this is due to a delay in maturation of chromatic perception, to a lack of attention, or some other cause. It has to be said, however, that Japanese educational discipline appears far more rigorous than the European, and that lack of attention would have to be demonstrated

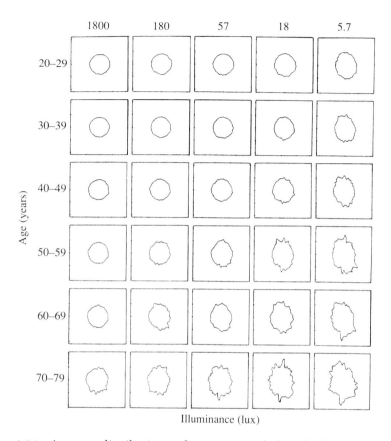

Fig. 4.24 Average distributions of errors recorded with the Farnsworth 100-hue test as a function of illuminance (horizontal) and age-range vertical. The age-related deterioration in perceived colour contrast at low levels of illuminance echoes a parallel observation on monochromatic contrast sensitivity reported by Sloane *et al.* (1988b). After Knoblauch *et al.* (1987).

experimentally, as is true of any other speculative explanation. Above all, it is desirable to use narrower age groups for this type of test, particularly in the region of the minimum.

Chips that were desaturated served in a study by Bowman *et al.* (1984), designed to compare the association between error and age with the functions obtained when conventional, i.e. more saturated, chips are used. The function for desaturated stimuli lay above the conventional one: not surprisingly, such stimuli led to greater numbers of errors at all ages. This result is explicable in terms of lenticular senescence because the chromaticities of non-spectral

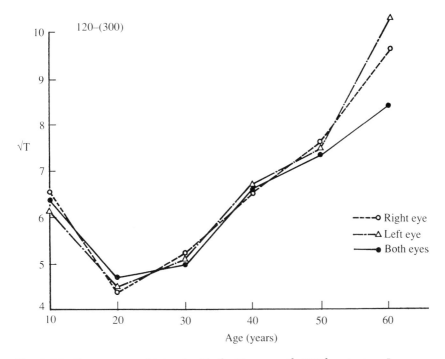

Fig. 4.25 Error scores obtained with the Farnsworth 100-hue test on Japanese observers, age-groups being shown along the abscissa. Data were obtained for each eye separately and both eyes combined. After Noyori *et al.* (1987).

stimuli vary with the transmission characteristics of pre-retinal filters, but the hypothesis has not been tested. It would be erroneous to think that dominant wavelengths could be equally affected by a filter acting on saturated and desaturated stimuli respectively: the effect of a filter progressively decreases from the centre of a chromaticity diagram to its periphery, i.e. toward the spectrum locus.

An interesting slant on how chromatic processing may vary with age has been provided by a study on the so-called unique hues by Schefrin and Werner (1990). A unique hue is a percept based on chromatic memory, and one of the main reasons for its acceptance by a considerable proportion of workers in the field of colour vision is that it can yield reproducible results. In a sense the hues are prejudged and defined as (i) that yellow which is neither orange nor greenish, (ii) that green which is neither yellow nor blue, and (iii) that blue which is neither green nor violet. If an observer is presented with equiluminant spectral stimuli on either side of the likely wavelength giving rise to the unique hue, he or she can produce a percentage response curve: for example, unique yellow would be deemed to be located at that spectral location at which a stimulus was judged equally often orange and green.

Neither unique blue nor unique yellow were found to vary when determined at three very moderate luminance levels, namely 0.7, 2.2, and 7.1 cd/m². Unique green, however, moved from an average wavelength of between 510–514 nm at the age of 13 years to toward 501–505 nm at 74 years. Chromatic processing being thought at the moment to involve inputs from the principal short-wavelength mechanism S into both the yellow-blue and the red-green channels of the chromatic response system, the deduction made by Schefrin and Werner from these results is that signals from S are selectively reduced with advancing years in the yellow-blue but not in the red-green channel. A possible alternative might be that changes occur in the yellow-blue channel as regards the mutual interaction of responses from peripheral sources.

4.8.2 Some results on patients with age-related maculopathies

The group of causes leading to the progressive condition of senile or age-related macular degeneration is receiving a great deal of attention, but this is not the place to discuss its pathology in any detail. However, as mentioned in Chapter 3, the presence in the retina of drusen, a frequent correlate of senescence, often appears to be a forerunner. Broadly speaking, the condition occurs in two forms, namely the wet and dry types. The former is being treated at present with laser coagulation which helps to arrest its progress.

The disease process is usually bilateral, but the onset in the two eyes is not necessarily synchronous. Once symptoms have appeared in one eye it has therefore become possible to search for early signs in the other eye. Alterations in colour vision are amongst these signs, and Applegate *et al.* (1987) have traced them longitudinally in three Caucasian women, aged 53, 66 and 73 years. In the last patient the diagnosis of a small detachment of the pigment epithelium (Stages III–IV, Sarks 1976) was followed in an examination with the Farnsworth 100-hue test by the appearance of a pronounced tritanopic ('blue-blind') defect. This turned out to be short-lived also in patient number 1, not because of a subsequent improvement in the condition, but because of a later increase in the number of errors in other spectral regions. Measurements of the spectral sensitivities confirmed this in a comparison with normal data. It is worth noting that the chromatic signs precede the deterioration in visual acuity; Sarks used the latter faculty in order to link functional changes with the histopathology of the retinal pigment epithelium. It would seem to follow that the earlier loss of colour vision is likely to be associated with other organic changes, which may not reside in the retina.

The loss of central function was mapped also by Smith *et al.* (1988) who used an anomaloscope with a field size variable within the limits of 0.5–8 degrees.

Given the instrumental constants, the green/red ratio of the stimuli required for a match of the 589 nm (yellow) standard decreased with field size in normal 20–40 year old observers using central fixation. The major change occurred over the first four degrees, being negligible over the remainder. For the smallest field size, patients typically either produced a lower green/red ratio than did the normals or else they were altogether unable to produce any measurement. In severe cases this inability extended to larger field sizes. The reduction in the green/red ratio can be taken to mean that there is a relative loss, predominantly of receptors, sensitive to long wavelengths. The reason is that the need for a stronger green stimulus (i.e. a large green/red ratio) betokens a comparatively low sensitivity of receptors responding to medium wavelengths and vice versa. In some cases the ratio was found to be inverted, i.e. there was a relative loss of medium-wavelength sensitivity.

4.9 Resumé

Some of the sensory changes appear to reflect a pattern which runs counter to the notion that senescence is accompanied by a continuous loss of function. There is evidence to show that foveal absolute thresholds, contrast thresholds, error sums in chromatic sorting tests, and other variables in fact decrease in early life, reach a nadir at some point and proceed on an upward path only later. The low points occur frequently in the fourth or even fifth decade, but the chromatic turn-round appears to be the earliest of all of them. It is possible that this type of variation in functions depending on contrast perception may be explicable in terms of a single rise-and-fall mechanism. But it is unlikely that the systematically earlier chromatic events can be encompassed by it. Some of these minima may be adventitious. For example, near ultraviolet radiation can cause fluorescence of both the retinal pigment epithelium (Chapter 3) and the crystalline lens (Chapter 2). They penetrate the young human eye relatively easily and so may cause the young retina to fluoresce (Weale 1991c). As the senescent lens absorbs these radiations, lenticular fluorescence may replace its retinal predecessor. Both types of fluorescence may cause a haze and so be undesirable; but there seems to be a period during the fifth decade when one has decreased sufficiently and the other has not become too obnoxious so that at least the aversion from light containing ultraviolet radiation is minimal.

It is possible that the optima observed in the variation of contrast measurements with age may be due to a similar physical explanation, but the different time-scales make it improbable. Nonetheless there appear to be sufficient instances in the senescence of visual functions to support the idea that they do not peak in youth, not even in early adulthood, but in maturity at a time when, in the wild, this would have been of paramount biological importance.

5. Coda

5.1 Correlation or coincidence?

A fair amount of evidence has been adduced above to support the view that several aspects of human vision follow the type of trapezoid or paraboloid variation with age which was discussed hypothetically in Chapter 1. That development, growth, and senescence of biological structures are likely to follow some such course is not altogether surprising. It is also to be expected that physiological functions will run along a similar path. What needs consideration is the relation of peak development and optimal performance to the individual's life in general, and the course of the decline in particular.

The rise-and-fall pattern is not observed at the retinal level (see Chapter 3), as follows also from a study specifically devoted to a comparison between retinal and cortical performance (Wright *et al.* 1985). Whereas the amplitudes of the a- and b-waves of the electro-retinogram show systematic age-related falls, the amplitude of the difference between the N2–P2 waves of the evoked response drops sharply from the age of 10 years to a minimum at 30 years and then rises gently to a plateau maintained during the second half of life. Lack of control of retinal illumination would modify both measures equally, and hence does not affect the issue. The absence of any difference between the results for the sexes contrasts with the observation that the latent period of the P25-wave decreases to a well-marked minimum during the fourth decade for women, and the fifth for men (Simpson and Erwin 1983).

The existence of peaks of visual performance, as determined by subjective tests has been reported by a number of observers, but Owsley and Burton (1992) have recently expressed doubts as regards their reality. In their own study of contrast sensitivity for two age-groups separated by several decades the age-related loss was very small. It remains to be seen whether this important difference between their results and those of a large number of other investigators is due to crucial refinements in experimental technique or to other causes. It is, for example, always difficult to decide whether, in one's choice of observers, one should probe the summit of the distribution function characterizing each age-group or skate alone the optimal extremes of ever-widening Gaussian curves. Should one look for what is typical or for the best that has evolved (p. 4)?

Owsley and Burton used the aforementioned method based on the projection of interference fringes on the retina. It will be recalled that this minimizes vitiating effects due to imperfect refraction. If the use of such stimuli leads to the conclusion that the human visual system shows comparatively small age-related alterations, but stimuli comparable with normal physiological ones equally reliably reveal significant changes, then the former result has to be considered as being of outstanding interest but of potentially limited applicability. Our eyes have evolved in the light of the sun, not that of the laser.

Appreciable variances notwithstanding, certain trends have been confirmed on a number of occasions. Amongst them one finds that the resolving power of the eye varies with age approximately as shown in Fig. 5.1. Reference to Fig. 2.8 will help to explain Fig. 5.1(*a*). The dashed lines represent extreme estimates of age-related variations of accommodation. The two points in the upper horizontal line indicate the range of the age of puberty, and those in the central one stand for double these figures. It will be recalled that they provide estimates of the ages of individuals whose eldest offspring will reach puberty when their parents are approximately twice as old as their children. The relevant theory (p. 61) indicates that accommodation may perhaps have evolved in such a manner as to enable everyone to work at close quarters at least up to this latter age limit. It was also shown that the probability of this occurring was tied to the six-fold value of the variance of accommodative measures, which accounts for the expression 6σ.

The synchrony between the interval elapsing between the parental and filial periods of puberty on the one hand, and the duration and temporal position of the optimum of the resolving power of the eye on the other is noteworthy. It is probable that many of the other peaks of visual performance coinciding with this period are governed by the maturation and decline of contrast vision.

However, because some of the summits are climbed appreciably later (see above), it is, as ever, important to pinpoint possible physical factors before the much harder task of identifying biological effects is attempted.

The preference or otherwise for artificial lighting provided by fluorescent tubes offers an instructive, if highly subjective, example (Weale 1991*c*). Volunteers in a number of age groups performed simple visual tasks when exposed to lighting with or without radiations containing near ultraviolet light (UVA). They were asked to express a preference for either, but 'don't knows' were allowed. In the event, the latter formed a small fraction of the total examined. Over 50 per cent of all the responses were in favour of lighting containing UVA, but about 40 per cent were against it. What is interesting is that of these 40 per cent the minority were in the 50–60 year group. There was a sharp rise of the negative response towards the younger age-groups and a much smaller one toward the elderly: a parabola described the data with greater precision ($p = 0.01$) than did a rectilinear regression.

The rationale of the study was based on the belief that, as the crystalline lens fluoresces progressively more with advancing years, light with UVA would be less acceptable to the old than to the young. But, as we have just seen, the opposite was observed. A possible explanation is to be sought in the fact that

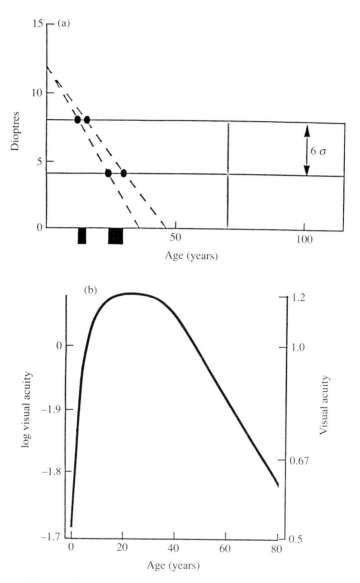

Fig. 5.1 *a* The amplitude of accommodation as a function of age with the left-hand dashed line based on the assumption that the pubertal age is 12 years, and the right-hand one that it is 18 years. See text for an explanation of the significance of 6σ. *b* A representation of the age-related variation of (the log of) visual acuity.

the retinal receptors and vitamin A fluoresce when irradiated with UVA. The latter may well reach the younger retina when the UVA absorbances of the crystalline lens and the cornea are still sufficiently low so as to admit this part of the spectrum to the retina. The resulting fluorescence may hence be obnoxious to a significant part of the population. As the lens absorbance increases, this untoward effect is reduced, but may experience a resurgence when lenticular fluorescence has increased sufficiently to form a mild haze in its turn (p. 102). However, such an adventitious parabolic effect is secondary to other facets of senescence and unlikely to form part of the pattern of evolution.

5.2 Vital statistics

Before trying to examine whether the decline of this or that of our visual faculties can be related to a general pattern of senescence we ought to take a brief look at some matters of life and death.

Life expectancy has increased appreciably even during this century: Olshansky *et al.* (1990) believe that before long it is probably going to reach a figure of 85 years for women at the time of their birth, and that this may well represent a maximum. This means that half the women will reach this age, and probably half of all men an age somewhat lower. Consequently a high percentage of each sex will live longer than this, and Olshansky *et al.* also hazard the guess that the human life span is unlikely to exceed some 120 years. Life span means the maximum age ever likely to be reached.

In relation to human development in general, and to the devolution of function in particular, this raises numerous questions, some of which were touched upon earlier. One fundamental point to remember is that our genetic make-up evolved to cope with existence 'in the wild'. Comfort (1979) and other writers state that the probability of survival **P(surv)** in such circumstances decreases exponentially with age **t**, i.e.

$$\mathbf{P(surv)} = \exp(-\mathbf{k}\mathbf{t}) \tag{5.1}$$

It is indeed found that the survival of animal species in the wild approximately obeys this relation, which implies that a given cohort is reduced by a constant fraction every so many years. Figure 5.2 shows that estimates of mortality made for the Ancient Romans differ from such a representation much less than is true of more recent survival curves (Fig. 5.3). The constant **k** has some biological significance, and it is worth examining this even though the human ability to survive has evolved from the wild to such an extent that eqn 5.1 no longer suffices to describe it.

It was noted on p. 85 that the magnitude and duration of the accommodative ability of the young eye seem excessive for what is useful in the interests of the

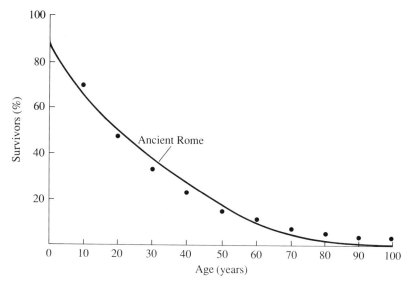

Fig. 5.2 Fractional survival as a function of age. The curve shows an estimate of mortality in Ancient Rome. The dots represent an exponential:
$$y = 102.\exp(-0.037y).$$

survival of the species, but found that a consideration of evolutionary economics (Chapter 1) may provide a plausible explanation. It is possible that the potential for survival to approximately 120 years, which appears to exceed overt biological needs, may likewise disguise results of evolutionary pressures which ensure basic biological objectives. The constant **k** seems to play such a role. Some elementary concepts relating to survival may help to illustrate this.

Let us assume that, in the wild, individuals are exposed to numerous hazards which they can survive with probabilities $p(i)$, $p(j)$, $p(k)$ etc., varying with the hazard. These are the fractions of a population exposed at the beginning of a year to hazards i, j, k, etc. and which has survived them when it ended. The hazards are independent from one another, because they are associated with the elements, enemies, diseases, etc. It follows that **P(surv)**, the overall probability of survival, is given by

$$\mathbf{P(surv)} = \mathbf{p(i).p(j).p(k)} .... = \Pi\mathbf{p(s)} \qquad (5.2)$$

This shows that, if one of the factors on the right-hand side drops to zero, the left-hand side obviously equals zero.

Now in every case,

$$p = 1 - q$$

where **q** is the fraction of a population exposed to a hazard at the start of a year which it has not survived by its end. Given that, in the wild, there are many different hazards, eqn 5.2 becomes

$$P(surv) = [1 - q(i)].[1 - q(j)].[1 - q(k)].$$

If this is the situation at the end of the first year of exposure to such hazards, after **t** years

$$P(surv) = \{[1 - q(i)].[1 - q(j)].[1 - q(k)]...\}^t$$

The substitution of

$$1 - q = \exp(-q)$$

leads to only a small error when **q** is small. It follows that

$$P(surv) = \{\exp - [q(i) + q(j) + q(k) + ...]\}^t$$

or, as above, $$P(surv) = \exp - \Sigma q(i).t \qquad (5.3)$$

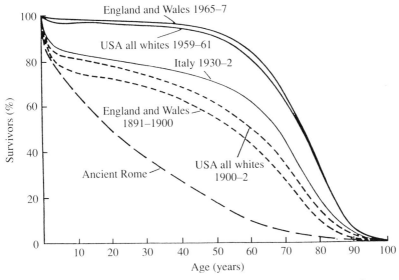

Fig. 5.3 Survival curves for various populations and various historical periods. With an improvement in the control of the environment and a reduction in infant mortality, fractional survival rises, and the 'wild' exponential form is replaced by a more nearly rectangular. This is described as a compression of mortality (into the higher age-groups). After Walford (1981).

In words, an exponential decay of the probability of survival can be seen as the result of members of a cohort succumbing in a chance fashion to random life-threatening insults which are independent of the individual's age. The chance of survival may be large or small without affecting the validity of the argument. This formulation, however, involves a gross simplification, because, although the hazards may not be changing throughout life in the wild, the individual's vulnerability to many of them decreases if the young one survives long enough to grow and to become mobile. For example, a small wild animal may attack a baby, but shrink from attacking a child. Again, a baby has a large ratio of body surface to volume, and, even if thermoregulation did not take a year or two to evolve, it loses heat at a far greater rate than is true of a larger individual: in the same climatic conditions, mice shiver more than elephants. However, it has to be remembered that the simple exponential curve of Fig. 5.3 describes the probability of survival of non-human species within certain limits, and their early vulnerability also decreases during the early stages of life.

The assumption of a progressive reduction in vulnerability to external hazards up to the age of 25 years, which may well coincide with the peak of our physique (Fig. 1.12), can be shown to modify the early shape of the exponential survival curve (Fig. 5.2), but the matter need not be pursued here any further.

Equation 5.3 describes only exogenous hazards on the assumption of an invariant vulnerability. But at all times an individual is also subject to life-threatening endogenous risks, and, if the early hazards have all been survived, these may become overwhelming singly or in multiple coincidental failures. This is one aspect of senescence. If it is taken into account it can be shown (Gompertz 1825) that in such circumstances, the chance of survival is given within certain limits by another set of expressions.

The probability of dying can then be expressed in a number of ways, for example

$$P(\text{mort}) = \exp-[\exp(g.t)] \tag{5.4}$$

$P(\text{mort})$ is the fraction of the population alive at age $t = -\infty$ to have died at the age t. The rate is determined by g. Differentiated with respect to time, eqn 5.4 yields R, the mortality pressure. This defines the number of people of a given age dying in the course of a year, expressed as a fraction of the number of those who were alive at its start.

This is precisely analogous to the definition of the incidence of an age-dependent disease, such as senile cataract: the incidence is the number of people in an age group who become affected in the course of a year, divided by the number in the same age group who were unaffected at the beginning of that year.

In other words, it is the number of actual cases per year divided by the number of possible ones.

Equation 5.4 implies that mortality pressure increases exponentially with age.

This is expressed conventionally (Comfort 1979) in the form of

$$\mathbf{R} = \mathbf{R}(0).\exp(\mathbf{g}t) \tag{5.5}$$

$\mathbf{R}(0)$ is the mortality pressure at birth and $\mathbf{g}$ the constant in eqn 5.4.

The limitations of the Gompertz formulation of mortality have often been emphasized (see Economos 1982), but it remains useful in the delineation of broad outlines in many different fields (see Easton 1988).

5.3 An anthropological aside

Our ability to survive before civilization helped to protect life must have been linked to our genetic make-up, and this will not yet appreciably reflect the changes in our life expectancy brought about more recently by human efforts. For example, the discovery of fire combats hazards resulting from the exposure to low temperatures. The invention of arms reduces those met with in attacks by wild beasts etc. The mortality of the young is reduced out of all proportion in comparison with that of older members of a cohort, at least in the first instance. This results in the gradual approximation of survival curves to functions of which eqn 5.4 (see Fig. 5.3) forms an example.

In order to obtain a model for the 'wild' situation, the aforementioned constant $\mathbf{k}$ is considered. A comparison of the eqns 5.1 and 5.3 shows that $\mathbf{k} = \Sigma\mathbf{q}(\mathbf{i})$, that is to say, $\mathbf{k}$ equals the sum total of the hazards, expressed as specific annual mortalities. Note that an analogous constant appears also in eqn 5.4, and its variation has an analogous effect on the values of $\mathbf{P}(\mathbf{mort})$. Since it appears in Gompertzian formulae, $\mathbf{g}$ is distinguished from the above $\mathbf{k}$ which appears in the exponential description of mortality.

The significance of $\mathbf{k}$ for the preservation of the species can be considered in extremely simplified anthropological terms. The numbers of a cohort diminish in the wild in accordance with eqn 5.3: in time it will be exterminated unless sufficient replacements are produced. However, not all losses are equally important. Those occurring after the termination of the reproductive age $\mathbf{t}(\mathbf{2})$ in particular of females (see p. 38 and Fig. 1.11) can be ignored from a purely biological point of view. On the other hand, all those occurring before this age have to be replaced during the period elapsing between puberty, $\mathbf{t}(\mathbf{1})$, and $\mathbf{t}(\mathbf{2})$.

Female fertility, however, is not uniform throughout this interval; it does not reach its maximum at the onset of puberty and is thought to tail off after the age of 35 years (Edwards 1980) and to drop to zero at about 50 years (Ginsburg 1991). These constraints can be allowed for by setting $t(1)$ to 15 years and $t(2)$ to 45 years (Chamberlain 1991) as the range of puberty lies between 12 and 18 years. It can be shown that an estimate can be made of the relation between k and WY, the number of fertile women-years.

Its value is linked to the average number N of children borne by one woman: this is estimated as 12 even today in basically agricultural societies. Before the onset of the first signs of civilization, in the absence of any senescence, and on the crudest of assumptions, with $k \cong 0.06$ to 0.08 one person in a thousand could have become a centenarian if losses before the end of the female reproductive period were to be made good so as to allow the numbers of a cohort to be kept at least constant. To allow for population growth, smaller rates of loss would have to be stipulated (see Hirsch 1980). Note that the exponential curve approximating to the estimate of Roman mortality in Fig. 5.2 has a $k = 0.037$. In practice, Methuselah notwithstanding, endogenous hazards made the appearance of centenarians virtually unheard of before the advent of preventive medicine and hygiene.

A similar calculation based on the Gompertz formula (eqns 5.4) can be made if the simplifying assumption is made that, in the wild, infant mortality is very high. Since this is regrettably still true in many parts of the so-called Third World, the assumption is hardly far-fetched in this particular connection. An anlaysis based on it leads to time-constants smaller than when the exponential formula is used. In fact it can be shown on the basis of data found in United Nations mortality statistics (Reading and Weale 1991) that g is small in populations with high infant mortality and vice versa. There is no record of any country with a time constant g greater than 0.144 (see p. 237) or smaller than 0.026. The latter approaches the range of theoretical values below which the survival of a population becomes improbable.

There is no pretence that the above considerations are introduced in order to offer a polished picture of population statistics. In a thoughtful analysis of the evolution of senescence, Hirsch (1980) has shown that what may need explaining is not a delay in evolution (as may perhaps be thought implicit in increasing longevity) but why the delay should evolve at all.

5.4 What limits life?

One other characteristic of the Gompertz equations needs to be considered before the above ideas are tentatively related to function in general and the eye in particular. The equations are expressible in terms of several different pairs of constants. We have already mentioned $R(0)$ and g, the mortality pressure at birth and its time constant respectively. It is also possible to use g and t', where t' is the age at which the mortality pressure $R = g$. Finally one can use $t(max)$

and **g**, where **t(max)** is the age at which **R** = 1 (and a very large part of the population has died). It follows from this and eqn 5.5 that the mortality pressure

$$\mathbf{R} = \exp\{g[t-t(m)]\} \tag{5.6}$$

and it can be shown that in the Gompertzian formulation the notional sum of hazards is inversely proportional to **g**, i.e. the steeper the slope of the plot of −ln**R** against age **t** (which determines **g**), the greater the chances of survival (cf. p. 231). It may be mentioned parenthetically that, contrary to a view sometimes held (see Comfort 1979), eqns 5.4 and 5.6 are equivalent.

On a comparative basis, **t(m)** may be looked on as a measure of the life span. Indeed, the United Nations data show that its largest value is unlikely to exceed 120 years, a value seen by Lestienne (1988) as in agreement with thermo-dynamic principles. Olshansky *et al.* (1990) estimate it as corresponding to the human life span because they believe 'a biological effect' to be in operation.

It was noted in Chapter 1 that there are many contenders for the guillotine of life, and some doubt was expressed as regards the biological need for specific genes for senescence. This sceptical approach is supported by the important observation (Nette *et al.* 1984) that the ability of DNA irradiated by ultraviolet radiation to repair itself steadily decreases with the donor's age. Equation 5.2 showed, not surprisingly, that the failure of one life-supporting component suffices to cause death. Nette *et al.* found that the regression describing the decline of the reparability **Y** of DNA as a function of age is given by

$$\mathbf{Y} = 78.4782 - 0.6032t \tag{5.7}$$

It is easily seen that **Y** drops to zero at the age of **t** ≅ 130 years. The spread of the data can make the value as low as 110 years and as high as about 200 years. When compared with contemporary survival curves (see Olshansky *et al.* 1990), eqn 5.7 decreases toward its limiting value too slowly to be envisaged in its present form as a controller for survival in the sense in which this was mooted in connection with eqn 5.2. It is, however, clear that a similar failure of repair processes, acting in a conjoint manner, could provide just the type of biological effect which Olshansky *et al.* envisage as a terminal to the human life span.

The fact that the views advanced in this section depend a great deal on inevitable extrapolation has already been stressed, and the deductions drawn from eqn 5.7 form no exception to this. That said, it may be noted that both this expression and the variations of the characteristics described in Fig. 5.4 below are expressed as linear functions and not as exponentials. If linearity persists in higher age groups hitherto left unexplored then it would be possible to think in terms of end-points as is being done in connection with eqn 5.7; this would be difficult if functions showed an unambiguous exponential or some cataclysmic decline (see Figs 1.9 and 1.11).

The above mechanism of DNA repair of lesions produced by electromagnetic radiation needs to be distinguished carefully from one which attributes senescence to an actual change in DNA (see DeLong and Poplin 1977). Nette *et al.* express no view on which part of the molecular structure may be involved in the process but only on the faculty for repair when damage has occurred. DeLong and Poplin say that, if DNA were to change so as to cause ageing, senescence would be a heritable attribute. This might be true if DNA were to change before the termination of the reproductive period. Any change thereafter would be without significance for the species. Thus while postreproductive changes in DNA could cause senescence, the loss of ability of the molecule to restore its constitution following an insult is a separate issue. It may be mentioned in passing that, so far, no one appears to have studied the age-related variation in the efficiency of mechanisms dealing with other types of damage, for example that caused by reactive oxygen species (Breimer 1991) or free radicals, etc.

5.5 Limiting functions

Chapter 1 introduced the notion of biomarkers, i.e. human morphological or functional characteristics which change systematically with age, and which are used by some authors as predictors of the probable duration of an individual's life, i.e. necro-markers. The preceding paragraphs have drawn attention to groups of variables which may be more relevant in this connection than others. They may incidentally provide an answer to an important and valid criticism of the whole idea of biomarkers (Adelman 1987), namely that they are of little use in the calculation of the elusive idea of a biological age and even less as prophets of death.

The notion that presbyopia can act as the latter has already been disproved (p. 59). The loss of accommodation has been known for some time to be complete between the ages of 50 and 60 years (in temperate climates), yet Danon *et al.* (1981) quote it as a component of a test battery for an age range between 21 and 83 years, and for good measure recommend it for inclusion in any test battery.

The group of functions worth considering are those which, by extrapolation, lead either to zero or to critically low values at the age associated with the end of the life span, for a number of reasons outlined above. For the time being it is unfortunately necessary to depend a great deal on extrapolation, because the bulk of relevant and interesting data have of necessity been recorded largely for age-groups still remote in time from that terminal. If, for example, the morphological or functional continuation of some entity depended on the intactness of DNA, and if the latter were generally to be found not to persist beyond 120–130 years, then that entity might be a suitable candidate for prediction.

The units wherein the variable is measured are without effect on the magnitude of this value. If the decrement is linear then the ordinate reaches zero value when the abscissa is equal to the ratio of the intercept and the slope of the regression: this is a function only of time. However, the variable may alternatively be expressed in terms of a coefficient defined as the percentage change per annum. This is likewise measured on a time scale, and is mathematically similar to the aforementioned mortality pressure or the incidence of age-related conditions.

A modified version of this idea is to express the variables as a percentage of a value measured for a fixed age, chosen as 30 years for example by Danon *et al.* (1981). The difference between the two figures is as follows. The coefficient is based on the value of the variable at the beginning of a year, and measures the change during the subsequent 12 months, and hence the change in the logarithm of the variable. If linear, this function implies an exponential decay of the basic variable. The percentage figure, however, relates the change to the value recorded for the age of 30 years, and will therefore tend to be smaller than the coefficient.

Figure 5.4 shows some interesting examples, involving an extrapolation of data quoted by Danon *et al.* Line b indicates that the velocity with which nerves conduct impulses decreases very slowly; neuronal failure is associated with cell death rather than with the atrophy of nerve fibres. It is therefore unlikely that the velocity of conduction of nerve impulses can fulfil a useful chronometric function. Its durability may well be a requisite for the development and maintenance of reflexes and memory the survival value of which in early life needs no emphasis.

In contrast the maximum breathing capacity drops to zero at an age no greater than 113 years. Similarly, renal blood flow reaches its statistical value of zero at maximally 130 years. Hand grip strength drops to zero for both men and women at not more than 123 years, if one extrapolates the data due to Hollingsworth *et al.* (1965). It is not surprising, however, that the cardiac index has greater reserves reaching an extrapolated zero value at up to almost 200 years: an intact heart excised from a body can beat even though the donor may be dead.

Attention was drawn in Chapter 3 to the increase in the putative incidence of cataracts, as expressed by numbers of operations (since there is little point in diagnosing a disabling cataract if nothing is going to be done about it). The functions follow Gompertz equations (Weale 1982*b*), and it is to be noted that the values of the slopes **g** are similar to those mentioned above in connection with mortality ($\cong 0.1 - 0.14$). This puts a new gloss on the observation that there is a correlation between cataracts and mortality (Hirsch and Schwartz 1983; Benson *et al.* 1988). While there is no proven causal relation, the fact that cataracts join the above variables which pinpoint the region around 120 years as a maximal endpoint is of considerable interest. The maintenance of lenticular transparence is biologically costly, as becomes evident when one considers the need for the preservation of an orderly quasi-crystalline lattice structure from the point of view of thermodynamics. The lenticular money runs out during the

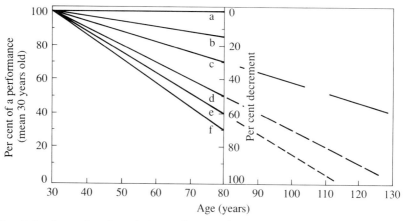

Fig. 5.4 Age-related variations of a number of physiological functions as measured in males. Peak performances were averaged from data for an age range of 20 to 35 years. (a) fasting blood glucose; (b) nervous conduction velocity; (c) (resting) cardiac index; (d) renal blood-flow; also vital capacity; (e) maximal breathing capacity; (f) maximal work rate; also maximal oxygen uptake. See text for details regarding the extrapolations.

twelfth decade of life, and, if the near simultaneity between this and the life span as given by the above-mentioned recent estimates is a coincidence, it is a remarkable one.

It is compounded by another extrapolation, namely one made from data on the age-related variation of free glutathione in the human crystalline lens (Harding 1970). The function of the compound is probably to protect the lens from free radicals such as O_2^+ and its role in the preservation of lenticular transparence is thought to be indispensable. A regression based on the linear part of Fig. 5.5 puts the level of the compound in the lens near zero at not later than about 116 years. It will be recalled that an analogous extrapolation applied to a function describing light scattered by the lens reached its terminal value at 113 years. This correlation between the age-related decay of glutathione on the one hand and both the physiological (p. 237) and pathological decreases in lenticular transparency on the other also raises the question of whether there are environmental influences on the concentration of glutathione. It is possible that the human life span is not the same all over the world (Reading and Weale 1991), but insufficient data are available to enable one even to speculate on links between a hypothetical variation in glutathione concentration, incidence of cataract, mortality, and variations in other physiological data. What is needed is experimental data, in particular on tissues from donors living in countries not renowned for the prosecution of biological research.

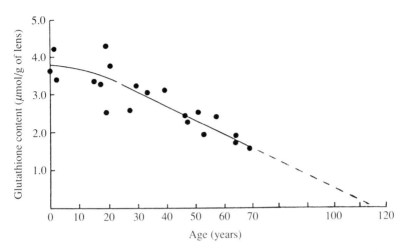

Fig. 5.5 The lenticular content of glutathione as a function of age. See text for the significance of the extrapolation. Data due to Harding (1970).

In contrast, the retina, a nervous tissue, seems to have greater stamina. The stability of absolute thresholds lasting into the 80s has been reported by several workers (see p. 175). Moreover, no matter whether one accepts Owsley and Burton's more optimistic and well-documented estimate of a very slow pace in the age-related decline in contrast sensitivity or the rather brisker pace reported by McGrath and Morrison (1981), Nameda *et al.* (1989), and others (see Weale 1982*a*), the average logarithm of visual contrast discrimination (for the highest frequencies) extrapolated to the 120 year region points to a statistical value of as much as approximately 0.25 of the value for 40 years. The spread of existing data may well accommodate a significant chance of the value dropping to 0.1, which implies legally defined blindness. But by the same token the value may be of the order of 0.4. The difficulty one is faced with is that the problem of distinguishing between retinal senescence and photic wear and tear (p. 112) is still to be resolved. Furthermore, the course of demyelination of Gennari's line (Fig. 3.1) may provide a cerebral as distinct from a retinal substrate for this change.

Since the human species has spent much of its recent history in adaptation to daylight, notwithstanding the fact that several of ocular attributes point to a nocturnal life in the long distant past, one would expect evolutionary pressures to have acted accordingly. It is therefore conceivable that both on account of the observed incidence of senile cataract and on that of the decline of photopic contrast discrimination the end of our visual lives may coincide with that of our lungs, of our kidneys, and our ability to maintain a mechanical entity.

5.6 The endpoint: is senescence programmed?

In these pages the bias has not been in support of the view that human senescence is programmed. Reasons for this have been advanced (see Chapter 1), but it is only right to try to see if the outcome of evolutionary pressures as described here may not perhaps have given rise to the illusion that a programme may exist after all. If it is accepted that mutations are accidental, then changes in the human genome are likely to take place in small steps. Otherwise additional adaptive changes would be unlikely to buttress any new equilibrium between individual and environment. Moreover, one change on its own may have to wait for others before a significant change in anatomy or function can occur. The brain cannot increase its size if the skull does not become larger, and, at the same time, vascularization does not evolve to accommodate an increased blood supply — a problem, incidentally, that does not appear to be fully resolved as yet.

At any one time, such a group of advances form the nibbling edge of evolutionary quantum leaps, and create the impression that they are co-ordinated, and *ipso facto* programmed.

The biological costs of maintaining structures and functions can perhaps be viewed in a similar way. Given that they support the continuation of the species, they will have evolved like any other biological characteristic, and the observed results will have ensued. A number of them are likely to be marginal precisely in the sense that they contribute to the balance between survival and extinction (p. 233). They may form the genomic cadre of the group from which we ultimately derive the notion of the life span.

Such an argument may answer the oft repeated regret that it is futile to seek a single pattern which might govern morphological and functional senescence. What modern molecular biology may therefore well lead us to ask is whether there are perhaps certain sets of functions which share, not a common ancestry, but a linked destiny. A number of studies have indicated (see pp. 20, 41–2) that each species possesses, encoded in its genome, some biological limit to its life span. One might therefore indeed expect different declining physiological functions to converge in time toward some approximately fixed common point which such a period defines. The senescence of human vision appears to be following one such path.

5.7 Resumé

There are some age-related properties of the human visual system which are non-linear and which reach an extreme in mid-life. Others, related in general to the perception of stimulus differences, as is true of contrast and of colour vision, reach an optimum earlier, namely during the third or fourth decades. If one adopts an evolutionary point of view, this becomes understandable, since, in the wild, the visual system had to be optimal at about this period of life in view of the need for the protection and rearing of offspring. There are, however, also some age-related functions which change in a monotonic manner. The constants describing their variation may be the result of evolutionary pressures which helped to ensure a certain level of performance essential for survival and crucial for the continuation of the species. The circumstance that they may have, as it were, outlasted life in the historic past is perhaps attributable to any other solution being biologically more costly.

Modern techniques may make it possible for life spans for all species to be established. It may then transpire that certain vital functions have been subject to evolutionary pressures only just strong enough for their duration to be orchestrated up to the end of this genetically determined time.

References

The numbers in italics refer to pages on which the authors are quoted.

Abernethy, J.D. (1979). The exponential increase in mortality rate with age attributed to wearing-out of biological components. *J. Theor. Biol.* **80**, 333–54. [*8*]

Abramov, I., Hainline, L., Lemerise, E., and Brown, A.K. (1985). Changes in visual functions of children exposed as infants to prolonged illumination. *J. Amer. Optom. Assoc.* **56**, 614–19. [*163*]

Abrams, J.D. (1964). Biomicroscopy of the transilluminated iris. *An. Inst. Barraquer*, **5**, 39–88. [*167*]

Adams, A.J., Wong, L.S., Wong, L., and Gould, B. (1988). Visual acuity changes with age: some new perspectives. *Amer. J. Optom. Physiol. Opt.* **65**, 403–6. [*206*]

Adefule, A.O. (1983). Presbyopia in Nigerians. *East Afr. Med. J.* **60**, 766–72. [*60*]

Adelman, R. (1987). Biomarkers of aging. *Exp. Gerontol.* **22**, 227–9. [*23, 43, 236*]

Alaku, O. and Steinbach, J. (1982). Effects of season of birth and age on eye lenses weight in the humid equatorial tropics. *Growth*, **46**, 22–5. [*64*]

Alexander, R.A. and Garner, A. (1983). Elastic and precursor fibres in the normal human eye. *Exp. Eye Res.* **36**, 305–15. [*74*]

Alexandridis, E. (1971). *Pupillographie*, Huthig, Heidelberg. [*82*]

Allen, M.J. and Vos, J.J. (1967). Ocular scattered light and visual performance as a function of age. *Amer. J. Optom.* **44**, 717–27. [*103, 105*]

Aloj Totaro, E., Cuomo, V., and Pisanti, F.A. (1986). Influence of environmental stress on lipofuscin production. *Arch. Geront. Geriatr.* **5**, 343–9. [*11, 149*]

Alpern, M., Ching, C.C., and Kitahara, K. (1983). The directional sensitivity of retinal rods. *J. Physiol. (Lond).* **343**, 577–92. [*201*]

Alpern, M., Kitahara, H., and Fielder, G.H. (1987). The change in colour matches with retinal angle of incidence of the colorimeter beams. *Vision Res.* **27**, 1763–78. [*201*]

Alphen, G.W.H.M. van, Robinette, S.L., and Macri, F.J. (1962). Drug effects on ciliary muscle and choroid preparations in vitro. *Arch. Ophthal.* **68**, 81–93. [*71*]

Andley, U.P. (1987). Photodamage to the eye. *Photochem. Photobiol.* **46**, 1057–66. [*164*]

Applegate, R.A., Adams, A.J., Cavender, J.C., and Zisman, F. (1987). Early color vision changes in age-related maculopathy. *App. Opt.* **26**, 1458–62. [*224*]

Arden, G.B. and Weale, R.A. (1954). Nervous mechanisms and dark adaptation. *J. Physiol. (Lond).* **125**, 417–26. [*172*]

Aufderheide, K.J. (1984). Cellular aging: an overview. *Monogr. Devl. Biol.* **17**, 2–8. [*28, 29*]

Aylward, G.W., Jeffrey, B.G., and Billson, F.A. (1990). Normal variation and the effect of age on the parametric analysis of the intensity-response series of the scotopic electroretinogram, including the scotopic threshold response. *Clin. Vision Sci.* **4**, 353–62. [*170, 171*]

Bacon, R. (1896). *Opus majus.* Vol. **II**. Clarendon Press, Oxford. [*49*]

Balazsi, A.G., Rootman, J., Drance, S.M., Schulzer, M., and Douglas, G.R. (1984). The effect of age on the nerve fiber population of the human optic nerve. *Amer. J. Ophthal.* **97**, 760–6. [*139, 140*]

Ball, K.K., Beard, B.L., Roenker, D.L., Miller, R.L., and Griggs, D.S. (1988). Age and visual search: expanding the useful field of view. *J. Opt. Soc. Amer.* **5**, 2210–19. [*213*]

Ball, K., Owsley, C., and Beard, B. (1990). Clinical visual perimetry underestimates peripheral field problems in older adults. *Clin. Vision Sci.* **5**, 113–25. [*193, 194*]

Ballard, F.J. and Read, L.C. (1985). Changes in protein synthesis and breakdown rates and responsiveness to growth factors with ageing in human lung fibroblasts. *Mech. Ag. Dev.* **30**, 11–22. [*28*]

Bamba, M. (1987). Particular features of the correction of presbyopia in Africa. In *Presbyopia*, (ed. L. Stark and G. Obrecht), pp. 30–31. Fairchild Publications, New York. [*60*]

Banks, M.S. (1980). The development of visual accommodation during early infancy. *Child Dev.* **51**, 646–66. [*81*]

Barbe, M.F., Tytell, M., Gower, D.J., and Welch, W.J. (1988). Hyperthermia protects against light-damage in the rat retina. *Science* **241**, 1827–20. [*167*]

Barlow, H.B. (1957). Increment thresholds at low intensities considered as signal/noise discriminations. *J. Physiol. (Lond).* **136**, 469–88. [*170*]

Bartosz, G., Grzelinska, E., and Wagner, J. (1982). Aging of the erythrocyte. XIV. ATP content does decrease. *Experientia*, **38**, 575. [*4*]

Bazan, H.E.P., Bazan, N.G., Feeney-Burns, L., and Berman, E.R. (1990). Lipids in human lipofuscin-enriched subcellular fractions of two age populations. *Invest. Ophthal. Vis. Sci.* **31**, 1433–43. [*129, 146*]

Bellamy, D. (1986). Cell death and the loss of structural units of organs. In *The biology of human ageing*, (ed. A.H. Bittles and K.J. Collins). Cambridge University Press. [*29*]

Ben-Sira, I., Weinberger, D., Bodenheimer, J., and Yassur, Y. (1980). Clinical method for measurement of light backscattering from the in vivo human lens. *Invest. Ophthal. Vis. Sci.* **19**, 435–7. [*105*]

Benson, W.H., Farber, M.E., and Caplan, R.J. (1988). Increased mortality rates after cataract surgery. *Ophthalmology*, **95**, 1288–92. [*10, 237*]

Beregi, E., Regius, O., and Rajczy, K. (1991). The lymphocytes in elderly individuals and centenarians. *Arch. Gerontol. Geriatr.* Suppl.2, 515–18. [*17*]

Bermbach, G., Mayer, U., and Naumann, G.O.H. (1991). Human lens epithelial cells in tissue culture. *Exp. Eye Res.* **52**, 113–19. [*64*]

Bernstein, F. and Bernstein, M. (1945). Law of physiologic aging as derived from long range data on refraction of the eye. *Arch. Ophthal.* **34**, 378–88. [*10, 59*]

Bessems, G.J.H. and Hoenders, H.J. (1987). Distribution of aromatic and fluorescent compounds within simple human lenses. *Exp. Eye Res.* **44**, 817–24. [*102*]

Bettelheim, F.A. and Ali, S. (1985). Light scattering of normal human lens III. Relationship between forward and back scatter of whole excised lenses. *Exp. Eye Res.* **41**, 1–9. [*105*]

Beutler, E. (1986). Planned obsolescence in humans and in other biosystems. *Persp. Biol. Med.* **29**, 175–9. [*3–5*]

Bleeker, J.C., van Best, J.A., Vrij, L., van der Velde, E.A., and Oosterhuis, J.A. (1986). Autofluorescence of the lens in diabetic and healthy subjects by fluorophotometry. *Invest. Ophthal. Vis. Sci.* **27**, 791–4. [*103, 104*]

Bobak, P., Bodis-Wollner, I., Guillory, S., and Anderson, R. (1989). Aging differentially delays visual evoked potentials to checks and gratings. *Clin. Vis. Sci.* **4**, 269–74. [*121, 122*]

Bochow, T.W., West, S.K., Azar, A., Munoz, B., Sommer, A., and Taylor, H.R. (1989). Ultraviolet light exposure and risk of posterior subcapsular cataracts. *Arch. Ophthal.* **107**, 369–72. [*109*]

Bone, R.A. and Sparrock, J.M.B. (1971). Comparison of macular pigment densities in human eyes. *Vision Res.* **11**, 1057–64. [*138*]

Bone, R.A., Landrum, J.T., Fernandez, L., and Tarsis, S.L. (1988). Analysis of the macular pigment by HPLC: Retinal distribution and age study. *Invest. Ophthal. Vis. Sci.* **29**, 843–9. [*137, 138*]

Borkan, G.A. and Norris, A.H. (1980). Assessment of biological age using a profile of physical parameters. *J. Geront.* **35**, 177–84. [*5*]

Boulton, M., McKechnie, N.M., Breda, J., Bayly, M., and Marshall, J. (1989). The formation of autofluorescent granules in cultured human RPE. *Invest. Ophthal. Vis. Sci.* **30**, 82–9. [*146*]

Boulton, M., Docchio, F., Dayhaw-Barker, P., Ramponi, R., and Cubeddu, R. (1990). Age-related changes in the morphology, absorption and fluorescence of melanosomes and lipofuscin granules of the retinal pigment epithelium. *Vision Res.* **30**, 1291–303. [*146–50, 153*]

Bowdler, A.J., Dougherty, R.M., and Bodler, N.C. (1981). Age as a factor affecting erythrocyte osmotic fragility in males. *Gerontology*, **27**, 224–31. [*4*]

Bowman, K.J., Collins, M.J., and Henry, C.J. (1984). The effect of age on performance on the panel D-15 and desaturated D-15. A quantitative evaluation. In *Colour vision deficiencies*, (ed. G. Verriest), pp. 227–31. Dr W Junk, the Hague. [*222*]

Braddick, O., Atkinson, J., French, J., and Howland, H. (1979). A photorefractive study of infant accommodation. *Vision Res.* **19**, 1319–30. [*81*]

Breimer, J.H. (1991). Repair of DNA damage induced by reactive oxygen species. *Free Rad. Res. Comm.* **14**, 159–71. [*236*]

Brewitt, B. and Clark, J.I. (1988). Growth and transparency in the lens, an epithelial tissue, stimulated by pulses of PDGF. *Science*, **242**, 777–9. [*42*]

Bridges, C.D.B. and Yoshikami, S. (1970). The rhodopsin-porphyropsin system in freshwater fishes − 1. Effects of age and photic environment. *Vision Res.* **10**, 1315–22. [*21*]

Brilliant, L.B., Grasset, N.C., Pokhrel, R.P., Kolstad, A., Lepkowski, J.M., Brilliant, G.E.O. *et al.* (1983). Associations among cataract prevalence, sunlight hours, and altitude in the Himalayas. *Amer. J. Epidemiol.* **118**, 250–64. [*109*]

Brock, M.A. (1985). Biological clocks and aging. *Rev. Biol. Res. Ag.* **2**, 445–62. [*11, 21*]

Brown, E.V.L. (1938). Net average yearly changes in refraction of atropinized eyes from birth to beyond middle life. *Arch. Ophthal.* **19**, 719–34. [*52*]

Brown, N. (1972). Quantitative slit-image photography of the lens. *Trans. Ophthal. Soc. UK.* **921**, 303–17. [*70*]

Brown, N. (1973). The change in shape and internal form of the lens of the eye on accommodation. *Exp. Eye Res.* **15**, 451–9. [*76, 83*]

Brown, N. (1974). The change in lens curvature with age. *Exp. Eye Res.* **19**, 175–83. [*66, 70, 71*]

Brown, W.T. and Wisniewski, H.M. (1983). Genetics and human aging. *Rev. Biol. Res. Aging*, **1**, 81–99. [*31*]

Brückner, R. (1967). Longitudinal research on the eye. *Geront. Clin.* **9**, 87–95. [*57, 63*]

Brückner, R., Batschelet, E., and Hugenschmidt, F. (1987). The Basel longitudinal study on aging (1955–1978). *Docum. Ophthal.* **64**, 235–310. [*59–69, 81*]

Buchanan, J.H. and Sidhu, J. (1986). Autofluorescence and ageing: changes in ribosome accuracy and lysome function. *Mech. Ag. Dev.* **36**, 259–67. [*13*]

Buckinhgam, T., Whitaker, D., and Banford, D. (1987). Movement in decline? Oscillatory movement displacement thresholds increase with ageing. *Ophthal. Physiol. Opt.* **7**, 411–13. [*215*]

Buell, S.J. and Coleman, P.D. (1979). Dendritic growth in the aged human brain and failure of growth in senile dementia. *Science*, **206**, 654–856. [*117*]

Bugiani, O., Salvarani, S., Perdelli, F., Mancardi, G.L., and Leonardi, A. (1978). Nerve cell loss with aging in the putamen. *Eur. Neurol.* **17**, 286–91. [*116*]

Burch, P.R.J. and Jackson, D. (1976). Molecular mechanisms of ageing. *Gerontology*, **22**, 206–11. [*24*]

Burns, E.M., Kruckeberg, T.W., Comerford, L.E., and Buschmann, T.M. (1979). Thinning of capillary walls and declining numbers of endothelial mitochondria in the cerebral cortex of the aging primate, *Macaca nemestrina. J. Geront.* **34**, 642–50. [*125*]

Burns, E.M., Kruckeberg, T.W., and Gaetano, P.K. (1981). Changes with age in cerebral capillary morphology. *Neurobiol. Ag.* **2**, 285–91. [*125*]

Cagianut, B. (1978). Zur Verteilung der Augendruckwerte in der Normalbevölkerung. *Klin. Mtsbl. d. Augenheilk.* **173**, 290–5. [*56*]

Caird, F.I., Hutchinson, M., and Pirie, A. (1965). Cataract extraction in an English population. *Brit. J. Prev. Soc. Med.* **19**, 80–4. [*110*]

Calder III, W.A. (1982). The relationship of the Gompertz constant and maximum potential lifespan to body mass. *Exp. Geront.* **17**, 383–5. [*41, 42*]

Calderini, G., Bellini, F., Consolazione, R. Dal Toso, Milan, F., and Toffano, G. (1987). Reparative processes in aged brain. *Gerontology*, **33**, 227–33. [*117*]

Campbell, F.W. (1957). The depth of field of the human eye. *Optica Acta*, **4**, 157–64. [*51, 52*]

Campbell, F.W. and Green, D.G. (1965). Optical and retinal factors affecting visual resolution. *J. Physiol.* **181**, 576–93. [*61, 62, 201, 208*]

Carroll, J.P. (1982). On emmetropization. *J. Theor. Biol.* **95**, 135–44. [*57*]

Chalmers, J.H., Morrison, J.D., Ogg, A., and Reilly, J. (1985). The effects of ageing on the human visual evoked response. *J. Physiol.* **367**, 27P. [*121*]

Chamberlain, G. (1991). Vital statistics of birth. *Brit. Med. J.* **303**, 178–81. [*234*]

Chatterjee, A., Milton, R.C., and Thyle, S. (1982). Prevelence and aetiology of cataract in Punjab. *Brit. J. Ophthal.* **66**, 35–42. [*109*]

Choe, B.-K. and Rose, N.R. (1976). In vitro senescence of mammalian cells. *Gerontology*, **22**, 89–108. [*16, 26*]

Clemmesen, V. and Luntz, H. (1976). Lens thickness and angle-closure glaucoma. *Acta Ophthalm.* **54**, 193–7. [*69*]

Clemmesen, V. and Olurin, O. (1985). Lens thickness in Western Nigeria. *Acta Ophthalm.* **63**, 274–6. [*69*]

Cogan, D.G. (1963). Development and senescence of the human retinal vasculature. *Trans. Ophthal. Soc. UK.* **83**, 465–89. [*125*]

Coleman, D.J. (1970). Unified model for accommodative mechanism. *Amer. J. Ophthal.* **69**, 1063–79. [*83*]

Coleman, P.D. and Flood, D.G. (1986). Dendritic proliferation in the aging brain as a compensatory repair mechanism. *Progr. Brain Res.* **70**, 227–36. [*71, 117*]

Collins, K.J. and Exton-Smith, A.N. (1986). Effects of ageing on human homeostasis. In *The biology of human ageing*, (ed. A.H.J. Bittles and K.J. Collins). Cambridge University Press. [*20*]

Collins, M. (1989). The onset of prolonged glare recovery with age. *Ophthal. Physiol. Opt.* **9**, 368–71. [*187, 199, 200, 201, 204*]

Collins, M. and Brown, B. (1989). Glare recovery and age related maculopathy. *Clin. Vis. Sci.* **4**, 145–53. [*203, 204*]

Collins, J.J., Brown, B., and Bowman, K.J. (1989). Peripheral acuity and age. *Ophthal. Physiol. Opt.* **9**, 314–6. [*187*]

Comfort, A. (1969). Test battery to measure aging rate in men. *The Lancet*, **ii**, 1411–5. [*43*]

Comfort, A. (1979). *The biology of senescence*. Churchill Livingstone, London. [*1, 229*]

Cooper, G.F. and Robson, J.G. (1969). The yellow colour of the lens of man and other primates. *J. Physiol.* **203**, 411–7. [*90, 91, 94*]

Corberand, J., Laharrague, P., and Fillola, G. (1987). Blood cell parameters do not change during physiological human ageing. *Gerontology*, **33**, 72–76. [*4*]

Cotman, C.W. and Scheff, S.W. (1979). Compensatory synapse growth in aged animals after neuronal death. *Mech. Ag. Dev.* **9**, 103–17. [*117*]

Cox, J.R. and Shalaby, W.A. (1981). Potassium changes with age. *Gerontology*, **27**, 340–4. [*5*]

Coyne, A.C. (1981). Age differences and practice in forward visual masking. *J. Geront.* **36**, 730–2. [*198*]

Crassini, B., Brown, B., and Bowman, K. (1988). Age-related changes in contrast sensitivity in central and peripheral retina. *Perception*, **17**, 315–22. [*213*]

Crawford, B.H. (1947). Visual adaptation in relation to brief conditioning stimuli. *Proc. Roy. Soc. B*, **134**, 283–302. [*196, 198*]

Crawford, K.S., Kaufman, P.L., and Bito, L.Z. (1990). The role of the iris in accommodation of rhesus monkey. *Invest. Ophthal. Vis. Sci.* **31**, 2185–90. [*71, 83*]

Cullinan, T. (1986). *Visual disability in the elderly*. Croom Helm, London. [*v*]

Curcio, C.A. (1986). Aging and topography of human photoreceptors. *J. Opt. Soc. Amer.* **3**, 59. [*131*]

Curcio, C.A. and Hendrickson, A.E. (1991). Organisation and development of the primate photoreceptor mosaic. *Progr. Ret. Res.* **10**, 89–120. [*127*]

Curcio, C.A., Sloan Jr., K.R., Packer, O., Hendrickson, A.E., and Kalina, R. (1987). Distribution of cones in human and monkey retina: individual variability and radial asymmetry. *Science*, **236**, 579–82. [*129, 131*]

Curcio, C.A., Kimberly, A.A., and Kalina, R.E. (1990). Reorganization of the human photoreceptor mosaic following age-related rod loss. *ARVD Abstracts*, **31**, 38. [*129, 132, 136, 139*]

Danon, D., Shock, N.W., and Marois, M. (1981). *Aging: a challenge to science and society*. Oxford University Press. [*236–8*]

Dartnall, H.J.A., Lander, M.R., and Munz, F.W. (1961). Periodic changes in the visual pigment of a fish. In *Progress in photobiology*, (ed. B.C. Christensen and B. Buchmann). Elsevier, Amsterdam. [*21*]

Daum, K.M. (1983). Accommodative dysfunction. *Docum. Ophthal.* **55**, 177–98. [*71*]

Davanger, M. (1975). The suspensory apparatus of the lens. The surface of the ciliary body. *Acta Ophthal.* **53**, 19–33. [*76*]

Davies, I. and Fotheringham, A.P. (1981). Lipofuscin – does it affect cellular performance? *Exp. Geront.* **16**, 119–25. [*13*]

Davies, I., Fotheringham, A., and Roberts, C. (1983). The effect of lipofuscin on cellular function. *Mech. Ag. Dev.* **23**, 347–56. [*11, 13*]

Davson, H. (1978). *The eye*. Vol. IIA. Academic Press, London. [*172*]

Dawkins, R. (1989). *The selfish gene*. Oxford University Press. [25]

Dell'Orco, R.T., Whittle, W.L., and Macieira-Coelho, A. (1986). Changes in the higher organisation of DNA during aging of human fibroblast-like cells. *Mech. Ag. Dev.* **35**, 199–208. [26]

DeLong, R. and Poplin, L. (1977). On the etiology of aging. *J. Theor. Biol.* **67**, 111–20. [14, 236]

Denlinger, J.L., Eisner, G., and Balazs, E.A. (1980). Age-related changes in the vitreous and lens of rhesus monkeys (*Macaca mulatta*). *Exp. Eye Res.* **31**, 67–79. [63]

Devaney, K.O. and Johnson, H.A. (1980). Neuron loss in the aging visual cortex of man. *J. Gerontol.* **35**, 836–41. [118, 119]

Dillon, J. (1984). Photolytic changes in lens protein. *Curr. Eye Res.* **3**, 145–50. [102]

Dillon, J. and Atherton, S.J. (1990). Time resolved spectroscopic studies on the intact human lens. *Photochem. Photobiol.* **51**, 465–8. [92]

Dobrin, P.B. (1978). Mechanical properties of arteries. *Physiol. Rev.* **58**, 397–460. [124]

Dolman, C.L., McCormick, A.Q., and Drance, S.M. (1980). Aging of the optic nerve. *Arch. Ophthal.* **98**, 2053–8. [120, 139]

Domey, R.G. and McFarland, R.A. (1961). Dark adaptation as a function of age: individual prediction. *Amer. J. Ophthal.* **51**, 1262–8. [172–4]

Donders, F.C. (1864). On the anomalies of accommodation and refraction of the eye. New Sydenham Society, London. [61, 81, 82]

Donovan, H.C., Weale, R.A., and Wheeler, C. (1978). The perimeter as a monitor of glaucomatous changes. *Brit. J. Ophthal.* **62**, 705–8. [191]

Dorey, C.K., Wu, G., Ebenstein, D., Garsd, A., and Weiter, J.J. (1989). Cell loss in the aging retina. *Invest. Ophthal. Vis. Sci.* **30**, 1691–9. [129, 145, 156–8]

Doubal, S. (1982). Theory of reliability, biological systems and aging. *Mech. Ag. Dev.* **18**, 339–53. [8]

Drew, N.J. (1941). Norms of refraction. A partial historical survey of reported data. *Amer. J. Optom.* **18**, 97–111. [60]

Driscoll, W.G. and Vaughan, W. (1978). *Handbook of optics*. Section 2.35. McGraw Hill, London. [200]

Drucker, D.N. and Curcio, C.A. (1990). Retinal ganglion cells are lost with aging but not in Alzheimer's disease. *ARVO* **31**, 356. [139]

Duane, A.J. (1912). Normal values of the accommodation at all ages. *Amer. Med. Assoc.* **59**, 1010–13. [61, 81, 82]

Easton, D.M. (1988). Mathematical model of cardiac mechanogram rhythmicity (based on mollusc heart). *Comp. Biochem. Physiol.* **91C**, 91–8. [233]

Economos, A.C. (1982). Rate of aging, rate of dying and the mechanism of mortality. *Arch. Gerontol. Geriatr.* **1**, 3–27. [38, 233]

Edwards, R.G. (1980). *Conception in the human female*, p. 980. Academic Press, London. [234]

Eichhorn, G.L. (1979). Aging, genetics, and the environment: potential of errors introduced into genetic information transfer by metal ions. *Mech. Ag. Dev.* **9**, 291–301. [29, 161]

Eisner, A., Fleming, S.A., Klein, M.L., and Mauldin, W.M. (1987). Sensitivities in older eyes with good acuity: cross-sectional norms. *Invest. Ophthal. Clin. Sci.* **28**, 1824–31. [179]

Elliott, D., Whitaker, D., and MacVeigh, D. (1990). Neural contribution to spatio-temporal contrast sensitivity decline in healthy ageing eyes. *Vision Res.* **30**, 541–7. [214]

Elliott, D.B. (1987). Contrast sensitivity decline with ageing: a neural or optical phenomenon? *Ophthal. Physiol. Opt.* **4**, 415–19. [*213*]

Elliott, D.B., Whitaker, D., and Thompson, P. (1989). Use of displacement threshold hyperacuity to isolate the neural component of senile vision loss. *App. Opt.* **28**, 1914–18. [*215–18*]

Ellis, C.J.K. (1981). The pupillary light reflex in normal subjects. *Brit. J. Ophthal.* **65**, 754–9. [*82*]

Elsner, A.E., Berk, L., Burns, S.A., and Rosenberg, P.R. (1988). Aging and human cone photopigments. *J. Opt. Soc. Amer.* **5**, 2106–12. [*137*]

Enroth, C. (1952). The mechanism of flicker and fusion studied on single retinal elements in the dark-adapted eye of the cat. *Acta Physiol. Scand.* **27**, Suppl. 100. [*218*]

Farnsworth, P.N. and Shyne, S.E. (1979). Anterior zonular shifts with age. *Exp. Eye Res.* **28**, 291–7. [*78, 79*]

Feeney-Burns, L. and Ellersieck, M.R. (1985). Age-related changes in the ultrastructure of Bruch's membrane. *Amer. J. Ophthal.* **100**, 686–97. [*141, 143*]

Feeney-Burns, L., Hildebrand, E.S., and Eldridge, S. (1984). Aging human RPE: morphometric analysis of macular, equatorial and peripheral cells. *Invest. Ophthal. Vis. Sci.* **25**, 195–200. [*11, 145, 151, 155, 156, 159*]

Feeney, Burns, L., Burns, R.P. and Gao, C.-L. (1990). Age-related macular changes in humans over 90 years old. *Amer. J. Ophthal.* **109**, 265–78. [*125, 129, 131, 145*]

Feke, G.T., Zuckerman, R., Green, G.J., and Weiter, J.J. (1983). Response of human retinal blood flow to light and dark. *Invest. Ophthal. Vis. Sci.* **24**, 136–41. [*162*]

Fincham, E.F. (1937). *The mechanism of accommodation*. G. Pulman, London. [*66, 67, 76*]

Fincham, W.H.A. and Freeman, M.II. (1977). *Optics* (8th edn), ch. 9, 10. Butterworth, London. [*68*]

Fiorentini, A. and Maffei, L. (1973). Contrast in night vision. *Vision Res.* **13**, 73–80. [*211*]

Fisher, R.F. (1968). The variations of the peripheral visual fields with age. *Docum. Ophthal.* **24**, 41–67. [*187*]

Fisher, R.F. (1969*a*). The significance of the shape of the lens and capsular energy changes in accommodation. *J. Physiol.* **201**, 21–47. [*67, 80*]

Fisher, R.F. (1969*b*). Elastic constants of the human lens capsule. *J. Physiol.* **201**, 1–19. [*57, 67, 78, 80*]

Fisher, R.F. (1970). Senile cataract: A comparative study between lens fibre stress and cuneiform opacity formation. *Trans. Ophthal. Soc. UK.* **90**, 93–108. [*108*]

Fisher, R.F. (1971). The elastic constants of the human lens. *J. Physiol.* **212**, 147–80. [*7, 65, 67, 80*]

Fisher, R.F. (1973*a*). Presbyopia and the changes with age in the human crystalline lens. *J. Physiol.* **228**, 765–79. [*67*]

Fisher, R.F. (1973*b*). Human lens fibre transparency and mechanical stress. *Exp. Eye Res.* **16**, 41–9. [*67*]

Fisher, R.F. (1977). The force of contraction of the human ciliary muscle during accommodation. *J. Physiol.* **270**, 51–74. [*81, 82*]

Fisher, R.F. (1982). The vitreous and lens in accommodation. *Trans. Ophthal. Soc. UK.* **102**, 318–22. [*67, 79, 81*]

Fisher, R.F. and Pettet, B.E. (1973). Presbyopia and the water content of the human crystalline lens. *J. Physiol.* **234**, 443–7. [*54*]

Fixa, B., Komarková, O., and Nožička, Z. (1975). Ageing and autoimmunity. *Gerontologia*, **21**, 117–23. [*18*]

Flaye, D.E., Sullivan, K.N., Cullinan, T.R., Silver, J.H., and Whitelock, R.A.F. (1989). Cataracts and cigarette smoking. *Eye*, **3**, 379–84. [*109*]

Fledelius, H. (1981). Accommodation and juvenile myopia. *Docum. Ophthal.* **28**, 103. [*59*]

Fledelius, H.C. (1988). Refraction and eye size in the elderly. *Arch. Ophthalmologica*, **66**, 241–8. [*55*]

Flood, D.G. and Coleman, P.D. (1988). Neuron numbers and sizes in aging brain: comparison of human, monkey, and rodent data. *Neurobiol. Ag.* **9**, 453–63. [*112, 113*]

Flood, M.T., Haley, J.E., and Gouras, P. (1984). Cellular aging of human retinal epithelium in vivo and in vitro. *Monogr. Devl. Biol.* **17**, 80–93. [*159*]

Flügel, C., Lütjen-Drecoll, E., and Barány, E. (1990). Über strukturelle Unterschiede im Aufbau des Ziliarmuskels des Primatenauges. *Fortschr. Ophthal.* **87**, 384–7. [*77*]

Francis, A.A., Lee, W.H., and Regan, J.D. (1981). The relationship of DNA excision repair of ultraviolet-induced lesions to the maximum life span of mammals. *Mech. Ag. Dev.* **16**, 181–9. [*20, 27*]

Friedenwald, J.S. (1952). The eye. In *Cowdry's problems of aging*, (ed. A.I. Lansing). Williams & Wilkins, Baltimore. [*56*]

Friedman, D., Boltri, J., Vaughan Jr., H., and Erlenmeyer-Kimling, L. (1985). Effects of age and sex on the endogenous brain potential components during two continuous performance tasks. *Psychophysiol.* **22**, 440–52. [*114*]

Friedman, E. and Ts'O, M.O.M. (1968). The retinal pigment epithelium. *Arch. Ophthal.* **79**, 315–20. [*145*]

Frisén, L. and Frisén, M. (1981). How good is normal visual acuity? *Graefe's Arch. Klin. Ophthal.* **215**, 149–57. [*206*]

Fujishima, M. and Omae, T. (1980). Brain blood flow and mean transit time as related to aging. *Gerontology*, **26**, 104–7. [*123*]

Gareau, R., Goulet, H., Chenard, C., Caron, C., and Brisson G.R. (1991). Fluorescence studies on aged and young erythrocyte populations. *Cell. Molec. Biol.* **37**, 15–19. [*4*]

Gärtner, J. (1970). Elektronenmikroskopische Untersuchungen über Altersveränderungen an der Zonula Zinnii des menschlichen Auges. *Graefe's Arch. Klin. Exp. Ophthal.* **180**, 217–30. [*78*]

Gartner, S. and Henkind, P. (1981). Aging and degeneration of the human macula. I. Outer nuclear layer and photoreceptors. *Brit. J. Ophthal.* **65**, 23–8. [*129, 138, 145, 189*]

Gelfant, S. and Smith Jr., J.G. (1972). Aging: noncycling cells an explanation. *Science*, **178**, 357–61. [*27*]

Gershon, D. and Gershon, H. (1976). An evaluation of the 'error-catastrophe' theory of aging in the light of recent experimental results. *Gerontology*, **22**, 212–19. [*24*]

Gershon, H. and Gershon, D. (1970). Detection of inactive enzyme molecules in ageing organisms. *Nature*, **227**, 1214–17. [*24*]

Giess, M.C. (1980). Differences between natural ageing and radio-induced shortening of the life expectancy in Drosophila melanogaster. *Gerontology*, **26**, 301–10. [*9*]

Ginsburg, J. (1991). What determines the age at the menopause? *Brit. Med. J.* **302**, 1288. [*234*]

Girgus, J.S., Coren, S. and Porac, C. (1977). Independence of in vivo human lens pigmentation from u.v. light exposure. *Vision Res.* **17**, 749–50. [*100–1*]

Gleichen, A. (1921). *The theory of modern optical instruments.* HMSO, London. [*49*]

Goldmann, H. (1937). Studien über die Alterskernstreifen der Linse. *Arch. Augenheilk.* **110**, 405–14. [*57*]

Gomez-Ulla, F., Louro, O., and Mosquera, M. (1986). Macular dazzling test on normal subjects. *Brit. J. Ophthal.* **70**, 209–13. [*201, 202*]

Gompertz, B. (1825). On the nature of the function expressive of the law of human mortality and on a new mode of determining life contingencies. *Phil. Trans. Roy. Soc. (Lond.) A* **115**, 513–85. [*232*]

Good, P.I. (1975). Aging in mammalian cell populations: a review. *Mech. Ag. Dev.* **4**, 339–48. [*27*]

Gordon, R.A. and Donzis, P.B. (1985). Refractive development of the human eye. *Arch. Ophthal.* **103**, 785–9. [*67, 68*]

Gottesman, S.R.S., Hall, K.Y., and Walford, R.L. (1982). A thesis of genetic linkage of immune regulation and aging: the major histocompatibility complex as a supergene system. In *Developmental immunology: clinical problems and aging*, (ed. E.L. Cooper and M.A.B. Brazier). Academic Press, London. [*20*]

Green, D.G., Powers, M.K., and Banks, M.S. (1980). Depth of focus, eye size and visual acuity. *Vision Res.* **20**, 827–35. [*49*]

Gregor, Z. and Joffe, L. (1978). Senile macular changes in the black African. *Brit. J. Ophthal.* **62**, 547–50. [*165*]

Grey, R.H.B. (1978). Foveo-macular retinitis, solar retinopathy, and trauma. *Brit. J. Ophthal.* **62**, 543–6. [*164*]

Grimby, G. and Saltin, B. (1983). The ageing muscle. *Clinical Physiology*, **3**, 209–18. [*6, 8*]

Grimley Evans, J. (1988). Ageing and disease. In *Research and the ageing population*, (ed. D. Evered and J. Whelan). John Wiley, Chichester. [*10*]

Grinna, L.S. (1977). Changes in cell membranes during aging. *Gerontology*, **23**, 452–64. [*16*]

Grover, D. and Zigman, S. (1972). Coloration of human lenses by near ultraviolet photoxidized tryptophan. *Exp. Eye Res.* **13**, 70–76. [*100*]

Gsell, O.R. (1967). Longitudinal Gerontological Research over 10 years. *Geront. Clin.* **9**, 67–80. [*55*]

Gunkel, R.D. and Gouras, P. (1963). Changes in scotopic visibility thresholds with age. *Arch. Ophthal.* **69**, 4–9. [*175, 176*]

Haegerstrom-Portnoy, G. (1988). Short-wavelength-sensitive-cone sensitivity loss with aging: a protective role for macular pigment? *J. Opt. Soc. Amer.* **5**, 2140–44. [*138, 177, 178*]

Haegerstrom-Portnoy, G., Hewlett, S.E., and Barr, S.A.N. (1989). S cone loss with aging. In *Colour vision deficiencies IX*, (ed. G. Verriest). Kluwer, Dordrecht. [*178, 179*]

Halévy, H.S. and Landau, J. (1962). Hospitalized senile cataract in different Jewish communities in Israel. *Brit. J. Ophthal.* **46**, 285–90. [*110*]

Hall, T.C., Miller, A.K., and Corsellis, J.A.N. (1975). Variations in the human Purkinje cell population according to age and sex. *Neuropath. Appl. Neurobiol.* **1**, 267–92. [*20*]

Ham, Jr., W.T., Mueller, H.A., Ruffolo Jr., J.J., and Clarke, A.M. (1979). Sensitivity of the retina to radiation damage as a function of wavelength. *Photochem. Photobiol.* **29**, 735–43. [*162*]

Hamasaki, D., Ong, J., and Marg, E. (1956). The amplitude of accommodation in presbyopia. *Amer. J. Optom.* **33**, 3−13. [*61, 62, 81*]

Harding, J.J. (1970). Free and protein-bound glutathione in normal and cataractous human lenses. *Biochem. J.* **117**, 957−60. [*14, 238, 239*]

Harding, J.J. (1991). *Cataract − biochemistry, epidemiology and pharmacology.* Chapman & Hall, London. [*73, 90*]

Harding, J.J. and Rixon, K.C. (1980). Carbamylation of lens proteins: a possible factor in cataractogenesis in some tropical countries. *Exp. Eye Res.* **31**, 567−71. [*109*]

Harman, D. (1984). Free radical theory of aging: the 'free radical' diseases. *Age*, **7**, 111−31. [*13, 14*]

Harper, R.A., Kirkness, C.M., and Jay, B. (1988). Colour discrimination in pseudo-phakia. *Eye*, **2**, 382−9. [*221*]

Hart, R.W. and Setlow, R.B. (1974). Correlation between deoxyribonucleic acid excision-repair and life-span in a number of mammalian species. *Proc. Natl. Acad. Sci. USA*, **71**, 2169−73. [*20, 21*]

Hart, R.W. and Turturro, A. (1985). Review of recent biological research on theories of aging. *Rev. Biol. Res. Ag.* **2**, 3−12. [*32, 41*]

Hart, R.W., D'Ambrosio, S.M. and Ng, K.J. (1979). Longevity, stability, and DNA repair. *Mech. Ag. Dev.* **9**, 203−23. [*106, 127*]

Harvey, Jr., L.O. (1986). Efficient estimation of sensory thresholds. *Behav. Res. Meth. Instr. & Comp.* **18**, 623−32. [*170*]

Haug, H., Kühl, S., Mecke, E., Sass, N.L., and Wasner, K. (1984). The significance of morphometric procedures in the investigation of age changes in cytoarchitectonic structures of human brain. *J. Hirnforsch.* **25**, 353−74. [*118−21*]

Hayflick, L. (1965). The limited in vitro lifetime of human diploid cell strains. *Exp. Cell Res.* **37**, 614−36. [*9, 11, 22*]

Hayflick, L. (1985). Theories of biological aging. *Exp. Geront.* **20**, 145−59. [*11, 14, 17*]

Hecht, S., Shlaer, S., and Pirenne, M.H. (1942). Energy, quanta, and vision. *J. Gen. Physiol.* **25**, 819−40. [*172, 175*]

Heintel, H., Faust, U., and Faust, C. (1979). Altersabhängigkeit der P2-Amplituden schachbrettmusterevozierter Potentiale. *Zeits. EEG-EMG* **10**, 194−6. [*121*]

Helmholtz, H.v. (1855). Über die Akkommodation des Auges. V. *Graefes Arch. Ophthal.* **1/2**, 1−74. [*73*]

Helps, E.P.W. (1973). Physiological effects of ageing. *Proc. Roy. Soc. Med.* **66**, 815−18. [*10*]

Hemenger, R.P. (1984). Intraocular light scatter in normal vision loss with age. *Appl. Opt.* **23**, 1972−4. [*97, 210*]

Hemenger, R.P., Occhipinti, J.R., and Mosier, M.A. (1989). Ageing parameters of the ocular lens by scanning fluorophotometry. *Ophthal. Physiol. Opt.* **9**, 191−8. [*102*]

Hernandez, M.R., Luo, X.X., Andrzejewska, W., and Neufeld, A.H. (1989). Age-related changes in the extracellular matrix of the human optic nerve head. *Amer. J. Ophthal.* **107**, 476−84. [*140*]

Hess, C. (1911). Pathologie und Therapie des Linsensystems. Ch. 9. In *Graefe-Saemisch's Handbuch der gesammten Augenheilkunde*, Part 2. (3rd edn). Wilhelm Engelmann, Leipzig. [*94*]

Hess, R., Nordby, K., and Sharpe, L.W. (1990). *Night vision.* Cambridge University Press. [*170*]

Higgins, K.E., Jaffé, M.J., Caruso, R.C., and deMonasterio, F.M. (1988). Spatial contrast sensitivity: effects of age, test-retest, and psychophysical method. *J. Opt. Soc. Amer.* **5**, 2173−80. [*205*]

Hiller, R., Sperduto, R.D., and Ederer, F. (1983). Epidemiologic associations with cataract in the 1971–1972 National Health and Nutrition Examination Survey. *Amer. J. Epidemiol.* **118**, 239–49. [*109*]

Hirsch, H.R. (1980). Evolution of senescence: influence of age-dependent death rates on the natural increase of a hypothetical population. *J. Theor. Biol.* **86**, 149–86. [*234*]

Hirsch, H.R. (1986). The waste-product theory of aging: cell division rate as a function of waste volume. *Mech. Ag. Dev.* **36**, 95–107. [*22*]

Hirsch, R.P. and Schwartz, B. (1983). Increased mortality among elderly patients undergoing cataract extraction. *Arch. Ophthal.* **101**, 1034–7. [*10, 237*]

Hockwin, O., Weigelin, E., Laser, H., and Dragomirescu, D. (1983). Biometry of the anterior eye segment by Scheimpflug photography. *Ophthalm. Res.* **15**, 102–8. [*72*]

Hofstetter, H.W. (1965). A longitudinal study of amplitude changes in presbyopia. *Amer. J. Optom.* **42**, 3–8. [*60*]

Holliday, R. (1988). Toward a biological understanding of the ageing process. *Persp. Biol. Med.* **32**, 109–23. [*32*]

Hollingsworth, J.W., Hashizume, A., and Jablon, S. (1965). Correlations between tests of aging in Hiroshima subjects – an attempt to define 'physiologic age'. *Yale J. Biol. Med.* **38**, 11–26. [*237*]

Holmin, C. and Krakau, C.E.T. (1980). Visual field decay in normal subjects and in cases of chronic glaucoma. *Albrecht von Graefes Arch. Klin. Ophthalmol.* **213**, 291–8. [*193*]

Hoshino, M., Mizuno, K., and Ichikawa, H. (1984) Aging alterations of retina and choroid of Japanese: microscopic study of macular region of 176 eyes. *Jap. J. Ophthal.* **28**, 89–102. [*165*]

Howarth, P.A., Zhang, X.X., Bradley, A., Still, D.L., and Thibos, L.N. (1988). Does the chromatic aberration of the eye vary with age? *J. Opt. Soc. Amer.* **A5**, 2087–92. [*58*]

Hunziker, O., Abdel'Al, S., and Schulz, U. (1979). The aging human cerebral cortex: a stereological characterization of changes in the capillary net. *J. Geront.* **34**, 345–50. [*124*]

Hunziker, O., Abdel'Al, S., Frey, H., Veteau, M.-J., and Meier-Ruge, W. (1978). Quantitative studies in the cerebral cortex of aging humans. *Gerontology*, **24**, 27–31. [*123*]

Huttenlocher, P.R. and de Courten, C. (1987). The development of synapses in striate cortex of man. *Human Neurobiol.* **6**, 1–9. [*119*]

Hyams, S.W., Pokotilo, E., and Shkuro, G. (1977). Prevalence of refractive errors in adults over 40: A survey of 8102 eyes. *Brit. J. Ophthal.* **61**, 428–32. [*54*]

Hyman, L.G., Lilienfeld, A.M., Ferris III, F.L., and Fine, S.L. (1983). Senile macular degeneration: a case-control study. *Amer. J. Epidemiol.* **118**, 213 27. [*165*]

Ito, M., Hatazawa, J., Yamaura, H., and Matsuzawa, T. (1981). Age-related brain atrophy and mental deterioration – a study with computed tomography. *Brit. J. Radiol.* **54**, 384–90. [*115, 116*]

Itoh, M., Hatazawa, J., Miyazawa, H., Matsui, H., Meguro, K., Yanai, K., *et al.* (1990). Stability of cerebral blood flow and oxygen metabolism during normal aging. *Gerontology*, **36**, 43–8. [*121, 123*]

Iwasaki, M., and Inomata, H. (1988). Lipofuscin granules in human receptor cells. *Invest. Ophthal. Vis. Sci.* **29**, 671–9. [*129, 130*]

Iwase, A., Kitazawa, Y., and Ohno, Y. (1988). On age-related norms of the visual field. *Jap. J. Ophthal.* **32**, 429–37. [*189*]

Jacobs, N.A., Patterson, I.H., and Broome, I.J. (1987). The macular threshold: determination of population normal values. *Docum. Ophthal.* **49**, 137–42. [*177*]

Jaffé, G.J., Alvarado, J.A., and Juster, R.P. (1986). Age-related changes of the normal visual field. *Arch. Ophthal.* **104**, 1021–5. [*188–91*]

Jain, I.S., Prasad, P., Gupta, A., Ram, J., and Dhir, S.P. (1984). Senile macular degeneration in Northern India. *Afro-Asian J. Ophthal.* **3**, 23–5. [*166*]

Jay, J.L., Mammo, R.B., and Allan, D. (1986). Effect of age on visual acuity after cataract extraction. *Brit. J. Ophthal.* **71**, 112–15. [*211*]

Johnson, B.M., Miao, M., and Sadun, A.A. (1987). Age-related decline of human optic nerve axon population. *Age*, **10**, 5–9. [*140*]

Johnson, C. and Keltner, J.L. (1983). Incidence of visual field loss in 20000 eyes and its relationship to driving performance. *Arch. Ophthal.* **101**, 371–5. [*194*]

Johnson, C.A., Adams, A. J., Twelker, J. D., and Quigg, J.M. (1988). Age-related changes in the central visual field for short-wavelength-sensitive pathways. *J. Opt. Soc. Amer.* **5**, 2131–9. [*177–9*]

Johnson, C.A., Adams, A.J., and Lewis, R.A. (1989). Evidence for a neural basis of age-related visual field loss in normal observers. *Invest. Ophthal. Vis. Sci.* **30**, 2056–64. [*192, 193*]

Johnson, M. and Choy, D. (1987). On the definition of age-related norms for visual testing. *App. Opt.* **26**, 1449–54. [*206*]

Johnson, T.E. and McCaffrey, G. (1985). Programmed aging or error catastrophe? An examination by two-dimensional polyacrylamide gel electrophoresis. *Mech. Ag. Dev.* **30**, 285–97. [*24*]

Kahn, H.A., Leibowitz, H.M., Ganley, J. P., Kini, M.M., Colton, T., Nickerson, R.S., and Dawson, T.R. (1977). The Framingham Eye Study. I. Outline and major prevalence findings. *Amer. J. Epidemiol.* **106**, 17–32. [*207*]

Kamiya, S. (1987). Causes of refractive changes in myopia. *Ophthalm.* **34**, 56–75. [*56*]

Kato, H., Harada, M., Tsuchiya, K., and Moriwaki, K. (1980). Absence of correlation between DNA repair in ultraviolet irradiated mammalian cells and life span of the donor species. *Jap. J. Genetics*, **55**, 99–108. [*21*]

Katz, J. and Sommer, A. (1987). A longitudinal study of the age-adjusted variability of automated visual fields. *Arch. Ophthal.* **105**, 1083–6. [*191*]

Katz, M.L., Robison, W.G., and Dratz, E.A. (1984). Potential role of auto-oxidation in age changes of the retina and retinal pigment epithelium of the eye. In *Free radicals in molecular biology*, (ed. D. Armstrong). Raven Press, New York. [*11, 149*]

Katz, M.L., Drea, C.M., Eldred, G.E., Hess, H.H., and Robison Jr., W.G. (1986). Influence of early photoreceptor degeneration on lipofuscin in the retinal pigment epithelium. *Exp. Eye Res.* **43**, 561–73. [*157*]

Katz, M.L., Eldred, G.E., and Robison Jr., G. (1987). Lipofuscin autofluorescence: evidence for vitamin A involvement in the retina. *Mech. Ag. Dev.* **39**, 81–90. [*158*]

Katzman, R. (1988). Alzheimer's disease as an age-dependent disorder. In *Research and the ageing population*, (ed. D. Evered and J. Whelan). John Wiley, Chichester. [*32*]

Kauffman, R.G., Norton, H.W., Harmon, B.G., and Breidenstein, B.C. (1967). Growth of the porcine lens as an index to chronological age. *J. Animal Sci.* **26**, 31–5. [*64*]

Kay, C.D. and Morrison, J.D. (1987). A quantitative investigation into the effects of pupil diameter and defocus on contrast sensitivity for an extended range of spatial frequencies in natural and homatropinized eyes. *Ophthal. Physiol. Opt.* **7**, 21–30. [*210*]

Keunen, J.E.E., Van Norren, D., and Van Meel, G.J. (1987). Density of foveal pigments at older age. *Invest. Ophthal. Vis. Sci.* **28**, 985–91. [*135, 136, 180*]

Kilbride, P.E., Hutman, L.P., Fishman, M., and Read, J.S. (1986). Foveal cone pigment density difference in the aging human eye. *Vision Res.* **26**, 321–5. [*135, 137, 180*]

Kilbride, P.E., Alexander, K.R., Fishman, M., and Fishman, G.A. (1989). Human macular pigment assessed by imaging fundus reflectometry. *Vision Res.* **29**, 663–74. [*138*]

Killingsworth, M.C. (1987). Age-related components of Bruch's membrane in the human eye. *Graefe's Arch. Clin. Exp. Ophthal.* **227**, 406–12. [*144*]

Kirkness, C. and Weale, R.A. (1985). Does light pose a hazard to the macula in aphakia? *Trans. Ophthal. Soc. UK*, **104**, 699–702. [*183*]

Kirkwood, T.B.L. (1984). Towards a unified theory of cellular ageing. *Monogr. Devl. Biol.* **17**, 9–20. [*1, 20, 34*]

Kirkwood, T.B.L. (1988). The nature and causes of ageing. In *Research and the ageing population*, (ed. D. Evered and J. Whelan). Ciba Foundation Symposium 134; pp. 193–207, Wiley, Chichester. [*34*]

Kirkwood, T.B.L. and Holliday, R. (1986). Ageing as a consequence in natural selection. In *The biology of human ageing*, (ed. A.H. Bittles and K.J. Collins). Cambridge University Press. [*1, 3, 34–6*]

Kline, D.W. and Schieber, F. (1981). Visual aging: A transient/sustained shift? *Perc. & Psychophys.* **29**, 181–2. [*198*]

Kline, D.W., Ikeda, D.M., and Schieber, F.J. (1982). Age and temporal resolution in colour vision: Why do red and green make yellow? *J. Geront.* **37**, 705–9. [*198*]

Kline, D.W., Schieber, F., Abusamra, L.C., and Coyne, A.C. (1983). Age, the eye, and the visual channels: contrast sensitivity and response speed. *J. Geront.* **38**, 211–16. [*218*]

Kluxen, G. (1985). Klinische und experimentelle Untersuchungen an Alterskatarakten. *Fortschr. Med.* **103**, 243–6. [*108*]

Knoblauch, K., Saunders, F., Kusada, M., Hynes, R., Podgor, M., Higgins, K.E., and DeMonasterio, F.M. (1987). Age and illuminance effects in the Farnsworth-Munsell 100-hue test. *App. Opt.* **26**, 1441–8. [*221, 222*]

Koistinaho, J., Sorvaniemi, M., Alho, H., and Hervonen, A. (1986). Microspectro-fluorometric quantitation of autofluorescent lipopigment in the human sympathetic ganglia. *Mech. Ag. Dev.* **37**, 79–89. [*12, 160*]

Koretz, J., Handelman, G.H., and Brown, N.P. (1984). Analysis of human crystalline lens curvature as a function of accommodative state and age. *Vision Res.* **24**, 1141–51. [*70, 73*]

Korth, M., Horn, F., Storck, B., and Jonas, J.B. (1989). Spatial and spatiotemporal contrast sensitivity of normal and glaucoma eyes. *Graefe's Arch. Clin. Exp. Ophthal.* **227**, 428–35. [*207*]

Kragha, I.K.O.K. (1986). Does the discrepancy between retinoscopic and subjective refraction vary linearly with age? *Ophthal. Physiol. Opt.* **6**, 115–16. [*53, 60*]

Krause, U., Krause, K., and Rantakallio, P. (1982). Sex differences in refraction errors up to the age of 15. *Acta Ophthalm.* **60**, 917–26. [*60*]

Laatikainen, L. and Larinkari, J. (1977). Capillary-free area of the fovea with advancing age. *Invest. Ophthal. Vis. Sci.* **16**, 1154–7. [*125, 126*]

Lakowski, R. and Oliver, K. (1973). Effect of pupil diameter on colour vision test performance. *Mod. Probl. Ophthal.* **13**, 307–11. [*221*]

Lapidot, M.B. (1987). Does the brain age uniformly? Evidence from effects of smooth pursuit eye movements on verbal and visual tasks. *J. Gerontol.* **42**, 329–31. [*113*]

Larsen, J.S. (1971*a*). The sagittal growth of the eye. I. *Acta Ophthal.* **49**, 239–62. [*69*]

Larsen, J.S. (1971*b*). The sagittal growth of the eye. II. *Acta Ophthal.* **49**, 427–40. [*69*]

Laughrea, M. (1982). On the error theories of aging. *Exp. Gerontol.* **17**, 305–17. [*24*]

Lavery, J.R., Gibson, J.M., Shaw, D.E., and Rosenthal, A.R. (1988*a*). Refraction and refractive errors in an elderly population. *Ophthal. Physiol. Opt.* **8**, 394–6. [*53*]

Lavery, J.R., Gibson, J.M., Shaw, D.E., and Rosenthal, A.R. (1988*b*). Vision and visual acuity in an elderly population. *Ophthal. Physiol. Opt.* **8**, 390–93. [*206*]

Leech, S.H. (1980). Cellular immunosenescence. *Gerontology*, **26**, 330–45. [*17–19*]

Leenders, K.L., Perani, D., Lammerstma, A.A., Heather, J.D., Buckingham, P., Healy, M.J.R., *et al.* (1990). Cerebral blood flow, blood volume and oxygen utilization. *Brain*, **113**, 27–47. [*113, 115, 121, 123*]

Leibowitz, H.M., Krueger, D.E., Maunder, L.R., Milton, R.C., Kini, M.M., Kahn, H.A., *et al.* (1980). The Framingham Eye Study Monograph. *Surv. Ophthal.* Suppl. **24**, 335–610. [*166*]

Leonardo da Vinci (1513). Notebooks: cf. Richter, J.P. (1883). The literary works of Leonardo da Vinci. Sampson Low, Marston, Searle & Rivington, London. [*49*]

Leonardo da Vinci (1513) (1881). MS D 3v. Les manuscrits de Leonard de Vinci. Manuscrit A . . . M de la bibliothèque de l'Institut publiés par M.C. Ravisson-Mollien. Paris. [*49, 59*]

Lerche, W. (1967). Die Capillardichte in der menschlichen Retina unter Berücksichtigung altersbedingter Veränderungen. *Graefe's Arch. Klin. Exp. Ophthal.* **172**, 57–68. [*125*]

Lerman, S. (1988). Human lens fluorescence aging index. *Lens Research*, **5**, 23–31. [*103*]

Lerman, S. and Borkman, R.F. (1976). Spectroscopic evaluation and classification of the normal, aging and cataractous lens. *Ophthal. Res.* **8**, 335–53. [*92, 103, 154*]

Leske, M.C. and Sperduto, R.D. (1983). The epidemiology of senile cataract: A Review. *Amer. J. Epidemiol.* **118**, 152–65. [*109*]

Lestienne, R. (1988). On the thermodynamical and biological interpretations of the Gompertzian mortality rate distribution. *Mech. Ageing Dev.* **42**, 197–214. [*235*]

Leuba, G. and Garey, L.J. (1987). Evolution of neuronal numerical density in the developing and aging human visual cortex. *Human Neurobiol.* **6**, 11–18. [*118*]

Liang, J.N. (1990). Front surface fluorescence measurements of the age-related change in human lens. *Curr. Eye Res.* **9**, 399–405. [*97*]

Lightart, G.J., Corberand, J.X., Fournier, C., Galanaud, P., Hijmans, W., Kennes, B., Muller-Hermelink, H.K., and Steinmann, G.G. (1984). Admission criteria for immunogerontological studies in man: the Senieur protocoll. *Mech. Ag. Dev.* **28**, 47–55. [*4*]

Lightart, G.J., Corberand, J.X., Geertzen, H.G.M., Meinders, A.E., Knook, D.L., and Hijmans, W. (1990). Necessity of the assessment of health status in human immunogerontological studies: evaluation of the Senieur Protocoll. *Mech. Ag. Dev.* **55**, 89–105. [*17*]

Lindop, P.J. and Rotblat, J. (1961). Long-term effects of a single whole-body exposure of mice to ionising radiations. *Proc. Roy. Soc. B.* **154**, 332–49. [*8*]

Lintl, P. and Braak, H. (1983). Loss of intracortical myelinated fibers: a distinctive age-related alteration in the human striate area. *Acta Neuropathol. (Berl.)* **61**, 178–82. [*113, 114, 120, 121*]

Löpping, B. and Weale, R.A. (1965). Changes in corneal curvature following ocular convergence. *Vision Res.* **5**, 207–15. [*70*]

Lotmar, W., Goldmann, H., and Brückner, R. (1978). Zur Bestimmung zeitlicher Veränderungen der Papille bei normalen Erwachsenen. *Klin. Mtsbl. Augenheilk.* **173**, 480–86. [*140*]

Lovasik, J.V. (1983). An electrophysiological investigation of the macular photostress test. *Invest. Ophthal. Vis. Sci.* **24**, 437–41. [*202, 203*]

Lovett Doust, J.W. (1972). Influence of human ageing on aspects of the cerebral circulation. *Gerontologia*, **18**, 14–21. [*123*]

Lowe, R.F. (1970). Anterior lens displacement with age. *Brit. J. Ophthal.* **54**, 117. [*71*]

Lowe, R.F. and Clark, B.A.J. (1973). Radius of curvature of the anterior lens surface. *Brit. J. Ophthal.* **54**, 471–4. [*66, 70*]

Lumbroso, B. and Sciuto, V. (ed.) (1988). *L'occhio che invecchia.* Verduci, Rome. [*v*]

Lütjen-Drecoll, E., Tamm, E., and Kaufman, P.L. (1987). Functional morphology of rhesus monkey ciliary muscle during ageing. *Invest. Ophthal. Vis. Sci.* (Suppl.) 65. [*78*]

Lütjen-Drecoll, E., Tamm, E., and Kaufman, P.L. (1988). Age-related loss of morphologic responses to pilocarpine in rhesus monkey ciliary muscle. *Arch. Ophthal.* **106**, 1591–8. [*77*]

Lutze, M. and Bresnick, G.H. (1991). Lenses of diabetic patients 'yellow' at an accelerated rate similar to older normals. *Invest. Ophthal. Vis. Sci.* **32**, 194–9. [*99*]

Luyckx, J. (1966). Mesure des composantes optiques de l'oeil du nouveau-né par echographie ultrasonique. *Arch. Ophtal. Paris*, **26**, 159–70. [*56, 67*]

McBrien, N.A. and Millodot, M. (1986). Amplitude of accommodation and refractive error. *Invest. Ophthalm. Vis. Sci.* **27**, 1187–90. [*59*]

McEvedy, C. and Jones, R. (1978). *Atlas of world population history.* Allen Lane, London. [*86*]

McGrath, C. and Morrison, J.D. (1981). The effects of age on spatial frequency perception in human subjects. *Quart. J. Exp. Physiol.* **66**, 253–61. [*207–11, 219, 239*]

McLaren, D.S. (1982). Age-dependent changes in the effects of food toxins and other dietary factors on the eye. *Pharmac. Ther.* **16**, 103–42. [*30*]

Magoon, E.H. and Robb, R.M. (1981). Development of myelin in human optic nerve and tract. *Arch. Ophthal.* **99**, 655–9. [*120*]

Makrides, S.C. (1983). Protein synthesis and degradation during aging and senescence. *Biol. Rev.* **58**, 343–422. [*19, 27*]

Mann, D.M.A. and Yates, P.O. (1982). Accumulation of liproprotein pigments in nerve cells of British and Sri Lankan nationals. *Mech. Ag. Dev.* **18**, 151–8. [*11, 149, 160*]

Mann, D.M.A., Yates, P.O., and Stamp, J.E. (1978). The relationship between lipofuscin pigment and ageing in the human nervous system. *J. Neurol. Sci.* **37**, 83–93. [*11, 12*]

Mann, G.V., Shaffer, R.D., and Rich, A. (1965). Physical fitness and immunity to heart-disease in Masai. *Lancet*, **ii**, 1308–10. [*39*]

Marg, E. (1987). Presbyopia in man revisited. In *Presbyopia*, (ed. L. Stark and G. Obrecht), pp. 247–9. Fairchild Publications, New York. [*62*]

Marshall, J., Grindle, J., Ansell, P.L., and Borwein, B. (1979). Convolution in human rods: an ageing process. *Brit. J. Ophthal.* **63**, 181–7. [*127–9, 132*]

Martin, G.M. (1979). Genetic and evolutionary aspects of aging. *Fed. Proc.* **38**, 1962–7. [*30, 31*]

Martin, G.M., Ogburn, C.E., and Sprague, C.A. (1981). Effects of age on cell division capacity. In *Aging: a challenge to science and society*, (ed. D. Danon, N.W. Shock, and M. Marois). Oxford University Press. [*9*]

Massof, R.W., Choy, D., Sunness, J.S., Johnson, M.A., Rubin, G.S., and Fine, S.L. (1989). Foveal threshold elevations associated with age-related drusen. *Clin. Vis. Res.* **4**, 221–7. [*180*]

Mayer, M.J., Kim, C.B.Y., and Svingos, A. (1988). Foveal flicker sensitivity in healthy aging eyes. I. Compensating for pupil variation. *J. Opt. Soc. Amer.* **5**, 2201–9. [*210*]

Mayer, P.J., Bradley, M.O., and Nichols, W.W. (1987). The effect of mild hypothermia (34 °C) and mild hyperthermia (39 °C) on DNA damage, repair and aging of human diploid fibroplasts. *Mech. Ag. Dev.* **39**, 203–22. [*8, 9*]

Maynard Smith, J. (1962). The causes of ageing. *Proc. Roy. Soc. B* **157**, 115–27. [*8, 29*]

Maynard Smith, J. (1963). Temperature and the rate of ageing in poikilotherms. *Nature*, **199**, 400–2. [*26*]

Medawar, P.B. (1952). *An unsolved problem in biology*. H.K. Lewis, London. [*26, 32, 33*]

Medvedev, Z.A. (1972). Repetition of molecular-genetic information as a possible factor in evolutionary changes of life span. *Exp. Geront.* **7**, 227–38. [*3, 24–6*]

Megaw, J.M. (1984). Glutathione and ocular photobiology. *Curr. Eye Res.* **3**, 83–7. [*102*]

Meites, J., Goya, R., and Takehashi, S. (1987). Why the neuroendocrine system is important in aging processes. *Exp. Gerontol.* **22**, 1–15. [*17–20*]

Melamed, E., Lavy, S., Bentin, S., Cooper, G., and Rinot, Y. (1980). Reduction in regional cerebral blood flow during normal aging in man. *Stroke* **11**, 31–5. [*123*]

Mellerio, J. (1987). Yellowing of the human lens: nuclear and cortical contributions. *Vision Res.* **27**, 1581–7. [*90, 91, 94*]

Mergler, N.L. and Goldstein, M.D. (1983). Why are there old people. *Human Dev.* **26**, 72–90. [*vi*]

Mets, T., Bekart, E. and Verdonk, G. (1983). Similarity between in vitro and in vivo cellular aging. *Mech. Ag. Dev.* **22**, 71–8. [*23*]

Mikelberg, F.S., Drance, S.M., Schulzer, M., Yidegiligne, H.M., and Weis, M.M. (1989). The normal human optic nerve. *Ophthalmology* **96**, 1325–8. [*140*]

Millodot, M. (1976). The influence of age on the chromatic aberration of the eye. *Graefe's Arch. Klin. Exp. Ophthal.* **198**, 235–43. [*58*]

Millodot, M. and O'Leary, D. (1978). The discrepancy between retinoscopic and subjective measurements: effect of age. *Amer. J. Optom. Physiol. Opt.* **55**, 309–16. [*53*]

Miranda, M.N. (1979).The geographic factor in the onset of presbyopia. *Trans. Amer. Soc. Ophthal.* **77**, 603–21. [*60*]

Miranda, M.N. (1980). Environmental temperature and senile cataract. *Trans. Amer. Ophthal. Soc.* **78**, 255–62. [*109*]

Mordi, J. and Adrian, W.K. (1985). Influence of age on chromatic aberration of the human eye. *Amer. J. Optom. Physiol. Opt.* **62**, 864–9. [*58*]

Morrison, J.D. and McGrath, C. (1985). Assessment of the optical contributions to the age-related deterioration in vision. *Quart. J. Exp. Physiol.* **70**, 249–69. [*212–19*]

Morrison, J.D. and Reilly, J. (1986). An assessment of decision-making as a possible factor in the age-related loss of contrast sensitivity. *Perception*, **15**, 541–52. [*196*]

Muñoz, B., West, S., Bressler, N., Rosenthal, F.S., and Taylor, H.R. (1990). Blue light and risk of age-related macular degeneration. *Invest. Ophthal. Vis. Sci. ARVO*, **31**, 49. [*166*]

Murata, Y. (1987). Light absorption characteristics of the lens capsule. *Ophthalm. Res.* **19**, 107–12. [*89*]

Musk, P. and Parsons, P.G. (1987). Resistance of pigmented human cells to killing by sunlight and oxygen radicals. *Photochem. Photobiol.* **46**, 489–94. [*164*]

Nameda, N., Kawara, T., and Ohzu, H. (1989). Human visual spatio-temporal frequency performance as a function of age. *Optom. Vis. Sci.* **66**, 760–5. [*214–18, 239*]

Nandy, K. and Bourne, G.H. (1966). Effect of centrophenoxine on the lopofuscin pigments in the neurones of senile guinea-pigs. *Nature (Lond.)*, **210**, 313–14. [*11*]

Navarro, R., Mendez-Morales, J.A., and Santamaria, J. (1986). Optical quality of the eye lens surfaces from roughness and diffusion measurements. *J. Opt. Soc. Amer. A* **3**, 228–34. [*105*]

Nette, E.G., Xi, Y.-P., Sun, Y.-K., Andrews, A.D., and King, D.W. (1984). A correlation between aging and DNA repair in human epidermal cells. *Mech. Ag. Dev.* **24**, 283–92. [*20, 21, 27, 28, 235*]

Newsome, D.A., Huh, W., and Green, W.R. (1987). Bruch's membrane age-related changes vary by region. *Curr. Eye Res.* **6**, 1211–21. [*142*]

Nicak, A. (1986). Erythrocytes and age. Disintegration of erythrocytes by brilliant cresyl blue in correlation to age. *Physiol. Bohemosl.* **35**, 118–26. [*4*]

Niesel, P., Krauchi, H., and Bachmann, E. (1976). Der Abspaltungsstreifen in der Spaltlampenphotographie der alternden Linse. *Graefe's Arch. Klin. Exp. Ophthal.* **199**, 11–20. [*72*]

Nordby, K. and Sharpe, L.T. (1988). The directional sensitivity of the photoreceptors in the human achromat. *J. Physiol. (Lond.)* **399**, 267–81. [*201*]

Nordmann, J. (1973). Le noyau du cristallin. *Arch. Ophtal.* **33**, 81–6. [*54, 79*]

Noyori, S., Hamano, K., Tomonaga, M., and Ohta, Y. (1987). Farnsworth-Munsell 100 hue test. *Act. Soc. Ophthal. Jpn.* **91**, 298–303. [*221, 223*]

Ober, M. and Rohen, J.W. (1979). Regional differences in the fine structure of the ciliary epithelium related to accommodation. *Invest. Ophthal. Vis. Sci.* **18**, 655–64. [*76*]

Obstfeld, H. (1989). Crystalline lens accommodation and anterior chamber depth. *Ophthal. Physiol. Opt.* **9**, 36–40. [*69–71*]

Odom, J.V., Vasquez, R.J., Schwartz, T.L., and Linberg, J.V. (1989). Adult vernier thresholds do not increase with age; vernier bias does. *Invest. Ophthal. Vis. Sci.* **30**, 1004–8. [*207*]

O'Leary, D.J. and Millodot, M. (1979). Eyelid closure causes myopia in humans. *Experientia*, **35**, 1478–9. [*54*]

Olshansky, S.J., Carnes, B.A., and Cassel, C. (1990). In search of Methuselah: estimating the upper limits to human longevity. *Science*, **250**, 634–40. [*229, 235*]

Olson, C.B. (1987). A review of why and how we age: a defense of multifactorial aging. *Mech. Ag. Dev.* **41**, 1–28. [*15, 33*]

Orgel, L.E. (1963). The maintenance of the accuracy of protein synthesis and its relevance to aging. *Proc. Nat. Acad. Sci. USA*, **49**, 517–21. [*23*]

Orgel, L.E. (1973). Ageing of clones of mammalian cells. *Nature*, **243**, 441–5. [*24*]

O'Steen, W.K., Bare, D.J., Tytell, M., Morris, M., and Gower, D.J. (1990). Water deprivation protects photoreceptors against light damage. *Brain Res.* **534**, 99–105. [*167*]

Owsley, C. and Burton, K.B. (1992). Aging and spatial contrast sensitivity: underlying mechanisms and implications for everyday life. In *The changing visual system: maturation and aging in the central nervous system*, (ed. P. Bagnoli and W. Hodos). Plenum Press, New York, In press. [*95, 198, 226, 239*]

Owsley, C., Sekuler, R., and Siemsen, D. (1983). Contrast sensitivity throughout adulthood. *Vision Res.* **23**, 689–99. [*214, 215*]

Owsley, C., Gardner, T., Sekuler, R., and Lieberman, H. (1985). Role of the crystalline lens in the spatial vision loss of the elderly. *Invest. Ophthal.* **26**, 1165–70. [*210, 212*]

Parsons, P.A. (1978). The genetics of aging in optimal and stressful environments. *Exp. Geront.* **13**, 357–63. [*8–10*]

Parsons, P.G. and Hayward, I.P. (1985). Inhibition of DNA repair synthesis by sunlight. *Photochem. Photobiol.* **42**, 287–93. [*164*]

Pau, H. (1951). Zur Mechanik der akkommodativen Linsenverschiebung. *Graefe's Arch. Ophthal.* **151**, 565–73. [*81*]

Perkins, E.S. (1984). Cataract: refractive error, diabetes, and morphology. *Brit. J. Ophthal.* **68**, 293–7. [*109*]

Perkkiö, J. and Keskinen, R. (1985). The relationship between growth and allometry. *J. Theor. Biol.* **113**, 81–7. [*41, 42*]

Peters, W. (1987). Anomalies in the evolution of presbyopia in African tribes. In *Presbyopia*, (ed. L. Stark and G. Obrecht), pp. 28–29. Fairchild Publications, New York. [*60*]

Phair, J.P., Hsu, C.S., and Hsu Y.L. (1988). Ageing and infection. In *Research and the ageing population*, (ed. D. Evered and J. Whelan). John Wiley, Chichester. [*17*]

Plantner, J.J., Barbour, H.L., and Kean, E.L. (1988). The rhodopsin content of the human eye. *Curr. Eye Res.* **7**, 1125–9. [*131*]

Platt, D. (ed.) (1989) *Handbuch der Gerontologie*, Band 3, Augenheilkunde. Gustav Fischer, Stuttgart, New York. [*v*]

Pokorny, J., Smith, V.C., and Lutze, M. (1987). Aging of the human lens. *App. Opt.* **26**, 1437–40. [*40, 91*]

Polednak, A.P. (1978). Age changes in differential leukocyte count among female adults. *Hum. Biol.* **50**, 301–11. [*17*]

Pulos, E. (1989). Changes in rod sensitivity through adulthood. *Invest. Ophthal. Vis. Sci.* **30**, 1738–42. [*172, 176*]

Raeder, J.G. (1922). Untersuchungen über die Lage und Dicke der Linse im menschlichen Auge bei physiologischen und pathologischen Zuständen, nach einer neuen Methode gemessen. *Albr. v. Graefes Arch. Ophthal.* **110**, 73–108. [*69*]

Rao, C.M., Balasubramanian, D., and Chakrabarti, B. (1987). Monitoring light-induced changes in isolated, intact eye lenses. *Phtochem. Photobiol.* **46**, 511–15. [*102*]

Reading, V.M. (1968). Disability glare and age. *Vision Res.* **8**, 207–14. [*201*]

Reading, V.M. and Weale, R.A. (1991). A new analysis of United Nations mortality data. *Mech. Ag. Dev.* **57**, 25–48. [*8, 30, 234, 238*]

Reeb, O. (1957). 'Troland' und Stiles-Crawford Effekt. *Die Farbe* **6**, 73–7. [*221*]

Reim, M. (1984). The eye in the aging patient: cornea. In *Geriatrics*, (ed. D. Platt), pp. 310–25. Springer-Verlag, Heidelberg. [*7*]

Ripps, H. and Snapper, A.G. (1974). Computer analysis of photochemical changes in the human retina. *Comput. Biol. Med.* **4**, 107–22. [*132*]

Ripps, H. and Weale, R.A. (1976). Contrast and border phenomena. In *The eye*, (ed. H. Davson), Vol. 2A. pp. 131–84. Academic Press, London. [*63*]

Rivnay, B., Bergman, S., Shinitsky, M., and Globerson, A. (1980). Correlations between membrane viscosity, serum cholesterol, lymphocyte activity and aging in man. *Mech. Ag. Dev.* **12**, 119–26. [*15*]

Robert, Y., Gschwind, R., and Brückner, R. (1985). Fluctuations of light absorption of healthy papillae repeatedly photographed over a long period of time. *Ophthal. Res.* **17**, 154–62. [*140*]

Robson, J.G. (1966). Spatial and temporal contrast-sensitivity functions of the visual system. *J. Opt. Soc. Amer.* **56**, 1141–2. [*205*]

Rohen, J.W. and Rentsch, F.J. (1969). Der konstruktive Bau des Zonulaapparates beim Menschen und dessen funktionelle Bedeutung. *Graefe's Arch. Klin. Exp. Ophthal.* **178**, 1–19. [*74, 75*]

Roll, P., Reich, M. and Hofmann, H. (1975). Der Verlauf der Zonulafasern. *Graefe's Arch. Klin. Exp. Ophthal.* **195**, 41–7. [*74–6*]

Rosen, P., Woodhead, A.D., and Thompson, K.H. (1981). The relationship between the Gompertz constant and maximum potential lifespan; its relevance to theories of aging. *Exp. Geront.* **16**, 131–5. [*30*]

Rosenbloom, A. and Morgan, M.W. (ed.) (1986). *Vision and aging: general and clinical perspectives.* Butterworth, London. [*v*]

Ross, M.H. and Bras, G. (1973). Influence of protein under- and overnutrition on spontaneous tumor prevalence in the rat. *J. Nutr.* **103**, 94–63. [*30*]

Ruddock, K.H. (1963). Evidence of macular pigmentation from colour matching data. *Vision Res.* **3**, 417–29. [*138*]

Ruddock, K.H. (1965). The effect of age upon colour vision. II. Changes with age in light transmission of the ocular media. *Vision Res.* **5**, 47–58. [*94*]

Said, F.S. and Weale, R.A. (1959). The variation with age of the spectral transmissivity of the living crystalline lens. *Gerontologia*, **3**, 213–31. [*94, 98–101*]

Sample, P.A., Esterson, F.D., Weinreb, R.N., and Boynton, R.M. (1988). The aging lens: in vivo assessment of light absorption in 84 human eyes. *Invest. Ophthal. Vis. Sci.* **29**, 1306–11. [*97*]

Sandor, T., Albert, M., Stafford, J., and Kemper, T. (1990). Symmetrical and asymmetrical changes in brain tissue with age as measured on CT scans. *Neurobiol. Ag.* **11**, 21–7. [*114*]

Sanke, R.F. (1984). Relationship of senile ptosis to age. *Ann. Ophthalm.* **16**, 928–31. [*54*]

Saraux, H., Manent, J.-P., and Laroche, L. (1984). Erythropsie chez un porteur d'implant. *J. Fr. Ophtal.* **7**, 557–62. [*103*]

Sarks, S.H. (1976). Ageing and degeneration in the macular region: A clinico-pathological study. *Brit. J. Ophthal.* **60**, 324–41. [*165, 166, 203, 224*]

Saunders, H. (1986). A longitudinal study of the age-dependence of human ocular refraction-I. Age-dependent changes in the equivalent sphere. *Ophthal. Physiol. Opt.* **6**, 39–46. [*54–6, 58*]

Schadow, N. (1882). Beiträge zur Physiologie der Irisbewegung. *Graefe's Arch. d. Ophthalm.* **28/III**, 183–200. [*48*]

Schäfer, W.D. and Weale, R.A. (1970). The influence of age and retinal illumination on the pupillary near reflex. *Vision Res.* **10**, 179–91. [*82*]

Schefrin, B.E. and Werner, J.S. (1990). Loci of spectral unique hues throughout the life span. *J. Opt. Soc. Amer.* **7**, 305–11. [*223*]

Schmidt, S.Y. and Peisch, R.D. (1986). Melanin concentration in normal human retinal pigment epithelium. *Invest. Ophthal. Vis. Sci.* **27**, 1063–7. [*151, 160, 161*]

Schneider, E.L., Sternerg, H., Tice, R.R., Senula, G.C., Kram, D., Smith, J.R., and Bynum, G. (1979). Cellular replication and aging. *Mech. Ag. Dev.* **9**, 313–24. [*27*]

Schulz, U. and Hunziker, O. (1980). Comparative studies of neuronal perikaryon size and shape in the aging cerebral cortex. *J. Geront.* **35**, 483–91. [*113*]

Schwab, I.R., Dawson, C.R., Hoshiwara, I., Szuter, C.F., and Knowler, W.C. (1985). Incidence of cataract extraction in Pima Indians. *Arch. Ophthal.* **103**, 208–12. [*109, 110*]

Sealy, R.C., Sarna, T., Wanner, E.J., and Reszka, K. (1984). Photosensitization of melanin: An electron spin resonance study of sensitized radical production and oxygen consumption. *Photochem. Photobiol.* **40**, 453–9. [*163, 164*]

Sekuler, R., Kline, D., and Dismukes, K. (ed.) (1982). *Aging and human visual function*, Alan R. Liss, New York. [*v*]

Shinitzky, M. (1987). Patterns of lipid changes in membranes of the aged brain. *Gerontology*, **33**, 149–54. [*15*]

Shiose, Y. (1984). The aging effect on intraocular pressure in an apparently normal population. *Arch. Ophthal.* **102**, 883–7. [*56*]

Siebinga, L., Vrensen, G.F.J.M., De Mul, F.F.M., and Greve, J. (1991). Age-related changes in local water and protein content of human eye lenses measured by Raman spectroscopy. *Exp. Eye Res.* **53**, 233–9. [*54, 80*]

Sigelman, J., Trokel, S.L., and Spector, A. (1974). Quantitative biomicroscopy of lens light back scatter. *Arch. Ophthal.* **92**, 437–42. [*105*]

Siliprandi, N., Siliprandi, D., Zoccarato, F., Toninello, A., and Rugolo, M. (1979). Changes in mammalian mitochondria during aging. *Bull. Mol. Biol. Med.* **4**, 1–14. [*15*]

Silberkühl, W. (1896). Untersuchungen über die physiologische Pupillenweite. *Graefe's Arch. Ophthal.* **42**, 179–87. [*48*]

Silver, J. (1978). Cell death during development of the nervous system. In *Handbook of sensory physiology*, (ed. M. Jacobson), Vol. 9. Springer-Verlag, Berlin. [*20, 118*]

Simpson, D.M. and Erwin, C.W. (1983). Evoked potential latency change with age suggests differential aging of primary somatosensory cortex. *Neurobiol. Ag.* **4**, 59–63. [*226*]

Slataper, F.J. (1950). Age norms of refraction and vision. *Arch. Ophthal.* **43**, 466–81. [*52, 54, 56*]

Sliney, D.H. (1983). Eye protective techniques for bright light. *Ophthalmology*, **90**, 937–44. [*155*]

Sloane, M.E., Owsley, C., and Alvarez, S.L. (1988*a*). Aging, senile miosis and spatial contrast sensitivity at low luminance. *Vision Res.* **28**, 1235–46. [*172, 210*]

Sloane, M.E., Owsley, C., and Jackson, C.A. (1988*b*). Aging and luminance-adaptation effects on spatial contrast sensitivity. *J. Opt. Soc. Amer.* **5**, 2181–90. [*214–17, 222*]

Smith, V.C., Pokorny, J., and Diddie, K.R. (1988). Color matching and the Stiles-Crawford effect in observers with early age-related macular changes. *J. Opt. Soc. Amer.* **5**, 2113–21. [*44, 224*]

Sohal, R.S. and Wolfe, L.S. (1986). Lipofuscin: characteristics and significance. *Progr. Brain Res.* **70**, 171–83. [*146, 148, 160*]

Sohal, R.S., Svensson, I., Sohal, B.H., and Brunk, U.T. (1989). Superoxide anion radical production in different animal species. *Mech. Ag. Dev.* **49**, 129–35. [*14*]

Sohal, R.S., Svensson, I., Brunk, U.T. (1990). Hydrogen peroxide production by liver mitochondria in different species. *Mech. Ag. Dev.* **53**, 209–15. [*14*]

Sorsby, A., Benjamin, B., and Sheridan, M., with Stone, J. and Leary, G.A. (1961). *Refraction and its components during the growth of the eye from the age of three.* Med. Res. Coun. Special Rep. No. 301. HMSO, London. [*56, 57*]

Sperduto, R.D., Hiller, R., and Seigel, D. (1981). Lens opacities and senile maculopathy. *Arch. Ophthal.* **99**, 1004–8. [*166*]

Spritz, N., Singh, H., and Geyer, B. (1973). Myelin from human peripheral nerves. *J. Clin. Invest.* **52**, 520–3. [*120*]

Stanulis-Praeger, B.M. (1987). Cellular senescence revised: a review. *Mech. Ag. Dev.* **38**, 1–48. [*26–8*]

Stanulis-Praeger, B.M. and Gilchrest, B.A. (1986). Growth factor responsiveness declines during adulthood for human skin-derived cells. *Mech. Ag. Dev.* **35**, 185–98. [*28*]

Stark, L. (1985). Presbyopia in light of accommodation. In *Presbyopia*, (ed. G. Obrecht and L. Stark) pp. 264–74. Fairchild Publications, New York. [*83*]

Steinhaus, H. (1932). Untersuchungen über den Zusammenhang von Presbyopia und Lebensdauer und seine Bedeutung für die Akkommodation. *Arch. Augenh.* **105**, 731–60. [*10, 59*]

Stieve, R. (1949). Über den Bau des menschlichen Ciliarmuskels, seine Veränderungen während des Lebens und seine Bedeutung für die Akkommodation. *Anat. Anz.* **97**, 69–79. [*6, 71, 77, 84*]

Stiles, W.S. (1946). A modified Helmholtz line-element in brightness-colour space. *Proc. Phys. Soc.* **58**, 41–65. [*220*]

Stohs, S.J., El-Rashidy, F.H., Lawson, T., Kobayashi, R.H., Wulf, B.G., and Potter, J.F. (1984). Changes in glutathione and glutathione metabolizing enzymes in human erythrocytes and lymphocytes as a function of age of donor. *Age*, **7**, 3–7. [*4*]

Strehler, B.L., Mark, D.D., Mildvan, A., and Gee, M.V. (1959). Rate and magnitude of age pigment accumulation in the human myocardium. *J. Gerontol.* **14**, 430–39. [*11*]

Sturr, J.F., Church, K.L., and Taub, H.A. (1985). Early light adaptation in young, middle-aged, and older observers. *Percept. Psychophys.* **37**, 455–8. [*196, 197*]

Sturr, J.F., Church, K.L., Nuding, S.C., Van Orden, K., and Taub, H.A. (1986). Older observers have attenuated increment thresholds upon transient backgrounds. *J. Geront.* **41**, 743–7. [*197*]

Sturr, J.F., Van Orden, K., and Taub, H.A. (1987). Selective attentuation in brightness for brief stimuli and at low intensities supports age-related transient channel losses. *Exp. Ag. Res.* **13**, 145–9. [*195, 198*]

Sucs, S.I. (1974). Contribution à l'étude de l'adaptation à l'obscurité et la sommation spatiale. *Adv. Ophthal.* **28**, 206–326. [*176, 180*]

Sun, A.Y. and Sun, G.Y. (1979). Neurochemical aspects of the membrane hypothesis of aging. *Interdiscipl. Topics Geront.* **15**, 34–53. [*15, 16*]

Svanborg, A. (1988). The health of the elderly population: results from longitudinal studies with age-cohort comparisons. In *Research and the ageing population*, (ed. D. Evered and J. Whelan). John Wiley, Chichester. [*38, 40, 43*]

Swegmark, G. (1969). Studies with impedance cyclography on human accommodation at different ages. *Acta Ophthal.* **47**, 1186–206. [*77, 84*]

Takeda, S. and Matsuzawa, T. (1984). Brain atrophy during aging: A quantitative study using computed tomography. *J. Amer. Geriatr. Soc.* **32**, 320–520. [*116*]

Terry, R.D., DeTeresa, R., and Hansen, L.A. (1987). Neocortical cell counts in normal human adult aging. *Ann. Neurol.* **21**, 530–9. [*113, 116, 118*]

Thatcher, R.W., Walker, R.A., and Giudice, S. (1987). Human cerebral hemispheres develop at different rates and ages. *Science*, **236**, 1110−3. [*38, 39, 113, 114*]

The Italian-American Cataract Study Group. (1991). Risk factors for age-related cortical, nuclear, and posterior subcapsular cataracts. *Amer. J. Epidemiol.* **133**, 541−53. [*102*]

Till, R.E. (1978). Age-related differences in binocular backward masking with visual noise. *J. Geront.* **33**, 702−10. [*197*]

Till, R.E. and Franklin, L.D. (1981). On the locus of age differences in visual information processing. *J. Geront.* **36**, 200−10. [*199*]

Tollefsbol, T.O. and Cohen, H.J. (1986). Expression of intracellular biochemical defects of lymphocytes in aging: proposal of a general aging mechanism which is not cell-specific. *Exp. Geront.* **21**, 129−48. [*29*]

Tréton, J. and Courtois, Y. (1989). Evidence for a relationship between longevity of mammalian species and a lens growth parameter. *Gerontol.* **35**, 88−94. [*42*]

Trevor Roper, P.D. (1974). *The eye and its disorders*. Blackwell Scientific Publications, Oxford. [*6*]

Trick, G.L., Trick, L.R., and Haywood, K.M. (1986). Altered pattern evoked retinal and cortical potentials associated with human senescence. *Curr. Eye Res.* **5**, 717−24. [*202*]

Tulunay-Keesey, U., Ver Hoeve, J.N., and Terkla-McGrane, C. (1988). Threshold and suprathreshold spatiotemporal response throughout adulthood. *J. Opt. Soc. Amer.* **5**, 2191−200. [*215, 219*]

Tyler, C.W. (1973). Periodic vernier acuity. *J. Physiol. (Lond.)* **226**, 637−47. [*207*]

Ulshafer, R.J., Allen, C.B., and Rubin, M.L. (1990). Distributions of elements in the human retinal pigment epithelium. *Arch. Ophthal.* **108**, 113−17. [*161*]

Van Alphen, G.W.H.M. and Graebel, W.P. (1991). Elasticity of tissues involved in accommodation. *Vision Res.* **31**, 1417−38. [*80, 81*]

Van Best, J.A., Tjin A Tsoi, E.W.S.J., Boot, J.P., and Oosterhuis, J.A. (1985). *In vivo* assessment of lens transmission for blue-green light by autofluorescence measurement. *Ophthal. Res.* **17**, 90−95. [*98−100*]

Van Heyningen, R. (1973). The glucoside of 3-hydroxykinurenine and other fluorescent compounds in the human lens. In *The human lens − in relation to cataract*, (ed. K. Elliott and D.W. Fitzsimmons), pp. 151−68. Elsevier, Amsterdam. [*90*]

Van Kujik, F.J.G.M., Lewis, J.W., Buck, P., Parker, K.R., and Kliger, D.S. (1991). Spectrophotometric quantitation of rhodopsin in the human retina. *Invest. Ophthalm. Vis. Sci.* **32**, 1962−7. [*132*]

Van Meeteren, A. and Vos, J.J. (1972). Resolution and contrast sensitivity at low luminances. *Vision Res.* **12**, 825−33. [*201, 210, 211*]

Van der Zypen, E. (1975). Die Bedeutung der Altersveränderungen am Corpus ciliare des menschlichen Auges für die Presbyopie und die Kammerwasserzirkulation. *Verh. Anat. Ges.* **69**, 665−71. [*77*]

Vannas, S. and Teir, H. (1960). Observations on structures and age changes in the human sclera. *Acta Ophthalm. Copenh.* **38**, 268−79. [*56*]

Verriest, G. (1972). The relative spectral luminous efficiency in different age groups of aphakic eyes. *Die Farbe*, **21**, 17−25. [*180, 181*]

Verriest, G., Vandevyvère, R., and Vanderdomck, R. (1962). Nouvelles recherches se rapportant à l'influence du sexe, et l'âge sur la discrimination chromatique, ainsi qu'à la signification pratique des résultats du test 100 hue de Farnsworth Munsell. *Rev. Opt.* **41**, 499−509. [*221*]

Villermet, G.M. and Weale, R.A. (1972). Age, the crystalline lens of the rudd and visual pigments. *Nature*, **238**, 345−6. [*21*]

Vimal, R.L.P., Pokorny, J., Smith, V.C., and Skewell, S.L. (1989). Foveal cone thresholds. *Vision Res.* **29**, 66–78. [*172*]

Vogt, A. (1931). *Lehrbuch und Atlas der Spaltlampenmikroskopie des lebenden Auges*, Vol. II. Julius Springer, Berlin. [*98*]

Vrabec, F. (1977). Age changes of the human optic nerve head. *Graefe's Arch. Klin. Exp. Ophthal.* **202**, 213–36. [*139*]

Vrabec, F. (1986). 'Displaced nerve cells' in the human retina. *Graefe's Arch. Clin. Exp. Ophthal.* **224**, 143–6. [*139*]

Walford, R.L. (1981). Immunoregulatory systems and aging. In *Aging: a challenge to science and society*, (ed. D. Danon, N.W. Shock, and M. Marois), pp. 302–19. Oxford University Press. [*34, 231*]

Walford, R.L. (1983). Supergenes: histocompatibility; immunologic and other parameters in aging. In *Intervention in the aging process*, (ed. W. Regelson and F. Marott Sinex). Alan R. Liss, New York. [*17, 20*]

Walford, R.L. and Crew, M. (1989). How dietary restriction retards aging: an integrative hypothesis. *Growth Dev. Ag.* **53**, 139–40. [*34*]

Ward, P.A. (1987). The effect of spatial frequency on steady-state accommodation. *Ophthal. Physiol. Opt.* **7**, 211–17. [*62*]

Ward, P.A. and Charman, W.N. (1985). Effect of pupil size on steady state accommodation. *Vision Res.* **25**, 1317–26. [*62*]

Warnes, A. (1989). The ageing of populations. In *Human ageing and later life*, (ed. A. Warnes). Edward Arnold, London. [*8*]

Weale, R.A. (1959). Photochemical reactions in normal and cone-monochromatic retinae. *Opt. Acta*, **6**, 158–74. [*137*]

Weale, R.A. (1963). *The aging eye*. H.K. Lewis, London. [*42, 57, 60*]

Weale, R.A. (1970). The eye and measurement of ageing-rate. *Lancet*, **i**, 147. [*43*]

Weale, R.A. (1975). Senile changes in visual acuity. *Trans. Ophthal. Soc. UK*, **95**, 36–8. [*113, 207*]

Weale, R.A. (1980). A note on the possible relation between refraction and a disposition for senile cataract. *Brit. J. Ophthal.* **64**, 311–14. [*109*]

Weale, R.A. (1981). Human ocular aging and ambient temperature. *Brit. J. Ophthal.* **65**, 869–70. [*60*]

Weale, R.A. (1982a). *A biography of the eye: development, growth, age*. H.K. Lewis, London. [*v, 10, 43, 44, 48, 55, 63, 66, 77, 85, 90, 113, 132, 189, 239*]

Weale, R.A. (1982b). The age variation of 'senile' cataract in various parts of the world. *Brit. J. Ophthal.* **66**, 31–4. [*237*]

Weale, R.A. (1983). Transparency and power of post-mortem human lenses: variation with age and sex. *Exp. Eye Res.* **36**, 731–41. [*56, 67*]

Weale, R.A. (1985a). Human lenticular fluorescence and transmissivity, and their effects on vision. *Exp. Eye Res.* **41**, 457–73. [*98, 103, 104*]

Weale, R.A. (1985b). Retinal senescence. *Progr. Retinal Res.* **5**, 53–73. [*165*]

Weale, R.A. (1985c). Contrast thresholds and age. *J. Physiol.* **360**, 25P. [*205*]

Weale, R.A. (1986a). Sunglasses – an ocular hazard? *Brit. J. Ophthal.* **70**, 769–71. [*48*]

Weale, R.A. (1986b). Senescence and color vision. *J. Geront.* **41**, 635–40. [*220*]

Weale, R.A. (1986c). Real light scatter in the human crystalline lens. *Graefe's Arch. Clin. Exp. Ophthal.* **224**, 463–6. [*105, 106*]

Weale, R.A. (1987). Contrast sensitivity. In *Low vision – principles and applications*, (ed. G.C. Woo), pp. 45–55. Springer-Verlag, New York. [*210, 211*]

Weale, R.A. (1988). Age and the transmittance of the human crystalline lens. *J. Physiol.* **395**, 577–87. [*90, 92, 94*]

Weale, R.A. (1989*a*). Presbyopia toward the end of the 20th century. *Surv. Ophthal.* **34**, 15–30. [*60, 82*]

Weale, R.A. (1989*b*). Do years or quanta age the retina? *Photochem. Photobiol.* **50**, 429–438. [*11, 15, 90, 132, 146, 153–9*]

Weale, R.A. (1990). Evolution, age and ocular focus. *Mech. Ag. Dev.* **53**, 85–9. [*61, 86*]

Weale, R.A. (1991*a*). The lenticular nucleus, light, and the retina. *Exp. Eye Res.* **52**, 213–18. [*93, 156*]

Weale, R.A. (1991*b*). Effects of senescence. In *Limits of vision*, (ed. J.J. Kulikowski, V. Walsh, and I.J. Murray), Ch. 21, Vol. 5, *Vision and visual dysfunction*, (ed. J. Cronly-Dillon). Macmillan. Boca Raton, Florida. [*102, 205*]

Weale, R.A. (1991*c*). Personal preferences for fluorescent tubes with and without UVA. *Lighting Res. Technol.*, **23/4**, 171–3. [*225, 227*]

Weekers, R., Delmarcelle, Y., Luyckx-Bacus, J., and Collignon, J. (1973). Morphological changes of the lens with age and cataract. In *The human lens – in relation to cataract*, (ed. K. Elliott and D.W. Fitzsimons), pp. 25–40. Elsevier, London. [*69*]

Weiter, J.J. (1987). Phototoxic changes in the retina. In *Clinical light damage to the eye*, (ed. D. Miller). Springer, New York. [*11*]

Weiter, J.J., Delori, F.C., Wing, G.L., and Fitch, K.A. (1985). Relationship of senile macular degeneration to ocular pigmentation. *Amer. J. Ophthal.* **99**, 185–7. [*166*]

Weiter, J.J., Delori, F.C., Wing, G.L., and Fitch, K.A. (1986). Retinal pigment epithelial lipofuscin and melanin and choroidal melanin in human eyes. *Invest. Ophthal. Vis. Sci.* **27**, 145–52. [*15, 146, 151–4, 158*]

Werner, J.S. (1982). Development of scotopic sensitivity and the absorption spectrum of the human ocular media. *J. Opt. Soc. Amer.* **72**, 247–58. [*94, 97*]

Werner, J.S., Donnelly, S.K., and Kliegl, R. (1987). Aging and human macular pigment density. *Vision Res.* **27**, 257–68. [*137, 138*]

Werner, J.S. and Hardenbergh, F.E. (1983). Spectral sensitivity of the pseudophakic eye. *Arch. Ophthal.* **101**, 758–60. [*95, 96*]

Werner, J.S. and Steele, V.G. (1988). Sensitivity of human foveal color mechanisms throughout the life span. *J. Opt. Soc. Amer. A* **5**, 2123–30. [*181–4*]

Werner, J.S., Peterzell, D.H., and Schectz, A.J. (1990). Light, vision, and aging. *Optom. Vis. Sci.* **63**, 214–29. [*183, 185*]

West, S., Munoz, B., Emmett, E.A. and Taylor, H.R. (1989*a*). Cigarette smoking and risk of nuclear cataracts. *Arch. Ophthal.* **107**, 1166–9. [*109*]

West, S.K., Rosenthal, F.S., Bressler, N.M., Bressler, S.B., Munoz, B., Fine, S.L., and Taylor, H.R. (1989*b*). Exposure to sunlight and other risk factors for age-related macular degeneration. *Arch. Ophthal.* **107**, 875–9. [*166*]

Wilkins, A.J., Della Sala, S., Somazzi, L., and Nimmo-Smith, I. (1988). Age-related norms for the Cambridge low contrast gratings, including details concerning their design and use. *Clin. Vis. Sci.* **2**, 201–12. [*218*]

Williams, T.D. (1983). Aging and central visual field area. *Amer. J. Optom. Physiol. Opt.* **60**, 888–91. [*191, 192*]

Wing, G.L., Blanchard, G.C., and Weiter, J.J. (1978). The topography and age relationship of lipfuscin concentration in the retinal pigment epithelium. *Invest. Ophthal. Vis. Sci.* **17**, 601–7. [*11, 146, 151–9*]

Witten, M. (1983). A return to time, cells, systems and aging: rethinking the concept of senescence in mammalian organisms. *Mech. Ag. Dev.* **21**, 69−81. [*8*]

Witten, M. (1984). A return to time, cells, systems and aging. II. Relational and reliability theoretic approaches to the study of senescence in living systems. *Mech. Ag. Dev.* **27**, 323−40. [*8*]

Wooten, B.R. and Geri, G.A. (1987). Psychophysical determination of intraocular light scatter as a function of wavelength. *Vision Res.* **27**, 1291−8. [*106*]

Wright, C.E., Williams, D.E., Drasdo, N., and Harding, G.F.A. (1985). The influence of age on the electroretinogram and visual evoked potential. *Docum. Ophthal.* **59**, 365−84. [*210, 226*]

Wu, L. (1987). Study of aging macular degeneration in China. *Jap. J. Ophthal.* **31**, 349−67. [*166*]

Wu, L., Huang, Z., Wu, D., and Chan, E. (1985). Characteristics of the capillary-free zone in the normal human macula. *Jap. J. Ophthal.* **29**, 406−11. [*126*]

Yamaura, H., Ito, M., Kubota, K., and Matsuzawa, T. (1980). Brain atrophy during aging: a quantitative study with computed tomography. *J. Gerontol.* **35**, 492−8. [*115*]

Yap, M., Gilchrist, J., and Weatherill, J. (1987). Psychophysical measurement of the foveal avascular zone. *Ophthal. Physiol. Opt.* **7**, 405−10. [*127*]

Young, J.Z. (1968). *The brain*. Third Programme: 9th February. British Broadcasting Corporation, London. [*1, 10*]

Young, T. (1801). Bakerian Lecture. On the mechanism of the eye. *Phil. Trans. Roy. Soc.* **91**, 23−88. [*59, 79*]

Young, V.R. (1979). Diet as a modulator of aging and longevity. *Fed. Proc.* **38**, 1994−2000. [*30*]

Yu, B.P. (1985). Recent advances in dietary restriction and aging. *Rev. Biol. Res. Ag.* **2**, 435−43. [*29, 30*]

Zeimer, R.C. and Noth, J.M. (1984). A new method of measuring in vivo the lens transmittance, and study of lens scatter, fluorescence and transmittance. *Ophthal. Res.* **16**, 246−55. [*98*]

Zemcov, A., Barclay, L., and Blass, J.P. (1984). Regional decline of cerebral blood flow with age in cognitively intact subjects. *Neurobiol. Ag.* **5**, 1−6. [*123*]

Zglinicki, T.v. (1987). A mitochondrial hypothesis of aging. *J. Theor. Biol.* **127**, 127−32. [*14−16*]

Zigman, S. (1978). Ultraviolet light and human lens pigmentation. *Vision Res.* **18**, 509−10. [*101*]

Zrenner, E. and Lund, O.-E. (1984). Die erhöhte Strahlungsbelastung der Netzhaut nach Implantation intraokularer Linsen und ihre Behebung durch farblose Filtergläser. *Klin. Mbl. Augenheilk.* **184**, 193−6. [*95*]

Zs.-Nagy, I. (1978). A membrane hypothesis of aging. *J. Theor. Biol.* **75**, 189−95. [*15*]

Zs.-Nagy, I. (1979). The role of membrane structure and function in cellular aging: a review. *Mech. Ag. Dev.* **9**, 237−46. [*15*]

Index